THE
COCONUT
KETOGENIC
DIET

By
Dr. Bruce Fife

Piccadilly Books, Ltd.
Colorado Springs, CO

Every effort has been made to ensure that the information contained in this book is complete and accurate. However, neither the publisher nor the author is engaged in rendering professional advice or services to the individual reader. The ideas, procedures, and suggestions contained in this book are not intended as a substitute for consulting with your physician. Neither the publisher nor the author are responsible for your specific health or allergy needs that may require medical supervision and are not responsible for any adverse reactions to the recipes or procedures described in this book.

Piccadilly Books, Ltd.
P.O. Box 25203
Colorado Springs, CO 80936, USA
info@piccadillybooks.com
www.piccadillybooks.com

Library of Congress Cataloging-in-Publication Data

Fife, Bruce, 1952- author.
  The coconut ketogenic diet : supercharge your metabolism, revitalize thyroid function, and lose excess weight / by Bruce Fife, ND.
    pages cm
  Includes bibliographical references and index.
  ISBN 978-0-941599-94-8 (paperback)
  1. Coconut oil--Health aspects. 2. Fatty acids in human nutrition. I. Title.
  QP144.O44F5415 2014
  613.2'84--dc23
                              2014004856

Published in the USA

Contents

Chapter 1: **The Undiet Diet** 5

Chapter 2: **Big Fat Lies** 16

Chapter 3: **Are You In Need of An Oil Change?** 24

Chapter 4: **Cholesterol and Saturated Fat** 33

Chapter 5: **Good Carbs, Bad Carbs** 45

Chapter 6: **Carbohydrates Make You Fat** 61

Chapter 7: **Not All Calories Are Equal** 77

Chapter 8: **Eat Fat and Grow Slim** 85

Chapter 9: **Dietary Ketosis** 101

Chapter 10: **Is Your Thyroid Making You Fat?**............. 122

Chapter 11: **Iodine and Your Health** 133

Chapter 12: **Thyroid System Dysfunction** 152

Chapter 13: **Supercharge Your Metabolism** 165

Chapter 14: **Drink More, Weigh Less** 191

Chapter 15: **Low-Carb, High-Fat Eating Plan** 207

Chapter 16: **The Coco Keto Weight Loss Program** 230

Chapter 17: **Cooking the Keto Way** 258

Appendix: **Nutrient Counter** 282

References 296

Index 311

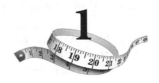

The Undiet Diet

EAT FAT AND LOSE WEIGHT: IS IT POSSIBLE?

Leah, 42, came to me complaining of a variety of problems: frequent migraine headaches, constipation, mood swings, irritability, depression, irregular menstruation, fatigue, and recurring yeast infections. Although she didn't mention it, Leah was overweight. She stood 5 feet 5 inches (1.65 m) and weighed 180 pounds (82 kg)—typical for many middle-age women nowadays.

Frustrated with doctors and medications, she had decided to seek help from someone experienced in alternative or natural medicine. As a nutritionist and naturopathic physician, my focus is helping people overcome health problems through safe, natural means, using diet and nutrition.

Leah indicated that she ate many refined white flour products (e.g., bread, rolls, pastry, crackers, etc.), breakfast cereals, and frozen and prepared foods, and snacked on sweets and chips. She assured me she ate healthfully because she avoided fat. She drank skim milk and ate low-fat foods; she chose lean cuts of meat and removed all visible fat. She avoided butter like the plague, using margarine in its place, and prepared meals with what she termed "healthy" vegetable oils. Although the prepared convenience foods she used often included small portions of vegetables, she rarely ate fresh produce. Leah's diet was typical of most people in our modern society—nutrient deficient and weight-promoting.

The first thing I did was to change her diet. I told her, "Don't eat anything that says low-fat or low-calorie, and get off the sweets and junk foods. Eat whole foods with butter and coconut oil, and don't be afraid of the fat in meats. Eat full-fat cheese, cream, and other dairy products. Eat fresh fruits and vegetables. Eat as much as much as you want, just don't overeat, and enjoy your new diet."

She was surprised. "Won't all this fat and rich food make me gain weight?" she asked.

"No," I replied. "You don't have to worry about your weight."

"Well, I do worry. I try to watch my calories and limit my fat intake."

"What I'm giving you is a way of eating that will improve your health. It provides your body with all the nutrients it needs to overcome the health problems you mentioned. And as you become healthier, you will also lose excess body fat."

"You mean I can eat delicious foods, gain better health, and lose weight at the same time?"

"Yes," I told her.

She returned for follow-up visits over the next several months. Each time she told me she was doing better and losing weight. She couldn't believe it. She was eating more rich, fatty foods than she ever had and was dropping pounds. In time, she reported that all of her symptoms had improved, and to her pleasant surprise, she lost 45 pounds (20 kg), dropping to a slim 135 pounds (61 kg). Now, several years later, she continues to follow my dietary recommendations and still maintains her slim figure.

When people come to see me, they usually are concerned with chronic health problems like Crohn's disease, diabetes, and arthritis. While treatment varies for each individual, the diet I recommend is basically the same—low in refined carbohydrates and rich in fresh produce, with plenty of healthy fats. I've had a great deal of success, especially with my diabetic patients. They are able to live normal lives without relying on medications and daily insulin injections.

Patients frequently comment, with delight, that they lose weight on my program. My main focus is to help people regain their health; losing weight is a natural consequence of that process. For many people, however, excess body fat is their primary concern. So I have tailored my health program specifically to address their concerns. This book is the result.

LOW-FAT DIETS MAY KILL YOU

"I hate diets. None of them have ever worked for me. I tried. I watched what I ate, cutting out all of my favorite foods and reducing calories. I felt deprived. I hated it. I was hungry all the time and felt miserable. I only lost a few pounds. It wasn't worth all the misery I went through. And once I stopped dieting, the weight came right back."

Does this sound familiar to you? It should. Most of us have tried dieting at least once in our lives. Why? Because most of us are overweight. Sixty percent of Americans are overweight; 30 percent are obese. One third of our children are now overweight. These figures are rapidly increasing. Fifty years ago, it was a problem for only a small percentage of the population. Now it's an epidemic. We're not alone. The same thing is occurring in Canada, Europe, and elsewhere.

Why are we gaining so much weight? We aren't eating that much more than we used to. In fact, we eat less fat now than ever before. Our grandparents got about 40 percent of their daily calories from fat. Today, we are averaging about 32 percent—a significant decrease. When you go to the grocery store, you're bombarded from every side with labels that read "Low-fat," "Non-fat," and "Low calorie." When you go to a restaurant, you can get diet soda and low-calorie or reduced-fat meals. Everything nowadays seems to be low- or non-fat. We've replaced saturated fats with polyunsaturated fats and fake fats. Sugar is being replaced by artificial sweeteners. We eat more low-fat, low-calorie foods now than ever before, yet we are fatter now than ever before. Why is that?

The simple answer is that low-fat diets don't work! They're not natural, they're not healthy, and in the long run they promote weight gain, not weight loss.

Research confirms this fact. The longest running study ever made on the relationship between diet and health is the Framingham study. The study began in 1948, was set up to continue throughout the lifetime of the volunteers, and is still going on today. The study included almost the entire population of Framingham, Massachusetts (population 5,127). After more than 40 years of research, the director of the study, Dr. William Castelli, admitted: "In Framingham, Mass., the more saturated fat one ate, the more cholesterol one ate, the more calories one ate, the lower the person's serum cholesterol...We found that the people who ate the most cholesterol, ate the most saturated fat, ate the most calories, weighed the least."[1] You would expect that the people who eat the least amount of saturated fat, cholesterol, and calories to weigh the least, but they don't, as revealed by the Framingham study.

It appears that if you want to lose weight, you need to avoid low-fat dieting. Trying to lose weight on a low-fat diet is a nightmare of deprivation and starvation. Many of us would rather die than go through the pain. There is a better way.

THE COCONUT KETOGENIC DIET

Which of the following best describes you? Are you a picky eater, habitual eater, recreational eater, or professional eater? Judging by our expanding waistlines, most of us are approaching the professional ranks.

When I first began showing people how to improve their health though diet and nutrition, I believed in the low-fat philosophy. I believed that restricting calories was the only way to lose weight and that eliminating as much fat as possible from the diet was the best approach. This is what I was taught in school. Meat and fat were something to avoid. Saturated fat and cholesterol were considered dietary villains capable of causing just about every ill, from heart disease and obesity to athlete's foot and hangnails, or so it seemed by the way saturated fats were criticized. We were led to believe that vegetable oils and margarine were much healthier.

I ate what I thought was a healthy diet and recommended it to my patients. Many people improved with the low-fat diet I recommended and they overcame their health problems, but for many others, progress was slow. At times it was frustrating; some people would not progress, or they would get better for some time and then digress.

The first clue that I needed to change my thinking about fats came when I attended a meeting with a group of nutritionists. During the meeting one member of the group stated that coconut oil was healthy and that we should all be using it. We were all dumbfounded by the comment. Coconut oil is a highly saturated fat, and saturated fat was believed to increase blood cholesterol, which in turn, was believed to promote heart disease.

We respected this member of our group so we listened to what she had to say. She backed up her statement by citing several studies published in medical journals. These studies showed that lab animals given coconut oil lived longer and developed fewer diseases than those given soybean, corn, or other vegetable oils. I also learned that coconut oil, in one form or another, was being used successfully to treat seriously ill hospital patients and speed recovery. Coconut oil also possesses superior nutritional qualities over other oils and, when added to baby formula, increases the survival rate of premature infants. For these reasons, it is commonly used in hospital intravenous solutions and commercial baby formulas.

When I left that meeting, I was curious. No, it was more powerful than that: I was determined—determined to find the truth. Maybe my thinking about fats, and particularly saturated fats, was all wrong. At that point, I made a commitment to find the answer. I began researching the medical literature, reading everything I could find on coconut oil, saturated fat, cholesterol, and vegetable oil. What I found was so remarkable that it changed my whole viewpoint of fats and oils.

Over the next several years, I began incorporating more saturated fats into my dietary program, especially coconut oil, and less and less vegetable oils. I started to see dramatic changes in patients that others had given up on. One of the biggest improvements was the loss in weight. People would add more fat, particularly saturated fat from coconut, into their diets and lose weight. I saw, just as the Framingham study demonstrated, that diets containing adequate fats, including saturated fat, produced better results than low-fat diets. When I say "better results," I mean everything improved—not just body weight, but cholesterol levels, blood sugar readings, blood pressure, and energy levels. Their overall health improved. Health problems they had before were alleviated.

8

People were losing weight without even trying. For some, all they did was substitute coconut oil for other oils they had been using and the pounds began melting off. They ate basically the same foods they had before but just made a simple oil change. That's exactly what happened to me.

Over the years, like most everyone else, I had been putting on extra weight. I ate what was considered a healthy, balanced diet. I used margarine and polyunsaturated vegetable oils instead of butter and natural saturated fats.

I was a bit overweight. I tried dieting. It was frustrating. It got to the point where I gave up hope of ever losing my spare tire and just accepted the fact I was overweight and I was going to stay that way. Clothes I had outgrown, but kept around for when I lost weight, were finally tossed out. "I'll never fit into those again," I said to myself.

That was before I learned about coconut oil. When I substituted coconut oil for all the vegetable oils I had been using, I began to lose weight. The weight came off slowly but steadily, and after about six months, I had lost nearly 20 pounds! I didn't change my diet, only the oils that I used. And the weight has stayed off. It's many years now, and I am at my ideal weight for my height and bone structure. I did this by eating more fat than I ever did before.

I instructed patients to eat fatty meats and full-fat dairy. I also had them cut down on carbohydrate-rich grains and cereals and eat more vegetables. When I had people eat healthy foods and use the right types of oils, excess weight seemed to melt off. I began to focus on developing a diet designed specifically to help people lose excess weight as well as improve overall health. That is what this book is all about.

From this discovery came a system of weight loss like none other. I call it the Coconut Ketogenic Diet or simply, the Coco Keto Diet. I don't really like calling it a "diet" because it's more than that. It's not a temporary diet you go on just to lose a few pounds. It's a lifestyle change.

In fact, some people don't even consider it a diet at all, at least not like the typical calorie-restricted, low-fat diets. The eating guidelines in this program allow you to eat until you're satisfied. And it's not all rabbit food either. You get to eat a variety of delicious foods—steaks, shrimp, pork, eggs, cream, cheese, creamy sauces and gravies, and, of course, coconut. You don't starve. That's one of the big advantages of this program. You eat foods that fill you up and keep you satisfied until your next meal. It's almost like an "undiet." You get to enjoy eating and you lose weight! You could call it The Undiet Diet.

There are three phases to this program: an induction phase, a weight loss phase, and a maintenance phase. The induction phase introduces you to low-carb eating and prepares you and your body for the remarkable changes that are about to occur. The second, or ketosis phase, is where you lose most of your unwanted body fat and achieve better overall health. The third phase transitions you to a healthy long-term, reduced carb eating plan that allows you to maintain your new body weight and level of health on a permanent basis.

Many weight loss programs are unhealthy. They may help you lose weight, but they are nutritionally unbalanced, setting the stage for new health problems in the future. The risks are too high. But with this program, you can enjoy food, lose excess weight, and gain better health. I've had a great deal of success with this program in helping people reverse the effects of diabetes, relieve various digestive disorders, clear up nagging skin problems, overcome chronic fatigue, stop recurrent candida infections, stabilize blood sugar, and bring relief from numerous other conditions.

The Coconut Ketogenic Diet is just as much a health-restoring program as it is a weight-loss program. So be prepared to notice some remarkable changes in your life.

If you are troubled by any of the following conditions, this program may help you:

Allergies	Heart/circulatory problems
Arthritis	High blood pressure
Asthma	Hypoglycemia
Brain fog/memory loss	Hypothyroidism
Candida	Insomnia
Chronic inflammation	Kidney disease
Constipation	Migraine headaches
Diabetes	Menstrual irregularity
Digestive problems	Nervousness/irritability
Fatigue/lack of energy	Osteoporosis
Frequent infections	Overweight/obesity
Gout	Reproductive problems
Gum disease	Skin disorders/dermatitis

WHY COCONUT?

Why does this program include the use of coconut? Because coconut is one of the world's healthiest foods—a superfood, in fact. For thousands of years people in Asia, Africa, Central America, and the Pacific Islands have relied on coconut as a major source of food. This is particularly true in the Pacific Islands, where other foods can be scarce. On some islands the only foods available are coconuts, taro root, and fish. Since the time the early explorers first landed on these islands, they noted that the Islanders were of exquisite physical stature and possessed superb health—far better than their own. Only after colonization by Europeans and the adoption of modern foods did conditions like obesity, cancer, heart disease, diabetes, arthritis, and others make their appearance.

The primary nutrient in coconut that sets it apart and makes it such a marvelous health food is the oil. This oil contains the secret to losing excess weight as well as gaining better health. Coconut oil has been described as the "World's Healthiest Dietary Oil." There is a mountain of historical evidence and medical research to verify this fact. I've documented much of this evidence in my book *The Coconut Oil Miracle*, which summarizes historical, epidemiological, and medical research on the nutritional and medicinal aspects of coconut oil. It also clearly refutes the negative publicity perpetuated by ill-informed writers.

Modern dietary studies on isolated island populations who maintain their traditional coconut-based diets have a complete absence of degenerative disease. Some island populations consume massive amounts of coconut and coconut oil and are the picture of good health.[2] In fact, many of these cultures regard coconut oil as a medicine and refer to the coconut palm as "The Tree of Life."

Once considered to be bad for the heart because of its saturated fat content, we now know that coconut oil is comprised of a special type of fat known as medium chain triglycerides (MCTs), which actually help to prevent heart disease. Yes, the fat in coconut oil can help protect you from heart disease. (This is documented in some detail in my book *Coconut Cures*, so I will not devote much space to it here.) If you don't believe me, go to any of the countries that rely heavily on coconut: Thailand, Fiji, the Philippines, many of the islands of the Pacific. Wherever you find people using coconut oil for everyday cooking, you will find heart disease to be extraordinarily low compared to those in the US.

In the coconut-growing regions of India, heart disease was almost unheard of. When the people there were told that coconut oil was bad for them, they switched to soybean and other vegetable oils. As a result, within ten years their rate of heart disease tripled! Likewise, obesity and diabetes are on the rise. When people remained on their traditional coconut-based diets, they were protected from many of these so-called "diseases of modern civilization."

A major study was done on two remote Pacific Islands—Pukapuka and Tokelau. The entire populations of the islands took part in the study. Coconut provided the main source of food for these people. They derived up to 60 percent of their daily calories from fat, mostly from coconut oil. The American Heart Association recommends no more than 30 percent of calories should come from fat and no more than 10 percent from saturated fat. Yet over 50 percent of this population's daily calories came from the saturated fat in coconuts. Despite eating all this fat, there was absolutely no evidence of heart disease, diabetes, cancer, or any other degenerative disease common in Western societies. Only when Islanders abandon their traditional coconut-based diet and take on the eating habits of Western countries, do they begin to develop the diseases of modern society.

11

If you stop for a moment and think about it, you will realize how silly it is to think of coconut oil as unhealthy. People have been using coconut oil as their major dietary oil for thousands of years; if it caused heart disease, or any other disease for that matter, it would be clearly evident in those populations, but it's not. Therefore, common sense tells us coconut oil is not harmful.

Unfortunately, because coconut oil has received a lot of bad publicity in the past, some misinformed writers and health care professionals still ignorantly criticize it as containing artery-clogging saturated fat. Such people are woefully behind the times and are only parroting what other misinformed writers have said. They need to read the new research, which now has been available for several years. If you hear anybody nowadays claim that coconut oil is unhealthy, and some still do, realize they are still in the dark ages of nutritional knowledge. Have them read *The Coconut Oil Miracle* or *Coconut Cures*. These books are fully documented, with references to the medical literature proving beyond doubt the many health benefits of this most remarkable food.

One of the unique characteristics about coconut oil is that, unlike other fats, it is not stored to any appreciable extent in the body as fat. It is metabolized completely differently from animal fats and vegetable oils. When we eat coconut oil, rather than storing it as fat, we convert it into energy. Coconut oil increases your energy and perks up your metabolism, which causes the body to burn calories at an accelerated rate. Yes, eating coconut oil can help you lose weight because it promotes the burning of calories. It not only burns up the calories it supplies itself, but also those of other foods as well. For this reason, it is appropriately called the world's only low-calorie fat! In addition, coconut oil boosts thyroid function. Many overweight people are that way because they have a sluggish thyroid—the gland that controls metabolism and body temperature. When they start eating coconut oil, their metabolism and thyroid function improves, and body temperature increases, becoming more normal. Weight loss becomes easier than it ever has.

Research has now confirmed that coconut oil is, without question, one of the most nutritious and healthful foods. That is why I instruct all my patients to incorporate it into their diets. I've seen amazing results, not just in weight loss, but in overcoming many health problems.

Here are a few comments from some of those who have experienced incredible changes in their health simply by adding coconut oil to their diets:

"Over the last 20 years I have been steadily and gradually gaining weight. You couldn't call me fat—but there I was, just too wobbly in all the wrong places. This year I decided to do something about it—finally. I went on a fruit diet. Nothing happened. I tried the cabbage soup diet (without the meat). Nothing happened. I fasted for a week. NOTHING HAPPENED!

That was when this book came into my hands—a godsend. I stopped fasting and began eating food again, but using coconut oil. After a few days

I weighted myself—I had lost 5 pounds! Since then I have lost a total of 24 pounds, and still losing steadily at about a pound a week, enjoying full meals."

Sharon

"The first week, I lost five pounds, and then two pounds a week after that. Getting ready in the morning used to be a chore—now I pop out of bed. I even wore a bikini this summer!…I feel great, and I'm actually eating a lot more now—and I have no fear of gaining weight."

Carine

"I've been taking about 1 or 2 tablespoons of virgin coconut oil per day for about 4 months now. I definitely notice a difference in my energy. It's steady through the day. No longer have the surges of ups and downs, especially that sleepy feeling after a meal. Obviously, my blood sugar must be steady."

Marty Ohlson

"I have been on a low-carbohydrate diet for the last 20 months and I have lost 52 pounds. I have about 10 pounds to go. I came across a statement in one book advocating a sugar-free lifestyle, and it said that coconut will help one get into ketosis. I was intrigued by that statement and so I purchased some coconut cream and oil and began to use them. I lost 2 pounds in a week (having lost only 4 pounds in the last six months, I was quite impressed). I shared this information with the low-carb newsgroup that I am on, and many of those members began to use the product and also lost weight; some of them had been on plateaus for a long time... Some also noticed an increase in energy as well as burning sensations that would indicate that their metabolism was up. Personally I get a sensation that I can only compare to a caffeine rush, although I haven't been a caffeine user for many years."

Gail Butler

"When I started, I weighed 316 and wore a size 52 pants. When I got on the scale this morning I weighed 256 for a total loss thus far of 60 pounds and I'm in 44's now…People that I work with intermittently comment on how much energy I have now. My 20-year-old son is doing this with me and has gone from 203 to 177 in three months. I don't count calories and in fact I think at any intake less than 2500-3000 I'd lose weight. I do figure out the calories every couple of weeks just to make sure I don't slip below 2000 a day. And I have a tendency to do that because I am never hungry anymore. With the fat intake at this level I am usually satiated for nine hours or so and find it very easy to inadvertently skip a meal if I get busy."

Chuck

"I was diagnosed with hypothyroidism... When I read your email about taking 3 teaspoons all at once, I decided it was worth a try. That was about 2:00 pm. About 20 minutes later, I went for a one-hour walk on very hilly terrain, and I could not help noticing how much energy I had, compared to three weeks ago, which was the last time I took that walk... At approximately 7:15 (some five hours after taking the 3 teaspoons of coconut oil), I took my temperature and to my amazement, it was 98.6° F. This is the first time in at least 15 years that my body temperature has been normal, unless I have the flu or some other illness. I cannot recall the last time that I have felt as good as I do right now. Thank you. I have renewed hope that I will be successful in losing the excess weight that has been preventing me from doing the many things that I love."

Rhea Lust

"It takes 3 teaspoons all at once to raise my body temperature. I usually run 97.1° F during the day. My new nut-balls recipe seems to be working too... These walnut-disappearing nut balls are delicious and they give me tons of energy. (I ate about 4 one-inch nut balls on an empty stomach as a snack.) Wondering where all this energy came from, I had a notion to take my temperature—98.6! Not only that, I have repeated the experiment several times this week and it works every time."

Marilyn Jarzembski

"I am a diabetic and I have taken myself off the meds the doctor wants me to take because I do not feel they are good for me long term. Last night I indulged myself with the coconut milk. I drank the whole can before bed. The amount of carbs was not real high, but it was an indulgence, so I was expecting my morning blood sugar to be somewhat high. What to my surprise, my morning blood sugars were much lower than normal. I try for fasting blood sugars of 110-120, but lately they have been around 140. This morning, they were 109. I am pleasantly surprised."

Alobar

"I have been on virgin coconut oil for the past two months (4 tablespoons daily) and feel better than I have in a long time! My energy levels are up and my weight is down. I am never hungry any more, and have incorporated a daily exercise routine, and have lost 20 pounds."

Paula Yfraimov

"I have lost a lot of weight recently (36 pounds in 5 months) and I use coconut and olive oil exclusively... I changed my diet to a low-carb program (nothing but meat, eggs, seafood, nonstarchy vegetables, fruit, nuts, and anything derived from these items, including coconut products). I do believe that coconut oil is part of the success because there have been times when I run out and will use only olive oil. During those times, I lose little or no weight."

Ann

"There are a few things I eat that boost my metabolism and many things that drain it. Coconut oil definitely boosts it. Taking a tablespoon of coconut oil is the quickest way I know of raising my temperature a whole degree within 45 minutes. It is really amazing."

Marilyn

"I am writing to express to you how happy I am with the use of coconut oil. I have been using it for all my cooking needs and have also been eating it by the spoonful. I also put it on my hair and use it in place of most hand and body creams. I am a 50-year-old overweight woman with chronic degenerative collagen vascular disorders. My energy level is improving. I am losing weight. My chronic pain is reducing. My skin and hair look much better and people are commenting on it. I can't thank you enough for telling the truth about coconut oil... Again thank you profusely!"

Janice W.

"I'm getting thinner by eating more fats. I am now down 31 pounds and I feel great! My husband's weight has dropped around 20 pounds and he is loving it too. Not eating wheat is certainly a factor in my continuing weight loss and improving health, but I have also made two radical changes when it comes to dietary fats. Firstly, I now eat at least three times the amount of fat I used to eat. That's right; I am eating more fat, not less. Secondly, the fats I am consuming are mostly saturated, with coconut oil at the top of the list, closely followed by butter and lard...I consume anything from 4 to 8 tablespoons a day."

Tracey T.

"I have been trying to lose weight since my hysterectomy a year ago. I was even starving myself, and nothing was happening. Then my mom mentioned that her boss had lost 10 pounds just by using coconut oil. I figured it couldn't hurt...In six weeks, I was 26 pounds smaller, I've tripled my energy, and I don't have to lie on the bed to zip my pants anymore!"

Abby

These are just a few of the many testimonials regarding the remarkable effects of adding coconut to the diet. The results are even more incredible when combined with a ketogenic eating plan, as you will learn in this book. Are you ready to lose excess weight and experience improved health and well-being? The following chapters will show you how.

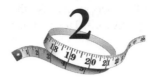

Big Fat Lies

LOW-FAT DIETS MAKE YOU FAT

The missing ingredient in most weight loss diets is fat. Yes, fat. Most other diets try to eliminate as much fat as possible—big mistake! Fat is the key to successful weight loss. As ironic as it may seem, you need to use fat to lose fat.

When people hear me say you need to eat more fat to lose weight and achieve better health, they look at me like I'm a nut. "Why, fat is bad for you," they say. "It makes you fat." Then when I tell them that the type of fat they should eat is predominately saturated, they gasp in horror. "Saturated fat causes heart disease!" I have to explain to them that over the years, advances in nutritional science have gone beyond the simple recommendations regarding saturated and unsaturated fats that we so commonly hear in the popular press. Popular diet books and the news media are usually years behind the advances made in science. Much of the dietary advice we have been given a few years ago has been proven wrong. One of these is the misconception that fat is unhealthy and should be avoided.

We now know that fat is a vital nutrient and must be present in the diet in order to maintain good health. That's why all major health organizations like the National Institutes of Health, The American Heart Association, and others recommend that we get 30 percent of our calories from fat rather than 20 or 10 percent as some extremists advocate.

Saturated fat in particular has received a lot of bad press in the past. What most people, including many health care professionals, don't understand is that there are many different types of saturated fat and they don't all act alike. Believe it or not, most of them don't raise blood cholesterol and are actually good for you. In fact, we need saturated fat in our diet to maintain good health. That is why health organizations don't say eliminate all saturated fat from your diet.

Eating fat, particularly saturated fat, is thought to be one of the ten deadly sins. Much of this misconception is fueled by the low-fat marketing efforts of the food industry. If a food is low in fat it means customers can eat more without guilt. The more we eat, the more we buy. The more we buy, the bigger the profits for manufacturers. The bigger the profits, the happier the food industry is. It's about money, not health. The low-calorie food craze hasn't accomplished a thing, except to make food producers rich and us fat. Yes, fat! People weigh more now than ever before.

In the United States, 60 percent of the population is now overweight; one in four adults is not merely overweight, but obese. A person is considered obese if weight is 20 percent or more than the maximum desirable weight for his or her height. According to the Centers for Disease Control and Prevention (CDC), the number of obese people in the US has exploded over the past two decades from 12 percent of the total population to 30 percent now. Even our kids are becoming fatter; as much as 25 percent of all teenagers are overweight. The number of overweight children has more than doubled in the past 30 years.

Over the past two to three decades, as the low-fat craze has been in full swing, obesity has increased by 70 percent in 18- to 29-year-olds. For people 30-39 years of age, it has increased 50 percent. All other age groups have likewise experienced a dramatic increase in weight.

We eat more low-fat foods than ever before but keep getting fatter and fatter. Low-fat dieting hasn't worked! Eating fat is not the problem.

LOW-FAT LIES

If you are one of the millions of people who have tried to lose weight on a low-fat diet and failed, don't blame yourself; give credit to the diet. Low-fat diets don't work. The whole theory behind them is flawed. Low-fat dieting requires radical and unpalatable changes that are almost impossible for most people to stay with for any length of time. For 30 years we have been cutting back on fat. The percentage of fat in the diet has dropped from about 40 percent to around 32 percent, yet we continue to gain weight. If you have tried to lose weight by removing fat from your diet, you have been a victim of a low-fat lie.

On the surface, the low-fat theory sounds logical. Of the three energy-producing nutrients—fat, protein, and carbohydrate—fat supplies the most calories. Gram for gram, fat contains over twice as many calories as either protein or carbohydrate. Therefore, if you replace protein or carbohydrate for fat in a meal, you can reduce the total number of calories while consuming basically the same volume of food. This much is true.

Unfortunately, it has led to the belief that the more fat you eliminate, the fewer calories you eat, and the fewer calories you consume the better. Weight loss is looked at as simply a problem of calorie consumption. That's why so many people, including health care professionals, have been misled.

The truth is, it just doesn't work that way. Common sense would tell you differently. Have you ever seen a large person eat salad every day and still gain weight? Or have you seen a thin person who eats fatty meats, gravies, and desserts and doesn't gain an ounce? Obviously, there is more to it than just calories. Other factors such as metabolism, nutrient content, and satiety are affected by the types of foods we eat and, consequently, influence our body weight. Losing or gaining weight is not simply a matter of calorie consumption.

The food industry would have you believe that body weight is simply a result of consuming too many calories. They promote this philosophy very aggressively. They sponsor studies, distribute educational materials to schools and health care professionals, write and publish articles, and send out news releases, all aimed at supporting their view. You can't pick up a general interest or health magazine nowadays without seeing articles on low-fat dieting. It's a popular subject on the radio and television. Books on the topic abound. The answer to our weight problem, we are led to believe, is conveniently provided by the food industry—eat less fat. They encourage us to buy leaner cuts of meat and low-fat, non-fat, and diet foods of every make and fashion. Their marketing strategy has worked. Grocery store shelves are jam-packed with such items. It's a very profitable multi-billion dollar business.

Leaner cuts of meat cost us more. Low-fat convenience foods are more expensive than natural foods like fresh fruits and vegetables. Sweets— cookies, cakes, pies, candy, ice cream—which common sense tells us are not exactly health or diet foods, are all too enticing. If they are low in fat, common sense goes out the window and we are given a license to eat without guilt. The consequence to all this is higher profits for the food industry and larger waistlines for us.

People won't keep eating foods they don't like. Fat gives food flavor. Low-fat foods lack flavor, so in order to make them more enticing to customers, manufactures must add more sugar, MSG, and other flavor enhancers. The result is a product that may have more total calories than the full-fat version and contain numerous chemical additives; both of which can have adverse affects on health and weight. While promoted as "healthy" alternatives to full-fat foods, in reality they are just the opposite.

We have been inundated with the low-fat mantra for so long that we equate "low-fat" with "healthy." Fat is treated as if it were a poison. We buy the leanest cuts of meat and trim off every ounce of fat. Our preferences are low- and non-fat foods in everything we buy. Our dinner plates are piled with sugar and starch, but heaven forbid if there is just the tiniest morsel of fat!

After years of being fed low-fat propaganda, we are led to believe that if a low-fat diet is good, a very-low fat diet must be better, and a no-fat diet must

18

be best of all. Many diet gurus such as Dr. Dean Ornish, Nathan Pritikin, and others have built empires off the low-fat hysteria. The low-fat myth extends through all corners of our society. Even our kids are brainwashed. In a poll conducted among schoolchildren, an incredible 81 percent thought that the healthiest diet possible was one that eliminated all dietary fat. Such a diet, however, would be a nutritional disaster.

FAT IS GOOD FOR YOU
Building Blocks
If you removed all the fat from your body you would have a lean, beautiful body, right?... Wrong! You would be reduced to a shapeless mass of protein and water lying in a puddle on the floor. You would resemble the Wicked Witch of the West after Dorothy doused her with a bucket of water.

Fat comprises a major structural component of every cell in your body. Fats make up the cell membrane—the skin that holds the cells together. Without fats, your cells would become puddles of water mixed with miscellaneous cellular debris. The cells in your heart, lungs, kidneys, and every other organ are dependent on fat to hold them together. Your brain is composed of 60 percent fat and cholesterol. To put it bluntly, a healthy, intelligent brain is full of fat.

Dietary fats are used not only to make structural components of cells, but also to make hormones and prostaglandins that control and regulate bodily functions. Vitamin D, estrogen, progesterone, testosterone, DHEA, and many other hormones are constructed out of cholesterol.

Hormones are the main regulators of metabolism, growth and development, reproduction, and many other processes. They play important roles in maintaining chemical balances within the body. Fat and cholesterol are used as building blocks for many hormones. If we had no cholesterol, we would have no sex hormones and, consequently, would be sexless. That is, there would be no male or female differentiation and reproduction would be impossible.

Likewise, prostaglandins, which are hormone-like substances made from fat, influence blood lipid concentrations, blood clot formation, blood pressure, immune response, and inflammation response to injury and infection.

A diet lacking in fat can seriously reduce the efficiency of your immune system and thus make you more susceptible to disease. The immune system not only protects us from infectious illnesses but from many degenerative conditions as well. Cancer, for example, is controlled by the immune system. Every one of us has cancerous cells in our bodies—yes, you, me, everybody. It's just a part of living. We don't all develop cancer, however, because our immune systems protect us. White blood cells roaming throughout our bodies attack and destroy cancerous cells, at least as long as the immune system

19

is functioning properly. If the immune system is depressed due to a lack of dietary fat or other nutrient deficiency, cancer is allowed to develop.

Without fat and cholesterol not only would you be a shapeless mass on the floor, and totally incapable of reproduction, you would be vulnerable to cancer and all manner of disease, and worst of all, you would be dead. Life would be impossible without fat.

Energy Source

Fat is fuel. Gasoline powers cars; fat powers our bodies. Fat is one of the three energy-producing nutrients. The other two are protein and carbohydrate. Our bodies use fat as a source of energy to power metabolic processes and maintain life. At least 60 percent of the body's energy needs are supplied by fat.

Every cell in our bodies must have a continual source of energy to function properly and maintain life. The body's first choice of fuel is carbohydrate. When there is adequate carbohydrate in the diet to meet energy needs, fat is put into storage inside fat cells. Excess carbohydrate and protein is converted into fat and also packed away into fat cells for use later. Between meals or during times of low food intake, fat is pulled out of storage and used to supply the body's ongoing energy needs.

Fat has more calories per gram than either carbohydrate or protein because it is a compact energy source that can be stored away and used later. Energy is measured in terms of calories. The body can store more calories (i.e., energy) as fat than it could as carbohydrate or protein. If the body stored protein instead of fat, you would look like a bloated pork sausage because your energy storage cells would double in size. So be thankful you store fat and not protein!

If you didn't have fat or adequate amounts of fat stored in fat cells, between meals and during prolonged periods of fasting, your body would resort to using protein, such as muscle tissue, for energy. Your body would literally consume itself to get the energy it needed to stay alive.

When you diet, it is important that you include fat in your meals. If you don't, your body will break down its own protein to supply its energy needs. You'll lose muscle mass. In extreme cases, such as starvation, organs are cannibalized to supply energy needs, which may cause permanent damage. Organ failure is the cause of death as a result of starvation.

Nutritional Source

It's a mistake to think of fat as a poison. On the contrary, it is an essential nutrient, just as much as protein, vitamin C, or calcium. We need fat in our diet to maintain proper health. Without fat in our diet, we would all sicken and die from nutrient deficiency.

Fats are composed of individual fat molecules called fatty acids. Two families of fat, known as omega-3 and omega-6 fatty acids, are considered

20

absolutely necessary for good health. Because of this, they are termed essential fatty acids. We must have them in the diet because the body cannot make them from other nutrients. These essential fatty acids are found in varying amounts in all foods—meat, fish, grains, and vegetables, as well as vegetable oils and animal fats. Avoiding fats or removing them from foods decreases the amount of essential fatty acids in the diet.

Without these fats, the body suffers from deficiency disease symptoms which include skin lesions, neurological and visual problems, growth retardation, reproductive failure, skin abnormalities, and kidney and liver disorders.

Fat is also necessary for the digestion and absorption of many other essential nutrients. For example, it is through the fatty portion of foods that we get our fat-soluble vitamins such as vitamins A, D, E, and K, as well as other important nutrients like beta-carotene. These nutrients cannot be absorbed without adequate fat in the diet.

One of the major problems with low-fat foods and low-fat diets is that they can create a nutrient deficiency. In order for your body to assimilate the fat-soluble vitamins, you need to have fat in your foods. If you don't eat enough fat, the vitamins pass right though the digestive tract without doing you a bit of good. For this reason alone, low-fat diets are dangerous.

Many of the fat-soluble vitamins function as antioxidants that protect you from free radical damage. Free radicals, which are highly reactive molecules that are continually being formed inside our bodies, are implicated as the cause, or at least a contributing factor, in most every known degenerative disease, including heart disease, cancer, and Alzheimer's. Free radical chemical reactions within our bodies cause the destruction of cells and their DNA. Many researchers believe that these reactions are the primary cause of aging. The more free-radical damage your body undergoes, the faster you age.

By reducing the amount of fat in your diet, you limit the amount of protective antioxidant nutrients available to protect you from destructive free-radical reactions. Low-fat diets speed the process of degeneration and aging. This may be one of the reasons why those people who stay on very low-fat diets for any length of time often look pale and sickly.

Carotenoids are fat-soluble nutrients found in fruits and vegetables. The best known is beta-carotene. All of the carotenoids are known for their antioxidant capability. Many studies have shown them, and other fat-soluble antioxidants such as vitamins A and E, to provide protection from degenerative conditions and support immune system function.

Vegetables like broccoli and carrots have beta-carotene, but if you don't eat any oil with them, you won't get the full benefit of their fat-soluble vitamins. If you eat a salad with low-fat dressing, you lose a good deal of the vitamins present in the vegetables. I often use a vinegar and water dressing. There is no fat in the dressing, but I always include nuts, avocado, cheese,

21

eggs, or other fat-containing foods to allow me to get the full benefit of the fat-soluble vitamins contained in the salad.

Another important nutrient that needs fat for proper absorption is calcium. How many people are deficient in calcium?... Lots. How many suffer with osteoporosis?... Lots. How many of these people eat low-fat foods? ... Lots. You can drink loads of non-fat milk and eat low-fat cheese and shovel down calcium supplements but still develop osteoporosis. Why? Because calcium needs fat to be absorbed. If you drink nonfat milk for the calcium, you are wasting your money. You need whole milk and full-fat cheese and other full-fat foods in order to absorb the calcium. Likewise, many vegetables are good sources of calcium. But in order to take advantage of that calcium, you need to eat them with butter and cream or other foods that contain fat.

Even your heart needs fat. This was shown in a study conducted by nutritionist Mary Flynn, Ph.D. Twenty subjects were given a diet with 37 percent of the calories from fat, and she measured their cholesterol and triglyceride levels. She then gave the same group a diet with less fat—25 percent of calories, but kept the total number of calories exactly the same by increasing carbohydrates. She found that low-fat diets lowered levels of good HDL cholesterol raised triglyceride levels, and basically left the levels of bad LDL cholesterol unchanged.[1] The overall effect was bad for the heart. You combine this with the fact that fat-soluble vitamins, such as vitamin E and beta-carotene, which help to protect against heart disease, are reduced in a low-fat diet, and you see that low-fat diets may actually promote heart disease—just the opposite from what the mainstream media leads us to believe. This is why many people who go on very low-fat diets become sick or develop intense food cravings. They need fat.

Nathan Pritikin advocated a very low-fat diet. Pritikin was a fanatic about keeping fat out of the diet. He claimed there was enough fat in lettuce and other vegetables to meet our body's needs. His diet limited fat consumption to a mere 10 percent of total calories. This is much less than The American Heart Association's recommendation of 30 percent. People lost weight, but they also developed health problems as a result of too little fat in their diet. Charles T. McGee, MD, describes patients who tried the Pritikin low-fat diet in his book *Heart Frauds*: "Pritikin Program patients become deficient in essential fatty acids after they have been on the diet about two years. These people entered the office looking gaunt, with skin that was dry, droopy, pale, gray, and flaky. Fortunately this complication was seldom seen because most people find it difficult to keep fat intake down to the 10 percent level without cheating."

Other Benefits

Fat has many important functions in the body. I have not mentioned all of them—just enough to show you how important they are in the diet. Researchers are discovering more benefits of dietary fat all the time. For example, in a study done at the University of Buffalo in 1999, female soccer players were able to perform longer at a higher intensity on a diet composed of 35 percent fat than on diets of 27 or 24 percent fat. This study showed that higher fat diets boost athletic performance.

Fat also helps regulate digestion and absorption of blood sugar, thus helping to prevent insulin resistance and diabetes. Without adequate amounts of fat in the diet, blood sugar levels can go out of control after eating a carbohydrate-rich meal.

Fat helps satisfy hunger longer so you don't eat as often, thus helping you to eat fewer calories. So eating fat helps you lose weight.

Fat keeps the skin soft and supple. Fat under the skin and fat working among the cells of the skin itself provides for good complexion and good skin tone.

Fat is essential for normal growth. It helps conserve important proteins, while carbohydrates tend to rob the body of proteins. Fat is also necessary for the proper growth and calcification of bones. People whose diet lacks sufficient fat are undersized.

Fat is helpful in controlling weight. You need to eat fat if you want to be slim.

As you see, fat is a very important component of our food. It is involved in a variety of functions throughout the body, many of which science has yet to fully understand.

Dietary fats, however, are not all alike. There are many different types of fats and each has a different effect on the body. Modern processing and food manufacturing have created some fats that are detrimental to your health and contribute to overweight and other health problems. So you must choose your fats wisely. In general, the more processing a fat or oil has undergone to reach the grocery store shelf, the less healthy it is. Fake fats like olestra and semi-fake fats like margarine and other hydrogenated vegetable oils are the most processed and the least healthy. Natural fats and oils—those that are easily extracted from their source with even primitive methods—such as olive oil, coconut oil, butter, and animal fats are the most beneficial.

I know this goes against popular opinion, but just because most people believe in something that is false doesn't make it true. Popular opinions are often wrong. Look at low-fat diets; they are still loudly proclaimed as the only way to lose weight, yet we know for a fact that in the long run they don't work.

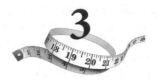

Are you In Need of An Oil Change?

FATS, TRIGLYCERIDES, AND FATTY ACIDS

Fat—the word often conjures up images of grotesque, greasy tissue hanging off of a slab of meat. Meat, however, isn't the only place we find fat. All living organisms have it. Animals have it, people have it, plants have it, even the tiniest organisms like protozoa and bacteria have it. Fat is an essential tissue to life. For this reason, fat in one form or another is found in all of our foods. And although most people like to eliminate it as much as possible, it constitutes an important part of our diet.

The terms "fat" and "oil" are often used interchangeably. Generally speaking, fats are solid at room temperature while oils remain liquid. You will often hear the term "lipid" in reference to fats and oils. Lipid is a general term that includes several fat-like compounds in the body. By far the most abundant and the most important of the lipids are the triglycerides. When we speak of fats and oils, we are usually referring to triglycerides. Two other lipids—phospholipids and sterols (which includes cholesterol)—technically are not fats because they are not triglycerides. But they have similar characteristics and are often loosely referred to as fats.

When you cut into a beefsteak, the white fatty tissue you see is composed of triglycerides. Cholesterol is also present, but it is intermingled within the meat fibers and undetectable to the naked eye. The fat that is a nuisance to us, the type that hangs on our arms, looks like jelly on our thighs, and makes our stomachs look like spare tires, is composed of triglycerides. The triglycerides make up our body fat and the fat we see and eat in animal foods. About 95 percent of the lipids in our diet from both plant and animal sources are triglycerides.

Triglycerides are comprised of individual fat molecules called fatty acids. The three general categories of fatty acids are saturated, monounsaturated, and polyunsaturated. All oils and animal fats consist of a mixture of these three fatty acids. To describe an oil as being saturated or monounsaturated is grossly oversimplifying the situation. No oil is purely saturated or polyunsaturated. Olive oil, for example, is often called "monounsaturated" because it is predominantly monounsaturated, but like all vegetable oils, it also contains some polyunsaturated and saturated fat as well. Lard as well contains saturated, monounsaturated, and polyunsaturated fatty acids. In fact, lard has a higher percentage of monounsaturated fat (47 percent) than saturated fat (41 percent). It is more accurate to refer to lard as a monounsaturated fat than as a saturated one.

Animal fats come from the flesh of animals and from milk and eggs. The vast majority of our vegetable oils come from seeds such as cottonseed, sunflower seeds, safflower seeds, and rapeseed (canola), but even grains (e.g., corn), legumes (e.g., soybeans and peanuts), and nuts (e.g., almonds, walnuts) are seeds. Coconut oil comes from the seed of the coconut palm. Some oils come from fruits (e.g., olive, palm, and avocado).

Like other oils, coconut oil contains a mixture of saturated, monounsaturated, and polyunsaturated fatty acids. However, it is predominately a saturated fat, 92 percent, in fact. The vast majority of this saturated fat is in the form of medium chain triglycerides (MCTs). This makes coconut oil unique among dietary fats. Most fats consist of long chain triglycerides (LCTs). Approximately 95 percent of all the fats in our diet consist of LCTs. Corn oil, soybean oil, olive oil, canola oil, lard, and most other common dietary fats are 100 percent LCTs. Butter and cream contain a very small amount of MCTs; coconut and palm kernel oils are the only significant dietary sources of MCTs. This is important, because most of the health-promoting and weight loss properties associated with coconut oil come from the MCTs. Since other oils don't have any appreciable amount of MCTs, they can't compare to coconut oil.

Generally, fats and oils found naturally in foods support good health and provide many essential nutrients. Not all fats, however, are of equal value in terms of weight management or health benefits. A healthy weight-loss diet must include an adequate amount of the right kind of fat.

If you were asked which oils are the healthiest, what would be your answer? If you responded to that question like most people, you probably would have said that polyunsaturated vegetable oils are the best and saturated fats are the worst. If this was your answer, than you have been deceived, just as most people are, including me at one time. Contrary to what the vegetable oil industry has led us to believe, the overconsumption of polyunsaturated oils carry far more health risks than do monounsaturated fats, saturated fats, or cholesterol. Although we need some polyunsaturated fats, we can get too much. If you are currently eating mostly polyunsaturated vegetable oils in your diet, you are in need of an oil change. In this chapter you will find out why.

REFINED AND UNREFINED OILS

Over the past century we have been in the midst of a revolution—a dietary revolution. Foods our ancestors have eaten, even thrived on for generations, have been pushed aside to make way for new, technologically advanced foods. One of the biggest changes that has taken place during this time is the type of oils we consume. Butter, lard, coconut oil, and other traditional fats have been usurped by highly refined, purified, and even chemically altered vegetable oils.

If you traveled to the mountains of northern Pakistan to visit the Hunza, you would find a people who relish butter and goat fat. If you went to rural China, you would find lard to be the dietary fat of choice. Among the Eskimos in Northern Canada and Alaska, seal oil is the traditional mainstay. In Thailand, coconut oil is used in all cooking. In India, ghee (clarified butter) and coconut oil are traditionally the preferred choices. In Italy and Greece, olive oil reigns supreme. Wherever traditional fats and oils are used, you will find them eating primarily saturated and monounsaturated oils of one type or another. What you won't find much of is polyunsaturated vegetable oils.

Oils have constituted an important part of the diet for generations. Those that were most popular were relatively easy to obtain using primitive methods of extraction. Animal fat was simply cut off the meat and rendered into oil by cooking. Butter was made from churning milk. Olive oil was squeezed out of the fruit by screw-type presses or pounded out using a wooden funnel and hammer. Vegetable oils from nuts and seeds were produced by the crushing action of wooden presses or stone rollers.

By far the most common oils used throughout history were animal fats, butter, coconut and palm oils, and olive oil. Some populations used vegetable oils more than others, but because of the difficulty of extraction, vegetable seed oils were not widely used and never contributed significantly to the human diet.[1]

Fats and oils have nourished mankind for generations. But the types of oils we consume now are much different than those that nourished our great-grandparents. We have moved away from using unrefined oils to highly refined and purified polyunsaturated oils.

With the invention of the hydraulic oil press and the use of chemical extraction agents, vegetable seed oils became more economical. As saturated fats began to be criticized for raising blood cholesterol, polyunsaturated vegetables oils became more popular. However, one of the drawbacks with using polyunsaturated vegetable oils is that they oxidize (go rancid) very quickly. Therefore, they need to be heavily refined and contain chemical

26

preservatives to retard spoilage. All of the common vegetable oils we see sold at the grocery store are of this type.

There are some vegetable oils that are produced using age-old traditional methods, without chemicals or high heat. The most popular is extra virgin olive oil. It retains its full flavor, color, aroma, and all its natural vitamins and minerals. Coconut oil is often produced by traditional methods or modern true cold-processing methods without the use of chemicals. It is sometimes referred to as virgin coconut oil to distinguish it from more refined oils; it retains a delightful coconut flavor and aroma. You can also find sesame, palm, almond, and other oils produced in a similar manner. The way to identifying truly unrefined oil is by taste and smell. The more an oil is processed and refined, the less flavor and aroma it retains. Oils high in saturated fats, like coconut oil, are very stable and even when they are heavily processed are still better choices than polyunsaturated oils.

Many oils have a very disagreeable flavor and must be deodorized to make them palatable. Soybean oil, for example, is one of these. Unprocessed soybean oil has a horrible taste and must undergo harsh processing and chemical treatments to remove its displeasing flavor and is, therefore, always highly processed.

HYDROGENATED VEGETABLE OILS

The process of hydrogenation was developed by the Proctor & Gamble company in 1907. Hydrogenation was an innovative new process that could transform a liquid vegetable oil into a solid fat that resembled lard. The first use of hydrogenation was to transform cheap cottonseed oil into a solid fat that could be used in place of lard and tallow in the making of soap and candles.

The success of their cheap imitation lard boosted company profits. It wasn't long before they reasoned that since hydrogenated cottonseed oil resembled lard, they could also sell it as a food. So in 1911 they introduced Crisco shortening. The name Crisco was derived from the words CRYStalized Cottonseed Oil. In order to encourage women to switch from using butter and lard to shortening, they distributed a cookbook and began publishing ads portraying Crisco as a more economical and healthier alternative to animal fats. The transformation away from animal fats and toward vegetable oils had begun.

Before long, margarine became available. Margarine was simply hydrogenated cottonseed oil mixed with flavoring and dye so as to resemble butter. Sales were modest at first but picked up during the Great Depression of the 1930s when people switched from using lard and butter to the cheaper shortening and margarine. Sales again made an upswing in the 1950s and 1960s as people suddenly became aware of the presumed dangers of animal fats. By 1957 more people were buying margarine than butter.

27

It is interesting that Proctor & Gamble and other vegetable oil companies sponsored much of the research which supposedly linked saturated fat and cholesterol with heart disease. In fact, Dr. Fred Mattson, one of scientists who worked for P&G, was instrumental in persuading the American Heart Association to accept the cholesterol theory of heart disease and was active in influencing governmental policy concerning dietary fats.

The process of hydrogenation begins with a refined vegetable oil. Nowadays, most hydrogenated oils are made from soybean oil. The oil is mixed with tiny metal particles—usually nickel oxide, which is very toxic and impossible to completely remove—that act as a chemical catalyst. Under high pressures and temperatures, hydrogen gas is squeezed into the oil and chemically bonded to the fat molecules. Emulsifiers and starch are then forced into the mixture to give it a better consistency. The mixture is again subjected to high temperatures in a steam-cleaning process to remove its horrible odor.

The hydrogenation process is now complete, but the resulting oil is a disgusting gray color, more like what you would expect to see in a jar of axle grease than food, so it is bleached to give it a more appetizing white appearance. The final result is hydrogenated vegetable oil or, as we see it on the store shelves, shortening. To make margarine, coal-tar dyes and chemical flavorings are added. This mixture is compressed and packaged in blocks or tubs, ready to be enjoyed on a slice of bread. Just knowing how margarine and shortening are made is enough to keep me from eating them.

In the process of hydrogenation, liquid vegetable oils become solid fats, and another thing with significant health implications happens: a new fatty acid, unlike those normally found in nature, is created. This is called the trans fatty acid. This toxic fatty acid is foreign to our bodies and can create all sorts of trouble.

"These are probably the most toxic fats ever known," says Walter Willett, MD, professor of epidemiology and nutrition at Harvard School of Public Health. Willett, who has researched the effects of trans fats on the body, disagrees with those who say that the hydrogenated fats found in margarine or shortening are less likely to raise cholesterol than the saturated fats found in butter: "It looks like trans fatty acids are two to three times as bad as saturated fats in terms of what they do to blood lipids."[2]

Studies now clearly show that trans fatty acids can contribute to atherosclerosis (hardening of the arteries) and heart disease. For example, swine fed a diet containing trans fatty acids developed more extensive atherosclerotic damage than those fed other types of fats.[3] In humans, trans fatty acids increase blood LDL (bad cholesterol) and lower the HDL (good cholesterol), both regarded as undesirable changes.[4] Trans fatty acids have been shown to raise blood cholesterol levels even more than saturated fat.[5] Since trans fat also lowers the good HDL cholesterol, unlike saturated fat, researchers now believe it has a greater influence on the risk of cardiovascular disease than any other dietary fat.[6]

28

The *New England Journal of Medicine* reported the results of a 14-year study of more than 80,000 nurses (New England Journal of Medicine November 20, 1997). The research, conducted the Harvard School of Public Health and Brigham and Women's Hospital in Boston, documented 939 heart attacks among the participants. Among the women who consumed the largest amounts of trans fats, the chance of suffering a heart attack was 53 percent higher than among those at the low end of trans fat consumption.

Another interesting fact uncovered by this study was that total fat intake had little effect on the rate of heart attack. Women in the group with the largest consumption of total fat (46 percent of calories) had no greater risk of heart attack than those in the group with the lowest (29 percent of calories).

The researchers said this suggested that limiting consumption of trans fats would be more effective in avoiding heart attacks than reducing overall fat intake. Unfortunately, about 10 percent of the fat in the typical Western diet is trans fat.

Trans fatty acids affect more than just our cardiovascular health. According to a study reported by Mary Enig, Ph.D., when monkeys were fed trans fat-containing margarine in their diets, their red blood cells did not bind insulin as well as when they were not fed trans fat.[7] This suggests a link with diabetes. Trans fatty acids have been linked with a variety of adverse health effects including cancer, ischemic heart disease, multiple sclerosis, diverticulitis, diabetes, and other degenerative conditions.[8]

Hydrogenated oil is a product of technology and may be the most destructive food additive currently in common use. If you eat margarine, shortening, or hydrogenated or partially hydrogenated vegetable oils (common food additives), then you are consuming trans fatty acids.

Many of the foods you buy in the store and in restaurants are prepared with or cooked in hydrogenated oil. Fried foods sold in grocery stores and restaurants are usually cooked in hydrogenated oil because it makes foods crispy and is more resistant to spoilage than ordinary vegetable oils. Many frozen processed foods are cooked or prepared in hydrogenated oils. Hydrogenated oils are used in making french fries, biscuits, cookies, crackers, chips, frozen pies, pizzas, peanut butter, cake frosting, and ice cream substitutes such as mellorine.

The liquid vegetable oils you buy in the store aren't much better. The heat used in the extraction and refining process also creates trans fatty acids. So that bottle of corn or safflower oil you have on the kitchen shelf contains trans fatty acids even though it has not been hydrogenated. Unless the vegetable oil has been "cold pressed" or "expeller pressed," it contains trans fatty acids. Most all of the common brands of vegetable oil and salad dressings contain trans fatty acids.

Liquid vegetable oils contain an average of 15 percent trans fatty acids. In comparison, margarine and shortening average about 35 percent, but some brands may run as high as 48 percent.

When monounsaturated and polyunsaturated oils are used in cooking, especially at high temperatures, trans fatty acids are formed. So even if you use cold pressed oil from the health food store, if you use it in your cooking, you are creating unhealthy trans fatty acids.

You might ask: does the amount of trans fatty acids that are produced when you heat oils at home pose any real danger? Studies show diets containing heat-treated liquid corn oil were found to produce more atherosclerosis than those containing unheated corn oil.[9] So, yes any unsaturated vegetable oil becomes toxic when heated. And even a small amount, especially if eaten frequently over time, will affect your health.

Saturated fats from any source are much more resistant to temperatures used in cooking, do not form trans fatty acids, and therefore, make much better cooking oils. Saturated fats are the safest to use in cooking. In an effort to create a cheap source of oil from polyunsaturated vegetable sources, modern technology has created a major health problem.

Under pressure from many health organizations and the public, the Food and Drug Administration (FDA) imposed a regulation requiring food manufactures to include the amount of trans fatty acids on the package labels. Before taking this step, however, they waited three years for the Institute of Medicine to study the issue.

After the study was performed, to everyone's surprise, the Institute of Medicine didn't give a recommendation as to what percentage of trans fats were safe to consume, as is often done with food additives, but flatly stated that no level of trans fats is safe. If you see a packaged food that contains hydrogenated oil, margarine, or shortening, don't touch it. If you eat out, ask the restaurant manager what type of oil they use to cook their food. If they say "vegetable oil," it almost definitely is hydrogenated vegetable oil; avoid it. The reason you can safely count on it being hydrogenated vegetable oil is because regular vegetable oil breaks down too quickly and becomes rancid. Restaurants like to reuse their oils as long as possible before they have to be tossed out. Ordinary vegetable oils have too short a life span.

FREE RADICALS

Research over the past few decades has identified a key player in the cause and development of degenerative disease and aging. That player is the free radical.

Simply stated, a free radical is a renegade molecule that has lost an electron in its outer orbit, leaving an unpaired electron. This creates a highly unstable and powerful molecular entity. These radicals will quickly attack and steal an electron from a neighboring molecule. The second molecule, now with one less electron, becomes a highly reactive free radical itself and pulls an electron off yet another nearby molecule. This process continues in a destructive chain reaction that may affect hundreds or even thousands of molecules.

Once a molecule becomes a radical, its physical and chemical properties change. The normal function of such molecules is permanently disrupted, affecting the entire cell of which they are a part. A living cell attacked by free radicals degenerates and becomes dysfunctional. Free radicals can attack our cells, literally ripping their protective membranes apart. Sensitive cellular components like the nucleus and DNA, which carry the genetic blueprint of the cell, can be damaged, leading to cellular mutations or death.

The more free radicals attacking our cells, the greater the damage and the greater the potential for serious destruction. If the affected cells are in our heart or arteries, what happens? If they are in the brain, what happens? If they are in our joints, pancreas, intestines, liver, or kidneys, what happens? Think about it. If the cells become damaged, dysfunctional, or die, can these organs fulfill their intended purpose at optimal levels, or do they degenerate?

Free-radical damage has been linked to the loss of tissue integrity and to physical degeneration. As cells are bombarded by free radicals, the tissues become progressively impaired. Some researchers believe that free-radical destruction is the actual cause of aging.[10] The older the body gets, the more damage it sustains from a lifetime accumulation of attack from free radicals.

Today some sixty or so degenerative diseases are recognized as having free radicals involved in their cause or manifestation.[10] Additional diseases are regularly being added to this list. The research that linked the major killer diseases such as heart disease and cancer to free radicals has expanded to include atherosclerosis, stroke, varicose veins, hemorrhoids, hypertension, wrinkled skin, dermatitis, arthritis, digestive problems, reproductive problems, cataracts, loss of energy, diabetes, allergies, failing memory, and many other degenerative conditions.

The more exposure we have to free radicals, the more damage occurs to our cells and tissues, which in turn increases our chances of developing the conditions listed above. We are exposed to free radicals from the pollutants in the air we breathe and from the chemical additives and toxins in the foods we eat and drink. Some free-radical reactions occur as part of the natural process of cellular metabolism. We can't avoid all the free radicals we encounter in our environment, but we can limit them. Cigarette smoke, for example, causes free-radical reactions in the lungs. Certain foods and food additives also cause destructive free-radical reactions that affect our entire body. Limiting your exposure to these free-radical-creating substances will reduce your risk of developing a number of degenerative conditions. In this regard, the types of oil you use have a very pronounced effect on your health.

When unsaturated oils oxidize (go rancid), they generate free radicals. The more unsaturated an oil is, the more easily it oxidizes. Therefore, polyunsaturated oils are much more vulnerable to oxidation than

31

monounsaturated oils, and monounsaturated oils are more vulnerable than saturated oils.

Heat, light, and oxygen act as catalysts to promote oxidation: the longer the exposure, the greater the degree of oxidation. Polyunsaturated oils when extracted from their source and exposed to heat, light, and oxygen, oxidize very rapidly. When you buy a bottle of soybean oil in the store, it has already begun to oxidize. Sitting on the store shelf exposed to light and heat (even room temperature) is enough to promote oxidation in a volatile oil. Once you bring it home and open the bottle, oxidation and free-radical formation accelerate. If you use the oil in any type of cooking, you greatly compound the problem by accelerating the formation of harmful free radicals.

Numerous studies, in some cases published as early as the 1930s, have reported on the toxic effects of consuming heated vegetable oils.[11] For this reason, you should never use polyunsaturated vegetable oils in cooking or baking. It's ironic that some people will buy "cold pressed" vegetable oils and go home and use them in cooking. Cold pressed oils oxidize just as rapidly as refined oils.

Monounsaturated and saturated oils do not oxidize as easily as polyunsaturated oils. They are much more stable for cooking purposes. Monounsaturated oils are safe to use for low-temperature cooking. Saturated fats, which are the most resistant to oxidation, can be used for all types of cooking even at high temperatures without harm, as long as they are not heated above their smoke point. Each oil has a different smoke point.

Refined vegetable oils are deceptive. You can't tell a rogue from a saint. They all pretty much look alike. They have been purified, deodorized, and stripped of all taste and character. When the oil begins to go rancid, it does not affect the smell or flavor.[12] You can eat a very rancid, highly oxidized oil and not even detect any difference, especially if the oil is combined with other foods as it normally is. The only time rancid oils produce an offensive smell and flavor is when they contain impurities such proteins or plant pigments. Free radicals attack these impurities and transform them into putrid-smelling substances. An oil that has been minimally processed and still contains some of its natural plant substances is more likely to produce an offensive smell than a highly processed and purified oil. You can eat rancid oil without realizing it.

Unsaturated oils that retain their natural flavor and aroma may go rancid in time. If the oil begins to taste a little off or sour, throw it out. However, polyunsaturated oils that have been deodorized and purified will not have any flavor or smell even when they go rancid. Don't use them. The best oils are those that have a pleasant, natural flavor.

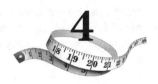

Cholesterol and Saturated Fat

THE CHOLESTEROL HYPOTHESIS OF
HEART DISEASE

I want to take you back in time. Back long before you were born. Not too far back, however—only far enough to meet face-to-face with your great-great-grandparents. The year is 1878. Why 1878? This was the year that a strange new disease was first documented in the medical literature. Dr. Adam Hammer, a British physician, described for the first time a previously unknown condition now referred to as a heart attack. Up to that time no cases of heart attack had ever been documented in the medical literature. Dr. Hammer reported that a patient had experienced crushing chest pain, then collapsed and died. An autopsy found that muscle tissue in the patient's heart had died, resulting in heart failure and death. Nowadays, the signs of heart attack are well known and common. Thousands of people die every single day from heart disease. It is the number one killer in the world. Statistically, your chance of dying from a heart attack is about one in three.

Why was heart disease so rare back then and why is it so common now? Many heart attack victims are only in their 30s and 40s. A century ago people could live to be 60, 70, and 80 years of age without dying from heart attacks. So it is not a disease caused by age. If you asked anyone on the street what causes heart disease, the most common answer you would receive is eating too much cholesterol and saturated fat. Is that really the cause of heart disease?

Let's go back to 1878. What types of fats and oils did they eat in those days? The oils in common use were lard (pig fat), tallow (beef fat), butter, coconut and palm oils, and to a lesser extent olive oil. They didn't have the technology then to produce to any great degree corn, soybean, safflower, and most other polyunsaturated oils. So our ancestors, who never heard of heart disease, ate mostly animal fats which are loaded with cholesterol and saturated fat. The effects on their health were clearly evident—heart disease, cancer, diabetes, obesity, and numerous other diseases of modern civilization were rare.

If cholesterol and saturated fat cause or even contribute to all of these health problems, as many claim, why after thousands of years in the human diet have they suddenly become toxic? Or have they? We've heard that cholesterol and saturated fat cause heart disease for so long and so often that we can repeat it in our sleep. But do they really? Both medical science and history say "no."

The cholesterol hypothesis of heart disease was first proposed in the 1950s by researcher Ancel Keys. Using data from six countries (United States, Canada, Australia, England, Italy, and Japan), Keys showed a correlation between fat consumption and death rate due to heart disease. The more fat consumed, the higher the heart disease death rate. Saturated fat was specifically identified as the primary culprit. Keys' cholesterol hypothesis was immediately hailed as the long sought for explanation for the rapid rise in heart disease deaths.

Keys' landmark study, however, was seriously flawed. He selected his data very carefully. He had available to him information from 22 counties but only used those that supported his hypothesis. Data from the other 16 countries did not support his hypothesis and even contradicted it. For instance, the death rate from heart disease in Finland was 24 times that of Mexico, even though fat consumption in the two countries was nearly identical. Another example: the heart disease death rate in the US is much higher than that of France even though the French consume a much higher amount of saturated fat and cholesterol. If you look at the dietary data from all countries available to Keys, you find there is no correlation between saturated fat consumption and heart disease. Regardless of this fact, doctors were desperate to find a reason for the sharp rise in heart disease over the first half of the 20th century and this theory supplied a convenient answer. Since there was no other theory at the time, Keys' hypothesis quickly gained acceptance and became the prevailing belief on the origin of heart disease.

Dr. Paul Dudley White is known as the father of cardiology—the study of the heart and its diseases. He graduated from medical school in 1910 and served as President Dwight D. Eisenhower's physician during his terms in office. As a young man, White wrote that he had an interest in a rare new disease that he had read about in the European medical literature. It was in 1921, 11 years after he began his practice, when he saw his first heart attack patient. At that time, heart attacks were extremely rare. By the 1950s, when he served as Eisenhower's physician, heart disease had become the nation's leading cause of death. Later in his career, and as the foremost authority in the world on cardiology and, consequently, heart disease, he was asked for his opinion about the theory that cholesterol and saturated fat cause heart disease. He stated that he couldn't support the theory because he knew it didn't fit the history of the disease.[1]

The graph below illustrates why saturated fat and cholesterol can't be the cause of heart disease. The number of heart attack deaths per 100,000 people are plotted over time in comparison to cholesterol and saturated fat intake. Note that cholesterol and saturated fat levels have remained essentially constant, but heart attack deaths have skyrocketed. There is clearly no correlation between heart disease and cholesterol or saturated fat consumption.[2]

From 1910 to 1920 heart disease deaths were fairly low, affecting only about 10 out of every 100,000 people per year. By 1930 the death rate jumped to 46 per 100,000 and by 1970 the rate reached 331 per 100,000. It is interesting to note that sugar consumption started to become more common at the beginning of the 20th century and has steadily increased along with the rate of heart disease. It would seem that there is a much stronger correlation between heart disease and sugar consumption than with saturated fat or cholesterol.

The food and drug industries have been very active in publicizing and promoting the theory that saturated fat and cholesterol cause heart disease. Since the 1950s they've been the primary financial sponsors in this area of study. Yet even after 60 years of research there is very little evidence to

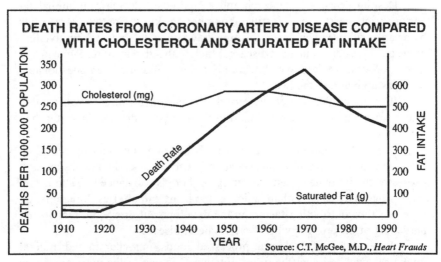

DEATH RATES FROM CORONARY ARTERY DISEASE COMPARED WITH CHOLESTEROL AND SATURATED FAT INTAKE

Source: C.T. McGee, M.D., *Heart Frauds*

From 1910 to 1970 deaths from coronary artery disease increased an incredible 3,010 percent, then began to decline. During this time, cholesterol and saturated fat intake remained fairly constant, indicating little correlation between cholesterol or saturated fat with heart disease.

35

support the belief that a diet low in cholesterol and saturated fat actually reduces death from heart disease or in any way increases one's life span.

The cholesterol theory or cholesterol hypothesis implies that animal fat consumption must have increased significantly since 1920 to correlate with the rise in heart disease, but in fact the consumption of butter and animal fats in America declined steadily during that period, while use of sugar and vegetable fats increased dramatically. During the 60-year period from 1910 to 1970, the proportion of traditional animal fat in the American diet declined from 83 percent to 62 percent, and butter consumption plummeted from 17 pounds per person per year to about 4 pounds. During the past 80 years, dietary cholesterol intake has increased only 1 percent. During the same period the percentage of dietary vegetable fat in the form of margarine, shortening, and processed oils increased about 400 percent. When you look objectively at all the facts, the cholesterol hypothesis doesn't hold up.

In an attempt to scare the public and promote the increased use of vegetable oils, animal fats are blamed for every disease under the sun. It is now the politically correct thing to do, even though there is very little evidence that animal fats cause any harm. Obesity, diabetes, cancer, heart disease—you name it and someone is claiming that saturated fat or cholesterol is somehow the cause. But again, the facts don't fit the theory.

VITAMIN AND MINERAL DEFICIENCY

Despite decades of research and a significant decrease in animal fat consumption, heart disease is still our number one killer. Continuous attempts by an army of researchers over this time have failed to show a definitive link between cholesterol and heart disease. Much to the dismay of researchers and their sponsors, studies have shown only a very mild and even questionable relationship between the two.

If saturated fats and cholesterol don't cause heart disease, what does? There are a number of factors found to tie into heart disease far better than these fats.

In the 1940s and 1950s, researchers Yudkin and Lopez discovered a link between consumption of refined sugar and heart disease. Sugar consumption depresses the immune system, lowering the body's resistance to bacteria and viruses that may cause inflammation in the heart and arteries. Inflammation is one of the contributing factors in the development of arterial plaque and hardening of the arteries, which leads to heart disease.

With the use of packaged, processed foods, our vitamin and mineral intake has declined over the years. Vitamin C is one of the nutrients that is depleted in processed foods. This vitamin is necessary to maintain integrity of connective tissue including those in the arteries. One of the signs of vitamin C deficiency is atherosclerosis (hardening of the arteries). The B vitamins, which have also declined in our food supply, are necessary in order to keep arteries strong and healthy. Research has shown that vitamin B deficiency is a major cause of atherosclerosis and heart disease.[3]

Heart disease has also been correlated with mineral deficiencies. Coronary heart disease rates are lower in regions where drinking water is naturally rich in minerals, particularly magnesium, which acts as a natural anticoagulant and aids in potassium absorption, thereby preventing heart rate irregularities. Vitamin D is also important in protecting the heart. It is essential for absorption of many minerals, particularly calcium and magnesium. Our bodies can manufacture vitamin D from cholesterol by the action of sunlight on the skin, but we are told to reduce our cholesterol consumption and our exposure to the sun in fear of developing skin cancer.

Excess sugar consumption also drains B vitamins needed to maintain healthy arteries. Research from the US Department of Agriculture indicates that fructose may be even more dangerous than sucrose (table sugar). Fructose, mainly in the form of high-fructose corn syrup, has become the sweetener of choice for soft drinks, snacks, and many so-called health foods.

In 1968 the death rate from heart attacks fell for the first time in over 40 years and has continued to slowly decline ever since. By 1990 the death rate had fallen to 194 per 100,000 people. Those who support the cholesterol hypothesis have not attempted to take credit for this decline because fat consumption has remained relatively constant the entire time. The reason why the death rate has fallen since the 1970s may be due to the increasing use of vitamin and mineral supplements. Nutritional deficiencies, which are probably a major contributor to heart disease, have somewhat lessened due to increased usage of vitamins and minerals.

Refined vegetable oils contain little nutritional value other than fatty acids. They are basically empty calories. These oils not only contribute no vitamins or minerals, but actually deplete the body's nutrient reserves and thereby promote deficiency. Polyunsaturated oils are highly unstable and oxidize very easily, both inside and outside the body. Oxidation of polyunsaturated oils creates destructive free radicals. Antioxidant nutrients such as vitamin A, vitamin E, Vitamin C, beta-carotene, zinc, selenium, and others are destroyed trying to fight off these free radicals. In this process the body can become deficient in these essential nutrients. The result is a condition called subclinical malnutrition, which can lead to physical degeneration and even promote obesity. It is no wonder that as vitamin sales have increased, heart disease rates have declined.

Another problem with polyunsaturated vegetable oils is the fact that the primary fatty acid they contain, linoleic acid, is transformed by the body into hormone-like substances called prostaglandins. In excess, these prostaglandins can have a negative effect on health. For example, they encourage blood clotting, constriction of arteries which narrows passageways, and inflammation, all of which contribute to heart disease. In addition, the free radicals these oils generate can damage the arteries, thereby initiating plaque deposits. It's no wonder that heart disease has risen along with the increase in vegetable oil consumption.

THE CHOLESTEROL MYTH

When we hear the word "cholesterol," the first thoughts that come to most people's minds are clogged arteries and heart disease. Cholesterol has almost become synonymous with heart disease. Everyone "knows" that cholesterol causes heart disease. You see it in the paper. You read about it in books. You hear it on television and the radio. They all loudly proclaim "High blood cholesterol causes heart disease." We hear it so much that it must be true. So many "experts" can't be wrong. Right?

We also know that saturated fat causes heart disease, don't we? That is what we read and that is what everyone says. Saturated fat has been labeled a villain because it can raise blood cholesterol levels too. And since saturated fat is much more abundant in our foods than cholesterol, it is considered by far the greater threat.

For years we have been told that cholesterol and saturated fat raise blood cholesterol and, therefore, cause cardiovascular disease. We hear this so often we are led to believe that there is a great deal of evidence supporting the cholesterol hypothesis. But actually, there has never been a study demonstrating that high blood cholesterol causes heart disease. Not a single one! In fact, the opposite is true. Numerous studies show that cholesterol does not cause clogged arteries or heart disease. People die of heart disease without having high blood cholesterol. Others with high blood cholesterol show no signs of cardiovascular disease—no plaque in arteries, no abnormal clotting, and blood pressure within normal ranges. If high blood cholesterol caused cardiovascular disease, then it would have to be present in all people who die from it. But it's not. This fact is clearly recognized.

Most cholesterol researchers will admit that high blood cholesterol does not cause heart disease. The drug industry has had a lot to do with creating a false impression because they sell billions of dollars worth of cholesterol-lowering drugs. Their cry that high blood cholesterol leads to cardiovascular disease has been so loud and so often repeated that we've been brainwashed into believing it. Throughout history, dubious political leaders have held to the philosophy that if you tell a lie often enough and loud enough, eventually everyone will accept it as truth, no matter how preposterous it may be. That is the situation we have with cholesterol.

"The cholesterol theory is not compatible with the history of coronary artery disease," says Charles T. McGee, MD, in his book *Heart Frauds*. "Dietary consumption of fats and cholesterol does not affect blood levels of cholesterol significantly in the vast majority of people. Many people with high blood cholesterol never experience coronary artery disease. People with low blood cholesterol can and do develop coronary artery disease. About one-third of the people who have a heart attack have a blood cholesterol level that is well within the range accepted as normal. Attempts to lower death rates from coronary artery disease with the American Heart Association diet have consistently failed. In addition, when drugs are given to try to lower blood cholesterol, overall death rates have gone up, not down as anticipated."[4]

In an attempt to prove the cholesterol hypothesis, researchers have worked for over sixty years trying to demonstrate that cholesterol and saturated fat cause heart disease. No study has been able to do this. The Framingham Heart Study which has monitored the health of nearly 5,000 people for several decades has shown that people who eat more saturated fat do not develop heart disease any more than anyone else.[5]

Heart surgeon, Michael DeBakey, performed a study using a large number of patients at Baylor University. He found that out of 1,700 patients who had atherosclerosis (clogged arteries), severe enough to require hospitalization, only 1 patient out of 5 had high blood cholesterol.[6] Dr. Harlan M. Krumholz reported in the *Journal of the American Medical Association* that people with higher cholesterol are not necessarily the most likely to have heart problems or die from heart disease. In a study, he monitored 997 people 65 years of age and older. Those with high cholesterol had the same rates of heart attack and death as those with normal levels. You would expect that as we age, more cholesterol will build up in the arteries and thus increase the risk of heart disease. Indeed, risk of heart attack does increase with age. However, research doesn't show any correlation between age and cholesterol.

For example, in a study where the mean age of the subjects was 79, the authors report finding "no evidence that an elevated level of cholesterol increased the risk of death or heart disease among this group."[7] Paul Addis and Gregory Warner, professors in the Department of Food Science and Nutrition at the University of Minnesota state: "The prevailing opinion, that atherosclerosis is simply an accumulation of cholesterol on arteries, has clearly shown to be erroneous. Therefore, the 'lipid hypothesis' has become less well accepted by serious researchers and has been replaced by a competing hypothesis, i.e. 'response-to-injury hypothesis.'"[8] Because of the many inconsistencies with the cholesterol hypothesis, it has often been called the cholesterol myth.

In 1950, coronary artery disease became our leading cause of death, and it still is today. Avoidance of cholesterol and saturated fat, the availability of cholesterol-lowering drugs, and eating foods low in cholesterol and saturated fats have not stopped the heart-disease epidemic. It should be obvious that something else, that is generally overlooked, is at the root of the problem.

CHOLESTEROL REGULATION

It is assumed that a diet high in cholesterol and saturated fat leads to high blood cholesterol. Saturated fat is included because it can be converted into cholesterol by the liver. The fat we eat, according to the cholesterol hypothesis, is directly responsible for the amount of cholesterol in our blood. The problem with this argument is that dietary consumption of fat has only a minor affect on our cholesterol levels. Why? Because the vast majority of the cholesterol in our blood does not come from our diet, but our liver. More than 80 percent of the cholesterol in our blood is manufactured in our own bodies.

To account for this fact, those who believe in cholesterol hypothesis claim that the saturated fat in our diet is automatically converted into cholesterol and that the more saturated fat we eat, the more cholesterol we have floating around in our bloodstream. The liver is depicted as a machine that blindly churns out as much cholesterol as it possibly can. The more saturated fat we eat, the more cholesterol it creates.

Such a scenario is inconsistent with human physiology. The liver produces and carefully regulates a balance of hundreds of compounds essential for growth, digestion, and protection. Blood cholesterol is not an accident that is easily influenced by diet. The liver doesn't just crank out chemicals, like cholesterol, for the fun of it. It does it for a specific reason. And the amounts are carefully controlled and monitored to achieve and maintain homeostasis, or chemical equilibrium. The liver carefully regulates the amount of cholesterol in our bodies, so it doesn't really matter how much saturated fat we eat; the liver will only manufacture the amount we need to maintain homeostasis. Everyone's body is different, so everyone has a different level of cholesterol with which the body is happy. This level is consistent (within a 5-10 percent margin) regardless of our diet and lifestyle.

The liver doesn't need saturated fat to make cholesterol. It can make it from other fats and even from sugar and carbohydrates.[9] So, the claim that saturated fat raises blood cholesterol while ignoring other fats and sugar is illogical and inaccurate. If not enough cholesterol is eaten, the liver will make it from other dietary sources. This is why even drastic decreases in dietary cholesterol intake have only a minor effect on blood cholesterol levels.[9]

Kilmer S. McCully, MD, a pathologist and medical researcher, has investigated the connection between diet and heart disease and cancer for over 30 years. He states, "The amount of cholesterol that is formed in the liver is carefully controlled and adjusted according to the needs of the different organs of the body. If the amount of cholesterol is increased in the diet, a healthy, well-functioning liver makes less cholesterol for the needs of the body. If the amount of cholesterol in the diet is decreased, the liver makes more cholesterol. In this way the body regulates very precisely how much cholesterol is produced for its needs."[3]

Each day the body churns out approximately 1,000 mg of cholesterol. In comparison, an average American man's daily cholesterol intake is only 327 mg and a woman's is 221 mg. Of the cholesterol we eat, only about one-third is absorbed through the intestines; the rest is excreted.

Theoretically, the dietary cholesterol that is absorbed by the body in a day would raise a man's blood cholesterol by some 163 mg/dl. However, this doesn't happen. Here's why. Instead of responding in a set way to a high-fat meal, the body has several options: the intestines can absorb large or small amounts of cholesterol; the liver can turn down its own cholesterol production; and the liver can also convert some of this cholesterol into bile acids ready for excretion. The degree to which these responses occur depends both on the cholesterol content of the meal and the genetic makeup of the person. Some people absorb more than others, but some excrete more.[10]

For most people the blood cholesterol level is determined more by heredity than it is by diet. However, drastic diets, toxins, infections, or drugs can upset the normal cholesterol balance. Lowering cholesterol will have little, if any, effect on your overall health. Lowering it too much can even be detrimental.

SATURATED FAT AND HEART DISEASE

Over the years, billions of dollars have been spent in research to prove the cholesterol hypothesis. However, to date no study has been able to provide this proof. Some studies seem to support the theory that saturated fat increases the risk of heart disease while others refute it.

When the results of studies are mixed, people can select the studies to support their personal beliefs. Those who promote the idea that saturated fat causes heart disease can find studies to back them up. On the other hand, those that don't believe saturated fat is harmful can find studies to support their view. Which is right?

Although the public usually hears only one side of the issue, this controversy has been raging within the medical community ever since Ancel Keys proposed the cholesterol hypothesis in the 1950s. While there have been many studies, they are not all of equal value. Some of these studies used relatively few participants, while others used much larger numbers. The accuracy and reliability of any study improves as the number of participants increases. Obviously, the results of a study involving 50,000 test subjects carries more weight than one involving only 1,000. One large study using 50,000 participants would produce far more reliable results than 10 small studies with a total combined number of only 10,000 participants. So the total number of studies is not an issue; the number of people in the studies is of more value. If all the subjects in these different studies were combined and evaluated in a single study, what would be the final outcome?

In order to come to a definitive conclusion, researchers at Harvard Medical School decided to combine the data from all of the previous studies on saturated fat and heart disease as if it were one gigantic study. Such a study

41

would give the most accurate results possible and since all studies would be combined, no single smaller study could refute the results. The researchers collected the data from the best designed studies over the past several decades and summarized the evidence. This meta-analysis study included data on nearly 350,000 subjects. The answer was finally found. The results of their analysis showed that saturated fat does not increase the risk of heart disease. Those people in these studies who ate the greatest amount of saturated fat had no more incidence of heart disease than those who ate the least.[11] People who feasted daily on bacon and eggs for breakfast and steak for dinner had no greater incidence of heart disease than vegetarians who avoided all saturated fats. This study showed beyond a reasonable doubt that saturated fats do not cause or even promote heart disease.

Since the publication of this landmark study in 2010, several newer studies comparing saturated fat consumption with other fats have confirmed the results—saturated fats do not promote heart disease.[12-13] In 2014 researchers at the University of Cambridge published another, more extensive meta-analysis. This study included data from 72 previous studies with more than 600,000 participants from 18 nations. The results of the Cambridge study confirmed those of the Harvard study—people who eat the most saturated fat have no more incidence of heart disease than those who eat the least. In fact, the study discovered that some forms of saturated fat actually protect against heart disease.[14] The evidence is now clear, saturated fats do not cause or even promote heart disease, and in some cases may even help prevent it.

WHY YOU NEED SATURATED FAT

Although we don't normally think of saturated fat as an essential nutrient, it is just as important to health as any other nutrient. In fact, saturated fat is an essential component of every cell in your body. Cell membranes are made of at least 50 percent saturated fat. This is necessary to give our cells the stiffness and integrity they need to function properly. If your cells don't get enough saturated fatty acids to maintain structural integrity, they become soft and leaky. This can lead to tissue degeneration and malfunction. Every organ in your body is made of specialized cells that are designed to perform a specific task. If the cells in any organ do not perform the function for which they were designed, the entire organ becomes dysfunctional. Kidney failure results because the cells die or fail to perform properly. Liver disease is the result of cells becoming dysfunctional. All diseases are cellular diseases.

Therefore, a healthy body requires healthy organs, which require healthy cells. Your cells need saturated fat to be healthy. Every cell in every organ of your body needs saturated fat—your brain, liver, kidneys, lungs, heart, etc. Your brain is especially important because it is composed of about 60 percent fat, much of it saturated.

Saturated fat is necessary for proper bone development and for the prevention of osteoporosis. Many people are eating low-fat diets, and especially low-saturated-fat diets, and taking huge amounts of calcium supplements, yet they still suffer from osteoporosis. For calcium to be effectively incorporated into the bones, at least 50 percent of the fats in the diet need to be saturated.[15] Vegetarians usually consume smaller amounts of saturated fat than nonvegetarians. The consequence is that vegetarians are at greater risk of osteoporosis. In a study of Seventh-Day Adventists, who are generally vegetarians, it was shown that they were more likely to suffer from hip fractures than nonvegetarians.[16] If you want to prevent osteoporosis you need to be eating saturated fat.

Saturated fats support the immune system and help keep you healthy.[17] It is the immune system that fights off infections and keeps you safe from cancer. Having an adequate amount of saturated fat in your diet will help protect you from these problems.[18] Saturated fats protect the liver from the toxic effects of alcohol, drugs, and other toxins.[19-20]

In the 1950s and 1960s when saturated fat was first being associated with elevated cholesterol, researchers began looking for other effects caused by saturated fat. They reasoned that if excessive consumption of saturated fat increased blood cholesterol, it may be associated with other undesirable conditions as well. Researchers began studying the link between saturated fat and cancer. What they found surprised them. It appeared that saturated fat had a protective effect against cancer rather than a causative one in comparison to other oils.[21] Further research showed similar results with several other conditions such as asthma, allergies, memory loss, and senility.[22]

Two of the consequences of heart disease are heart attacks and strokes. They are both caused by clogged arteries. In the case of a heart attack the coronary artery feeding the heart is blocked. Without oxygen the heart suffocates and dies. When the carotid artery that feeds the brain becomes blocked, a stroke occurs. Both human and animal studies have consistently shown that consumption of saturated fats actually protect against strokes (and heart disease in general).

Studies have consistently shown that high-fat diets *decrease* the risk of strokes, this is particularly true when the diet is high in saturated fat and cholesterol..[23-27] One notable long-term study out of Harvard involved 832 men aged 45 through 65 years who were initially free of cardiovascular disease. The study examined the association of stroke incidence with intake of fat and the type of fat over a span of 20 years. In conformity with other studies, intakes of saturated fat in comparison with polyunsaturated fat were associated with a reduced risk of ischemic stroke.[28]

A number of studies have shown that when people go on low-carb, high-fat diets, their bodies go through a transformation for the better. They lose excess body fat, cholesterol levels go down, HDL (good) cholesterol goes up, the cholesterol ratio decreases, C-reactive protein (an indicator of inflammation) goes down, blood sugars normalize, blood pressure improves, all of which indicate a reduced risk of heart disease as well as diabetes, dementia, cancer, and other degenerative conditions. Instead of contributing to heart disease, consuming saturated fat appears to protect against it, particularly when carbohydrate consumption is reduced.

The conclusion we come to is that it is okay to consume saturated fat and cholesterol-rich foods. Doing so will not increase your risk of suffering from heart attack or stroke but will reduce your risk as well as help you lose unwanted body fat and improve your overall health.

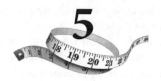

Good Carbs, Bad Carbs

SIMPLE AND COMPLEX CARBOHYDRATES

When you look at a hamburger what do you see? What makes a hamburger a hamburger? Most of us would see a skinny little meat patty stuck inside a bun with a dab of secret sauce and, if we're lucky, a pickle, diced onions, and a slice of tomato. If you were a dietitian you would view the meal differently. You would describe it in terms of its nutritional content: how much fat, protein, and carbohydrate it contains. The meat patty would represent the majority of the protein and fat. Fat would probably be included in secret sauce, since it would be mostly egg-based mayonnaise. The bun and veggies would comprise the carbohydrate.

The majority of the fat and protein in our diet comes from animal sources. Carbohydrate, on the other hand, comes from plants. The only significant animal source for carbohydrate is the lactose in milk. Next to water, carbohydrate is the most abundant substance found in plants. The wall that surrounds each plant cell and gives the plant structure and strength is made of carbohydrate. Plants also store carbohydrate, primarily in the form of starch, as a source of energy. Seeds use carbohydrate for energy during germination. While plants do contain some protein, fat, and other substances, carbohydrate, in one form or another, is by far the most abundant. Carrots are mostly carbohydrate; so are onions, potatoes, cucumbers, as well as crabgrass, oak trees, and petunias.

The plants with the highest amount of carbohydrate are grains, legumes, and tubers (root vegetables such as potatoes). These foods contain a high percentage of starch. Grains are of particular interest because in one form or another they constitute the vast majority of our diet. The grains in most common use have also been refined—stripped of most of their fiber, fat, protein, vitamins, and minerals—leaving almost pure starch. These are referred to as refined carbohydrates.

When you eat any plant food, you are really eating sugar. Why? Because carbohydrates are little more than sugar. All carbohydrates, whether they come from a grain of wheat, an artichoke, or a watermelon, are composed of simple sugars.

The technical name for sugar is saccharide. Saccharides form the building blocks for all carbohydrates. Carbohydrates come in different sizes; those that consist of a single molecule of sugar are called monosaccharides; those with two molecules of sugar are called disaccharides; and those forming long chains of sugar molecules are called polysaccharides.

Monosaccharides and disaccharides are referred to as sugars or simple carbohydrates. When eaten, they produce a sweet taste. Examples are glucose, fructose, sucrose, and lactose. When you eat fruit, the sweet taste comes from simple carbohydrates. Polysaccharides are called complex carbohydrates because they may contain hundreds or even thousands of sugar molecules linked together. Starches, for example, are composed of long chains of glucose molecules. Squash and beans don't taste sweet because most of the sugars are in the form of complex carbohydrates. During digestion complex carbohydrates are broken down into simple sugars.

Fiber, which is another complex carbohydrate, is also made of sugar. However, fiber is not broken down into individual sugars and provides little or no energy or calories. The sugar molecules are arranged in such a way as to form tight bonds. The human body does not possess the enzymes necessary to break these bonds. Consequently, fiber is essentially calorie-free and has none of the detrimental effects associated with sugar.

Fiber remains intact as it travels through the stomach and small intestine. When it finally reaches the large intestine (colon), bacteria there partially digest it and use it for their own nourishment. During this process the bacteria produce some vitamins and other nutrients that are absorbed and utilized by us. In this way, we form a symbiotic relationship with the bacteria where we both live together in a mutually beneficial way. We provide the bacteria a home and food, and they produce vitamins for our use.

High fiber foods, which include most fresh vegetables, can also be beneficial for weight loss. They provide bulk to fill the stomach and satisfy hunger, but provide no calories. Foods rich in fiber are generally also rich in vitamins, minerals, and other important nutrients that support good health.

Our bodies normally run on sugar. Sugar is the primary fuel that powers our cells. Now, before you get too excited and before you get the idea that the ideal diet is loaded with sugary foods like ice cream and cake, let me explain. Carbohydrates in themselves are not so much the problem; we obtain a lot of good nutrition from vegetables, nuts, and other carbohydrate-rich foods. It is the overconsumption of carbohydrates, particularly simple and refined carbohydrates, that is the problem. Foods rich in fiber and complex carbohydrates are considered the good carbs. Foods rich in sugar and refined carbohydrates are the potential troublemakers, and when eaten in excess become the bad carbs.

EAT YOUR VEGETABLES

Sugar and refined carbohydrates are the primary culprits that promote weight gain and obesity. In contrast, fresh vegetables and fruits are the good carbs. Study after study shows that diets rich in vegetables and fruits ward off disease and promote good health. Please note that vegetables are mentioned here before fruits because they are far more important to your health. Eating plenty of vegetables can help in your weight loss efforts and protect against diabetes, heart disease and stroke, control blood pressure, prevent some types of cancer, avoid painful digestive ailments, guard against cataract and macular degeneration, and protect the brain against neurodegeneration.

Vegetables and fruits are mostly water and are generally good sources of fiber, both of which can fill the stomach and satisfy hunger without adding any unwanted calories. For this reason, low-carbohydrate, low-sugar produce can aid in your weight loss efforts. Fresh produce is also a rich source of vitamins and minerals that promote good health.

Studies have consistently shown that diets rich in vegetables and other whole foods (fruits, whole grains, nuts, seeds) protect against degenerative disease. Reducing carbohydrate consumption by replacing it with vegetables, as well as fat and protein, improves health and protects against disease.[1]

Why are vegetables and other whole foods so good for us? Because they contain essential vitamins and minerals, along with a myriad of phytonutrients that nourish our bodies, protect us from disease, and keep us healthy. Phytonutrients are chemicals produced in plants that have vitamin-like characteristics. One of these is beta-carotene. Beta-carotene acts as an antioxidant and helps protect us from cancer and heart disease. It can also be converted into vitamin A, if the body needs it. Beta-carotene gives carrots, squash, and other vegetables their characteristic yellow and orange colors. Lycopene is another phytonutrient that has gained recognition lately for its ability to lower the risk of prostate cancer. It produces the red pigment in tomatoes, watermelon, and pink grapefruit. There are over 20,000 phytonutrients that have been identified in plant foods.

In the past, individual vitamins and minerals were thought to be adequate in curing health problems. We now know that while a single nutrient may be helpful, a variety of nutrients working together provides the greatest benefit. Nutrients work together in concert, like all the different instruments in a philharmonic orchestra together produce music. All of the instruments are needed to create the best sound. Likewise, a wide variety of nutrients is needed in the proper proportion, like that found in whole foods, to provide the health benefits scientists see in nutritional studies.

47

This is why it is better to eat food containing hundreds of phytonutrients than to take a vitamin tablet which only has a dozen or so. This is why it is better to eat bread made from whole wheat flour than white flour, which has had some 20 nutrients removed in the refining process. This is why fresh vegetables and fruits are superior to processed, packaged foods containing refined carbohydrates.

Most people will admit that they need to add more vegetables into their diets. But some people just don't care for vegetables. They were raised on white bread and pasta and other junk foods and never developed a taste for vegetables. Too often, vegetables are served more or less plain—maybe with a squeeze of lemon and a dash of salt—but without butter or any type of sauce in order to avoid adding fat into the diet. Adding sources of fat such as butter, cheese, cream, nuts, seeds, meat drippings, crumbled bacon, pieces of ham, and rich creamy sauces greatly improves both the nutritional value of the vegetables and their taste. When served this way, even the staunchest vegetable haters will love to eat their veggies. As you begin to add more vegetables into your diet, you will develop a greater liking for them, especially when they are prepared this way.

SUGAR, SUGAR EVERYWHERE

Throughout the vast majority of human history, sugar has been an insignificant part of the diet. For example, two hundred years ago people ate, on average, only about 15 pounds (6.8 kg) of sugar a year. During the latter half of the 1800s, as sugar refining technology improved, sugar consumption dramatically increased. By 1900 annual sugar consumption in the United States had risen to 85 pounds (38 kg) per year. Today we consume an average of about 160 pounds (72 kg) of sugar per year.

The current recommended daily maximum limit of added sugar is 8 teaspoons. Added sugar means table sugar, corn syrup, high-fructose corn syrup, honey, and others. It does not include the sugars found naturally in milk, fruit, and vegetables. One 12-ounce can of regular soda delivers nearly 10 teaspoons of added sugar. That means you are at or over your daily limit before you have eaten a single cookie or container of fruit-flavored yogurt or even some commercial tomato soups or salad dressings.

On average, we consume about 50 teaspoons (200 grams) of sugar every day! This is far above the 8 teaspoon recommended limit. Total carbohydrate consumption from all foods (fruits, vegetables, grains, beverages, etc.) for an averaged sized adult eating 2400 calories/day amounts to about 350 grams. If 200 grams of that is in the form of sugar, then nearly two-thirds of our total daily carbohydrate intake comes from empty calories with no nutritional value whatsoever, calories that drain nutrients from the body without replacing them, calories that cause the body to go into metabolic shock, leading to insulin resistance and weight gain.

Just because you don't add sugar to your foods or eat candy, doesn't mean you are not consuming massive amounts of the sweet poison. Sugar is found as an ingredient in thousands of "non-sweet" products. You will find it in processed meats, baked goods, cereals, catsup and barbecue sauce, peanut butter, spaghetti sauce, canned goods, and frozen foods; it's even added to canned and frozen fruits. It's hard to find a packaged, prepared food which doesn't contain sugar or some other sweetener. Even nonfood items like toothpaste, mouthwash, chewing gum, and vitamins contain sweeteners.

Today, sugars come in a variety of forms. Ingredient labels list the contents, starting with those that are the most predominant by weight followed in order to the least at the end. Sugar in one form or another is often listed multiple times. In many packaged products, although sugar may not be listed first, if you combined all the many forms of sugar under the name "sugar," it would be the first ingredient on the list.

We get additional sugar that comes naturally in foods. Fruits and especially fruit juices are loaded with sugar. If you include these hidden sources, your total daily sugar intake can be even higher than 200 grams that is added to our foods.

As sugar has increased in the diet over the years, other, more nutritious foods have been pushed out, setting the stage for nutritional deficiencies.

SUGAR'S EFFECT ON HEALTH

Studies show that excess consumption of sweet foods, particularly sugar-sweetened beverages, plays an important role in the epidemic of obesity and diabetes.[2] Diabetes is strongly associated with an increased risk of Alzheimer's disease, and evidence suggests it may also be a contributing factor in Parkinson's and other neurodegenerative diseases. Evidence is now emerging that shows a relationship between high sugar consumption and mental deterioration, learning difficulties, and memory loss.[3]

Researchers at the University of Alabama in Birmingham have shown that mice fed diets high in sugar develop the same amyloid plaque deposits in their brains and memory defects that characterize Alzheimer's disease. Over 25 weeks, one group of mice received a diet consisting of mouse chow and regular water. The other group ate the same chow, but drank a sugar water solution. The sugar-fed mice gained about 17 percent more weight over the course of the study. They also were more likely to develop insulin resistance, a hallmark of diabetes. In addition, these mice performed worse on tests designed to measure learning and memory retention. The brains of the sugar-fed mice also had substantially more plaque deposits, a common feature of Alzheimer's.[4]

The amount of sugar water consumed by the mice was equivalent to a human drinking five 12-ounce cans of regular soda a day. Five cans of soda contain about 210 grams of sugar. While most people don't drink five cans of soda every day, they do get sugar from other sources—fruit juice, candy, donuts, pancakes, coffee, pastry, ice cream, and even everyday foods like spaghetti, catsup, barbecue sauce, bread, and fruit—that can easily surpass 210 grams. On average, every man, woman, and child consumes about this much every day.

Of course, an infant or a child will consume less, and some people eat almost no sugar at all, so those adults who do eat sugar are consuming well over 210 grams daily. It is interesting that the memory defects and plaque deposits in the sugar-fed mice occurred after only 25 weeks. What happens in our brains after years of eating a high-sugar diet?

Eating sugar and starch elevates blood sugar levels. High blood sugar promotes the formation of destructive substances known as advance glycation end products (AGEs). Sugar in the blood tends to glycate or "stick" to proteins and fats, causing permanent damage to tissues and generating destructive free radicals. The accumulation of AGEs in the body is correlated with the process of aging. The more you accumulate, the more quickly you age. AGE accumulation is associated with chronic inflammation and insulin resistance, both hallmarks of diabetes. AGEs develop in the body whenever sugar or starch is consumed, regardless of the amount. The more sugar and starch consumed, the more AGEs are created.

The overconsumption of sugar leads to chronically high blood sugar levels and the development of insulin resistance. You don't have to be a diabetic to have insulin resistance. Anyone who has fasting blood sugar levels over 90 mg/dl (5.0 mmol/l) has some degree of insulin resistance. That includes most people who eat the typical Western-type diet high in sugar and refined grains.

Some of the damaged glycated proteins and fats can stick around for life, contributing to sagging skin, cataracts, and hardened blood vessels. But we are not completely defenseless against AGEs; the white blood cells of our immune system can remove some of these little troublemakers. They do this through a process biologists call phagocytosis. White blood cells engulf and digest AGEs, making them harmless. The same process is used on invading bacteria.

Sugar depresses the white blood cells' ability to phagocytize these harmful substances. Studies have shown that after a single dose of sugar, phagocytosis declines by nearly 50 percent and remains depressed for at least five hours.[5] If you eat a sugary meal, your immune system will be severely depressed and remain that way at least until your next meal. So if you eat pancakes or sugary breakfast cereal in the morning, drink a sugary soda with your lunch, and end your dinner with a bowl of ice cream, your immune system will be severely depressed all day long. You will be less able to remove AGEs and more susceptible to infection and cancer. Cancer cells feed on sugar. The more sugar you give them, the better they grow.[6]

Studies have shown that excessive sugar intake is associated with increased levels of C-reactive protein (CRP) a marker for inflammation. Inflammation is associated with a number of disease states including heart disease and diabetes. The list of problems that sugar can cause is virtually endless. It has been observed to aggravate asthma, mental illness, mood swings, personality changes, nervous disorders, heart disease, diabetes, gallstones, hypertension, senility, cancer, and arthritis. Sugar has an extremely detrimental effect on the endocrine system, which includes the adrenal glands, pancreas, and liver, causing the blood sugar level to fluctuate widely. Sugar is the leading cause of dental decay, gum disease, tooth loss, and obesity.

Other than the calories it supplies, sugar provides no nutritional value. It contains no vitamins, minerals, or other nutrients. It is a source of empty calories. It is, in fact, an anti-nutrient. It robs the body of nutrients vital to good health. The consumption of sugar causes the body to use up its supplies of calcium, potassium, thiamin, and chromium. Sugar competes with vitamin C for transportation into cells. Overconsumption of sugar can cause a vitamin C deficiency leading to subclinical scurvy. A disease that is subclinical means the condition is present but not yet advanced enough to be detectable through conventional diagnostic methods. Subclinical scurvy greatly increases the risk of heart attack, stroke, gum disease, infections, cancer, diabetes, and other health problems, including premature aging and death.

SUGARS AND SWEETENERS
Sucrose

The sweetener which we are all most familiar with, and which serves as the standard upon which all others are compared to, is white table sugar. Table sugar is 100 percent sucrose. It is the single most widely used sweetener. Regardless of the source, most natural and refined sweeteners are primarily sucrose. Brown sugar, corn syrup, honey, and maple syrup are all primarily sucrose.

You will often hear that natural sweeteners are better than refined. The only advantage that natural sweeteners have is that they are less processed and, therefore, retain some of their nutritional value, but it isn't much. The most commonly used natural sweeteners are raw honey, unrefined maple syrup, sucanat (dehydrated sugarcane juice), chopped dried dates, fruit juice concentrate, barley malt, brown rice syrup, and molasses. Like most sweeteners, these are made primarily of sucrose. Agave nectar or syrup, another product that is marketed as a natural sweetener, contains sucrose but is mostly fructose.

In addition to the sugars listed above, you may find others included on ingredient labels such as dextrin, dextrose, fructose, glucose, and maltodextrin. Some of these sugars differ slightly from sucrose, but they are all sugars and all are empty calories and promote the conditions described in the previous section. Whether you eat table sugar, honey, or molasses makes little difference. Sugar by any other name is still sugar.

Fructose

If you read ingredient labels you will frequently come across the word "fructose." Fructose is found in all types of foods from "health" foods and dietary supplements to junk foods and candy. Fructose once gained a reputation as a "good" sugar primarily because it doesn't raise blood sugar and insulin levels like table sugar does. For this reason, it has been the sugar of choice for many diabetics. Another reason for the popularity of fructose is because it is perceived to be more natural than sucrose and more healthful. It is often called "fruit" sugar, implying that its origin is from fruit rather than sugarcane or sugar beets and, therefore, is a less processed or more natural sweetener.

Unfortunately, most of this is untrue. Fructose is not, by any stretch of the imagination, a "natural" sugar, is not extracted from fruit, and is one of the last sweeteners a diabetic should ever use. The reason for much of this misinformation and its popularity is due to clever marketing tactics by the sugar industry. Fructose is preferred over sucrose as a sweetener by food producers for the simple reason that it is cheaper. Economics, not health, is the issue here. Fructose is much sweeter than sucrose and, therefore, can sweeten foods at less expense.

The biggest myth about fructose is that it is fruit sugar and comes from fruit. Fructose is not made from fruit. It comes from corn syrup, sugarcane, and sugar beets, just like any other sugar. The similarity between the names fructose and fruit helps to perpetuate this myth. I've heard many a health food and supplement salesperson claim their product was superior to others because it was made with fruit sugar, meaning fructose.

Fructose is one of the most extremely refined sugars in existence. One molecule of sucrose is composed of one molecule of fructose and one of glucose. The two chemically bonded together form sucrose. In order to make fructose, you must refine sugar cane or corn, down to sucrose first. Then you must process and refine it further, splitting the fructose and glucose apart. Fructose is so highly refined that it cannot be reduced into a simpler sugar. It's as refined as it gets. To say that fruit contains fructose is technically true. The natural sugar in fruit is mostly sucrose, and all sucrose, whether it comes from fruit or corn syrup, is 50 percent fructose.

Another problem with fructose is that while it doesn't affect blood sugar and insulin levels like sucrose, it has a more detrimental effect on insulin resistance, increasing the risk of a number of health problems like heart disease, high blood pressure, and diabetes. Studies on animals and humans have shown that consuming large amounts of fructose impairs the body's ability to properly handle glucose (blood sugar), which ultimately leads to hyperinsulinemia (elevated insulin levels), and the development of insulin resistance. This fact is so well established now, that researchers use fructose to intentionally induce insulin resistance to create high blood pressure and diabetes in laboratory animals. Some physicians are now claiming that the increased use of fructose in all our foods is largely responsible for the skyrocketing incidence of diabetes we have been experiencing over the past few years.

Fructose has also been shown to increase the rate at which fats in our body undergo peroxidation, which produces destructive free radicals. It adversely affects blood lipids and blood pressure, increasing risk of cardiovascular disease and interferes with nutrient absorption.[7]

Nutritionists have been aware of the health problems associated with sucrose for some time. Until recently, fructose was considered a much healthier alternative. As questions about the safety of fructose began to emerge, researchers wanted to know whether it was the fructose or the glucose in the sucrose that was causing the problems. An idea of just how bad fructose is, was revealed by a team of USDA researchers led by Dr. Meira Field. They conducted studies with two groups of healthy rats, one given high amounts of glucose in their food and one given high amounts of fructose. Researchers found no change among the animals in the glucose group. However, in the fructose group the results were disastrous. Young male rats were unable to survive to adulthood. They suffered from anemia, high cholesterol, and heart hypertrophy (their hearts enlarged until they ruptured). They also had delayed testicular development. Dr. Field explains that fructose in combination with copper deficiency in the growing animals interfered with collagen production. Collagen provides the protein matrix upon which all organs and tissues are built. In humans, copper deficiency is common among those who eat a lot of processed convenience foods, as most people tend to do. The rats' bodies more or less just fell apart. The females were not as severely affected, but they were unable to produce live young.

"The medical profession thinks fructose is better for diabetics than sugar," says Dr. Field, "but every cell in the body can metabolize glucose. However, all fructose must be metabolized in the liver. The livers of the rats on the high fructose diet looked like the livers of alcoholics, plugged with fat and cirrhotic."[8]

When sucrose is consumed, the glucose and fructose molecules are split apart. The glucose goes directly into the bloodstream where it is absorbed by the cells and used as fuel. Fructose, however, must be converted into glucose before it can be used by the cells. It does not circulate in the bloodstream but goes directly to the liver. Here it is converted into glucose and fatty acids. In fact, fructose is more likely to be transformed into fat than into glucose. Much of the fructose you eat is converted directly into fat and stored as body fat. This is why fructose does not raise blood sugar levels as high as sucrose and other sugars. But it does raise blood triglyceride (fat) levels, more so than eating fat does. The high amount of fat produced from fructose metabolism clogs the liver, leading to fatty liver disease that resembles the damage caused by alcohol abuse. Doctors call it non-alcoholic fatty liver disease to distinguish it from the disease caused by excessive alcohol consumption. In addition to the excess fat, fructose causes liver cirrhosis (inflammation) and fibrosis (scarring).[9-10]

Fructose, especially in the form of high-fructose corn syrup, is found in a wide range of foods and beverages, including fruit juice, soda, jam, desserts, cereal, bread, yogurt, salad dressings, ketchup, and mayonnaise. On average, Americans consume 60 pounds of high-fructose corn syrup per person every year. In the 40 years since the introduction of high-fructose corn syrup as a low-cost sweetener, rates of obesity have skyrocketed. According the Centers for Disease Control and Prevention (CDC), in 1970, around 15 percent of the US population met the definition for obesity; today, roughly one-third of American adults are considered obese. Some researchers believe that the dramatic increased use of fructose in manufactured foods is partly to blame.

All sweeteners are not equal when it comes to weight gain. Researchers at Princeton University have demonstrated that rats given access to high-fructose corn syrup gained significantly more weight than those with access to sucrose, even when their overall caloric intake was the same.[11] In addition to causing significant weight gain, long-term consumption of high-fructose corn syrup also led to abnormal increases in body fat, especially around the abdominal area. This makes sense since fructose is preferentially turned into fat by the liver.

"Some people have claimed that high-fructose corn syrup is no different than other sweeteners when it comes to weight gain and obesity, but our results make it clear that this just isn't true," says Dr Bart Hoebel, who specializes in the neuroscience of appetite, weight, and sugar addiction at Princeton. "When rats are drinking high-fructose corn syrup at levels well below those in soda pop, they're becoming obese—every single one, across the board. Even when rats are fed a high-fat diet, you don't see this: they don't all gain extra weight."

In the Princeton study the concentration of sugar in the sucrose solution was the same as that found in most soft drinks. However, the fructose solution was only half as concentrated as most sodas but still produced far greater weight gain and body fat accumulation in comparison.

In long term studies lasting over 6 months, the animals getting a diet with added fructose showed signs of a dangerous condition known in humans as the metabolic syndrome, which includes abnormal weight gain, significant increases in circulating triglycerides, and fat deposition, especially visceral fat around the belly. Male rats in particular ballooned in size. Animals with access to fructose gained 48 percent more weight than those eating a normal diet. Putting this into human terms, a 200 pound person would put on an additional 96 pounds! The rats weren't just getting fat; they were becoming obese.

Next time you read the ingredient label and see fructose, keep in mind that if you eat this product, fructose will end up as blubber around your middle.

Artificial Sweeteners

Even after all the processing and refining sugar goes through, it still retains calories. So scientists have created sweeteners with fewer calories. If real sugar wasn't bad enough, we can now "enjoy" artificial sugar—aspartame, saccharin, and such. Like sugar, these crystalline powders are just as addictive but even more detrimental to health. Yes, they contain fewer calories than sugar, but like any drug, they have undesirable side effects that range from headaches to death.

Artificial sweeteners look like sugar, taste like sugar, and can be used to sweeten foods just like sugar, but without the calories in sugar. In fact, compared to sugar, artificial sweeteners have almost no calories. Sounds like a dieter's dream, but in reality it's a nightmare. Artificial sweeteners have a dark side much more sinister than sugar.

Sugar, even as refined as it is, is still a product the body recognizes and can process, even though the processing causes the body a great deal of stress and drains nutrients. Artificial sweeteners, on the other hand, are strange new creatures the human body has never seen before and isn't programmed to handle safely or efficiently. This creates problems. While the materials that scientists use to make artificial sweeteners may come from "natural" sources, they are combined into unique chemicals that are unnatural and cause all types of mischief.

The most widely used artificial sweetener is aspartame. Aspartame is sold under the brand names NutraSweet, Equal, Spoonful, Equal-Measure, and AminoSweet. Discovered in 1965, it was approved for use as a food additive in the US in the early 1980s. The US Food and Drug Administration (FDA) allowed its use even under the heavy criticism by several scientists who warned of its dangers. Despite objections, approval was granted based on research funded by aspartame's manufacturer (Monsanto and its subsidiary, The NutraSweet Company).

Since its approval, aspartame has accounted for over 75 percent of the adverse reactions to food additives reported to the FDA. Many of these reactions have been serious enough to cause seizures and death. At least 90 different symptoms have been documented as being caused by aspartame. Some of these include headaches/migraines, dizziness, seizures, nausea, numbness, muscle spasms, rashes, depression, fatigue, irritability, tachycardia, insomnia, vision problems, hearing loss, heart palpitations, breathing difficulties, anxiety attacks, slurred speech, loss of taste, tinnitus, vertigo, memory loss, joint pain, and, believe it or not, weight gain.[12] In addition, aspartame has triggered or worsened brain tumors, multiple sclerosis, epilepsy, chronic fatigue syndrome, Parkinson's disease, Alzheimer's disease, birth defects, fibromyalgia, and diabetes.

Would any sane person knowingly eat a substance that caused or even contributed to these types of problems? The justification given to use aspartame is that this is a small price to pay in order to lose excess weight. The potential benefit it might have in helping people lose a few pounds is worth the risk, or so says the manufacturer and the doctors and researchers funded by them. Sure it's worth the risk for the people who benefit financially, but not for those people who lose their health in the process. It's interesting to note that one of the reported side effects of aspartame is weight gain! So why use it at all?

Aspartame is a relative newcomer compared to saccharin. Discovered in 1879, saccharin was the first of the artificial sweeteners. In 1937 cyclamate came on the scene. This was followed by aspartame in the 1960s and more recently acesulfame K and sucralose. These artificial sweeteners are many times sweeter than sugar. Saccharin has a sweetening power 300 times that of table sugar. Cyclamate is about 30 times as sweet as sugar and aspartame is 200 times sweeter. Gram for gram these sweeteners contain about the same number of calories as sugar, but since they are so much sweeter, only a fraction of the amount is needed for the same effect. This feature makes artificial sweeteners enticing for dieters. Their popularity has soared as waistlines have expanded.

Saccharin and cyclamate have fallen in stature since the late 1960s when it was discovered that they caused tumorous growths in laboratory animals. Cyclamate was banned in the US in 1970, although it has remained in limited use in the United Kingdom and Canada. In Canada it is only allowed as a tabletop sweetener on the advice of a physician and as an additive in medicines.

In 1977 a ban was also proposed for saccharin. Since it was the only remaining artificial sweetener in use at the time, many people opposed the ban, claiming the action was unfair to diabetics and the overweight. In response to the public outcry, the ban was put on hold. Instead, products containing saccharin are required to carry a warning which reads "Use of this product may be hazardous to your health. This product contains saccharin, which has been determined to cause cancer in laboratory animals." Saccharin, however, is banned completely in Canada.

Acesulfame K is of the same general chemical family as saccharin. It has the same potential drawbacks as saccharin in regards to cancer. Like saccharin, it also stimulates insulin secretion which makes it less desirable for diabetes.

The newest kid on the block is sucralose, known by the trade name Splenda. It is 600 times sweeter than sugar. This chemical sweetener is so alien to our bodies that the digestive system doesn't know what to do with it. It travels through the digestive tract without being absorbed. Thus it provides no calories and does not affect insulin or blood sugar levels and, therefore, is considered safe for diabetics. Sound too good to be true? Judging from the track record of all other artificial sweeteners, it is too good to be true.

It appears that Splenda has a very pronounced effect on the microflora of the gut and may play a role in causing irritable bowel disease (IBD).[13] The good bacteria in your gut supports health in many ways by producing important vitamins, maintaining pH balance, and supporting immune function, among other things. Splenda has been shown to reduce these good bacteria by as much as 50 percent. When the good bacteria are gone, what takes it place? Bad bacteria, viruses, and fungi, including candida, which can lead to a myriad of digestive complaints.

The main reason people use artificial sweeteners is to reduce total calorie consumption in an effort to control weight. Some people are so desperate to reduce calories that they ignore health warnings and consume artificial sweeteners anyway. They willingly take the risk of getting cancer or suffering from any number of discomforting symptoms just so they can enjoy sweet foods. Cravings for sweets can be very powerful. So powerful, in fact, that we throw good sense out the window and gamble with our health.

Artificial sweeteners are not the answer to weight problems and do not provide any real benefit. All sweets, including artificial sweeteners, keep sweet cravings alive and active. Sweet cravings drive us to seek out and consume sweet foods whether we are hungry or not.

Artificial sweeteners also give a false sense of security. We drink a diet soda and then feel it's okay to eat foods we shouldn't. The Aspartame Consumer Safety Network has reported that people who use artificial sweeteners actually gain more weight than those who avoid them.[14] If you're trying to lose weight or maintain your weight, artificial sweeteners are not the way to go; they aren't effective and can cause serious harm.

If you're not convinced that artificial sweeteners are harmful, and you're using them to control your weight, I recommend that you read *Excitotoxins: The Taste That Kills* by Dr. Russell L. Blaylock, a professor of neurosurgery at the Medical University of Mississippi. This book provides details on the medical research documenting the dangers of aspartame and other food additives.

Sugar Alcohols

Sugar alcohols are a group of carbohydrates that have a chemical structure similar to both sugar and alcohol, but technically are neither. They are not artificial sweeteners but are referred to as "sugar substitutes" because they do occur in nature and are found in small quantities in various fruits, vegetables, and other plants.

There are a number of sugar alcohols. The ones you will see most commonly used in foods are xylitol, erythritol, glycerol, mannitol, and sorbitol, with xylitol being the most widely used. The simplest sugar alcohols, ethylene glycol and methanol, are not used in foods. They are sweet tasting but notoriously toxic. They are the primary ingredient in antifreeze that makes it poisonous. The other sugar alcohols are considered safe.

Sugar alcohols are used in cakes, cookies, puddings, candies, ice creams, and other snack foods. These types of foods are often labeled "sugar-free" or "no sugar added." Sugar alcohols are commonly added to foods that contain artificial sweeteners because their sweetness can help mask the bitter aftertaste of these other products.

Xylitol is the most popular sugar alcohol because it has a sweetness comparable in intensity to sucrose, with only half the calories, and it looks similar to and can be used like sugar. The other sugar alcohols are slightly less sweet but contain about the same amount of calories as xylitol.

Unlike sugar, xylitol is not metabolized by oral bacteria and therefore does not contribute to tooth decay. For this reason, it is commonly added to toothpaste and sugarless chewing gum. None of the sugar alcohols are completely broken down in the digestive tract, so they are only partly absorbed. This is why they deliver fewer calories than sugar. Like other carbohydrates, they do raise blood sugar levels, although less so than sugar.

In comparison to aspartame, sucralose, and other artificial sweeteners, sugar alcohols are relatively safe. However, they are not entirely benign. The most common side effects include bloating, abdominal pain and cramping, diarrhea, and flatulence. These symptoms often occur when eaten in excess, but for some people a single serving can be an excess, bringing on severe cramping and diarrhea. Also, symptoms associated with preexisting digestive problems such as irritable bowel syndrome and celiac disease can be intensified.

Sugar alcohols are widely advertised as being "natural" sweeteners and safe to use, in moderation of course. Since they are found naturally in some fruits and vegetables, as well as birch tree bark, we are often lead to believe that they are simply extracted from these sources, however, this far from the truth. The amount of sugar alcohols found in these products is so minuscule that it is not economically feasible to extract them. Instead, manufactures synthesize them from the fibrous or woody portions of plants. Xylitol, for example, is made from hemicelluloses in corncobs and wood pulp. This material is mashed and processed using sulfuric acid, calcium oxide, phosphoric acid and other chemicals. The result is a crystalline product that is just as processed and refined as white sugar and just as "unnatural."

The major problem with sugar alcohols is that they provide a sweet taste that keeps sugar addictions alive and active. If you use sugar alcohols to sweeten foods, you will never break your sugar addition and will always craves sweets and other carbohydrates. Eating them will make it easier for you to cheat, become discouraged, and quit.

Although sugar alcohols do not affect blood sugar levels as much as sugar, they still affect it, and can block the release of fat from your fat cells, preventing weight loss. In carb sensitive people they can stop ketone production and prevent weight loss.

Stevia

Just when you were beginning to think that all sweeteners were probably bad, along comes stevia. Stevia is a different kind of sweetener. It's actually an herb that is native to South America. It's similar to artificial sweeteners in that it is many times sweeter than sugar with essentially no calories. Yet unlike other sweeteners, it appears to have no adverse health effects and is nonaddicting. Many consider it nature's sugar substitute.

Stevia comes from a small shrub that grows in Paraguay and Brazil, where it is known as the "sweet herb." Its leaves have a sweetness about 30 times greater than sugar. The Guarani Indians who live in the region have been using the herb for centuries. It is highly regarded among them as both a sweetener and as a medicine. It is used to sweeten beverages, to disinfect wounds, and as a tonic to improve digestion.

Ground or whole stevia leaf makes a good sweetener for herbal teas and strong beverages. Stevia used in leaf form is not practical for most other situations because it tastes too much like an herb. A more useable form is stevia extract. The extract is a concentrate of the phytochemicals (steviosides) which give the plant its sweetness. Stevia extract is 200 to 300 times sweeter than sugar and does not have a leafy taste. The extract is available in either a powder or liquid. Because of its sweetness, only a small amount is needed to sweeten foods. About ¼ to ½ teaspoon of stevia extract can replace one cup of sugar.

Stevia extract has been used as a sweetener in Japan, Taiwan, Korea, Paraguay, Brazil, and Israel for many years. Japan has been using it since the mid-1970s. Instead of aspartame they use stevia to sweeten low-calorie foods. It's used commercially in chewing gum, candy, soft drinks, juices, frozen desserts, and baked goods. Stevia makes up 50 percent of the high-intensity sweeteners used in Japan.

Is it safe? It seems to be. We know that it does not have the undesirable effects of sugar, nor does it pose the same health dangers as artificial sweeteners. Stevia has been used for centuries in South America and for the past 25 years in Japan and other countries without any noticeable harm. The Japanese consume the largest quantity of the sweetener in the world and have reported no ill effects. Extensive research and safety testing has been done on stevia. None of these tests have shown any harmful effects, even at very large doses normally given to lab animals. Few substances can make this claim.

Testing so far has shown the herb and extract to be non-toxic and beneficial as a means to help reduce calorie consumption. It does not affect blood sugar or insulin levels, so is safe for diabetics. It does not feed yeast like sugar so it is a perfect sweetener for candida sufferers. In many ways it is far superior to both sugar and artificial sweeteners.

It is difficult to overuse stevia. If you use too much, it produces a bitter, molasses-like aftertaste. So you use just enough to sweeten your foods without getting the strong aftertaste. This takes a little practice. I suggest you learn how to use it from one of the many stevia cookbooks that are available.

A little stevia is okay occasionally, but you need to be careful. For sugarholics, stevia can keep the sugar cravings alive. I've seen people who over use it and abuse it, even developing a tolerance to the bitter aftertaste. One such person gave me a sample of the stevia-sweetened water she was drinking and it almost knocked me over with its intense sweet-bitter taste. I've eaten plenty of foods and drinks sweetened with stevia, but this was way overboard. I couldn't imagine anyone enjoying it, but this person drank stevia sweetened water all day long. She also had a very difficult time losing weight.

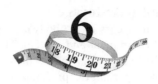

6

Carbohydrates Make You Fat

WHY CARBOHYDRATES MAKE YOU FAT

Have you ever tried to lose weight using the conventional method of calorie restriction and low-fat dieting? You ate lean cuts of meat, trimmed off even the tiniest morsel of fat, removed chicken skins, ate white meat only, abandoned whole eggs for egg whites, used skim milk and low-fat yogurt, ate baked potatoes and pasta without butter, salads without oil, had oatmeal and granola for breakfast, and low-fat, artificially sweetened brownies for dessert. To make sure you didn't overeat, you counted every calorie that passed through your lips. You did everything you were supposed to do and stuck with it because you were told this was the only way to lose weight.

Even though everybody was pleased with your efforts and praised you for eating healthfully, you weren't feeling any better. You lacked energy, tired easily, were constantly hounded by hunger, and your weight showed only modest improvement, if any at all. Despite your sincere effort, it was a struggle. Before long you were eating the way you had before you began the diet and before you knew it, all of your weight came right back. For all of your effort, you accomplished nothing except feeling miserable and perhaps getting fatter.

The reason for your failure was not that you lacked willpower or that you weren't following the program properly, the problem was the program itself. Any diet that restricts fat without limiting carbohydrates is bound for failure. The truth of the matter is that eating carbohydrates is what make us fat, not eating fat. You will never be able to lose excess weight and successfully keep it off using a diet that has no restriction on carbohydrates. The very nature of carbohydrates makes it impossible. Let's look at the major reasons why carbohydrates make us fat.

Insulin Secretion and Fat Storage

Carbohydrate eaten in excess of the body's caloric needs *always* turns into fat. The same is not true for fat and protein. The body can use fat and protein to produce energy but prefers to use them as building blocks for cells and tissues, enzymes, hormones, prostaglandins, and other products important for health. In fact, you don't even need carbohydrate in your diet, but you must have fat and protein or you would die.

The sole purpose of carbohydrate is to produce energy. What isn't used to satisfy immediate needs is converted into either glycogen or fat and stored for use later. Both glycogen and fat are compact forms of fuel that can be pulled out of storage whenever additional energy is needed.

Carbohydrate is not an essential nutrient. There are essential fatty acids (fats) and essential amino acids (proteins), but there is no such thing as an essential carbohydrate. If there were no source of carbohydrate in your diet, your body would utilize fat and protein to satisfy all its energy needs. There have been many populations that have thrived on a carbohydrate-free diet. The most notable being the Eskimo whose traditional diet consisted entirely of meat and fat.

You can gain unwanted weight from eating carbohydrates even if you eat no fat at all. The flab on your waist and arms did not get there from eating steak and eggs, it got there from eating bread, donuts, cake, and soda. The nutrients from the steak and eggs went to building muscle and bone, not fat.

You can eat much more fat and protein without packing it away in storage because they can be used for other important purposes. Our bodies are designed to either burn or store carbohydrate (glucose). Glucose is the primary fuel that powers our cells. However, the cells cannot absorb glucose directly out of the bloodstream. The hormone insulin is needed to unlock the door on the cell membrane to allow the glucose to enter. After a meal, carbohydrates are converted into glucose and released into the bloodstream. As blood glucose levels rise, a signal is sent to the pancreas to secrete insulin. The action of insulin allows the cells to absorb the glucose and lower blood glucose levels. As blood sugar drops, insulin secretion slows down.

Our blood glucose levels rise and fall according to how often we eat and what we eat. The range in which blood glucose rises and falls is carefully regulated through the secretion of insulin and other hormones. When blood glucose levels are low, fatty acids are released from our fat cells. Like glucose, fatty acids can be burned to produce energy.

When a person is on a low-calorie diet or fasting, blood glucose levels are low, so the body relies heavily on stored fat to provide most of its energy. As fatty acids are released and burned, weight is reduced. This is why we lose weight and body fat on a diet. However, the rate of weight loss is heavily influenced by the types of foods in the diet.

Insulin not only shuttles glucose into the cells, but also triggers the conversion of glucose into fatty acids and shuttles them into the fat cells.

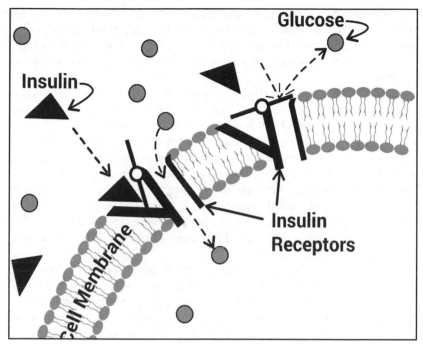

Insulin is necessary for glucose to enter the cells.

Insulin is a fat storage hormone. The more insulin you have coursing through your bloodstream, the more fat is deposited in your fat cells. When blood insulin levels are high, your body stores fat and you gain weight. Every time you eat carbohydrate, blood sugar levels rise, triggering the release of insulin and the storage of fat. Eating fat and protein have very little effect on blood glucose levels and therefore, do not stimulate much of an insulin response, and do not encourage fat storage.

High insulin levels not only stimulate the production of fat but prevent or limit the release of fat from storage around the body. When you eat carbohydrates, you must cut calories down exceptionally low in order to trigger the release of fat. Any carbohydrate in the diet will stimulate insulin secretion, which will prevent or retard fat release. By removing carbs from your diet, you limit insulin, which will allow stored fat to be released and weight to decline.

Whenever you eat foods containing carbohydrates, including carrots, tomatoes, apples, and other fruits and vegetables, blood glucose and insulin levels rise. This is why some people on high-carb, reduced-calorie diets can gain weight eating nothing but rabbit food. Even if calories are limited, consuming carbohydrate will raise blood insulin levels, promoting fat storage. This is why a person can limit their total daily calorie intake to 1,000 calories or less eating salads and grains and still gain weight.

Foods rich in sugar and starch trigger the greatest insulin response, and therefore, have the greatest effect on fat storage. This is why bread, pasta, potatoes, donuts, pancakes, candy, soda, fruit juice, pizza, and other high-carb foods promote weight gain more than low-carb foods rich in fat and protein.

Technically speaking, the body can take the tiny amount of glycerol in fats and convert it into glucose. However, the amount of glucose derived from glycerol is so small that it is insignificant. Likewise, up to 50 percent of the protein you eat can also be converted into glucose. However, this only happens if you eat an excessive amount of protein, the excess is converted into glucose. This is one of the reasons why people can gain weight on low-carb, high-protein diets. Although they restrict their carbohydrates, they load up on meat and eggs to satisfy their appetites. Eating too much meat will raise blood glucose and, consequently, blood insulin levels. If you tried a low-carb, high-lean protein diet in the past and gained weight or had difficulty losing it, this is probably the reason why.

Since fat is not converted into glucose in any appreciable amount, it does not cause or trigger insulin release. If you ate a high-carb, low-fat meal containing 500 calories, your body would respond by quickly pumping out a high amount of insulin, promoting fat synthesis and storage. However, if you ate a low-carb, high-fat meal containing the same number of calories, your body would release only a tiny amount of insulin and consequently there would be no fat synthesis or storage. Whenever you eat carbs, you promote fat storage. When you eat fat, you do not.

It makes sense to fill up on fatty foods, while limiting carbohydrate and protein. The most effective weight-loss diet is one that encourages the consumption of ample fat, adequate but not too much protein, and very little carbohydrate. Total calorie consumption should also be limited to encourage fat mobilization from fat cells.

Insulin Resistance

We are led to believe that most people gain weight simply because they eat too much food; in other words, they are gluttons that cannot control their appetites. This, however, is not always true. Many, if not most, overweight people do not eat any more than normal weight people. Overweight individuals have a metabolic propensity to store body fat. Their problem is not gluttony, but metabolism. Almost all overweight people are carbohydrate sensitive—that is, they readily convert the carbohydrates that they eat into body fat.

A normal weight individual can eat 200 or 300 grams of carbohydrate a day with little effect on body weight. A carbohydrate sensitive person, on the other hand, consuming the same total number of calories may gain weight eating less than 100 grams of carbohydrate. A carbohydrate sensitive person is metabolically programmed to store carbohydrates as body fat. A low-calorie carbohydrate based diet is not going to be successful in the long run. In order to lose weight on such a diet, the dieter must restrict calories to unsustainably low levels. Hunger and malnutrition will get the better of them and they will eventually loosen up their restrictions and regain the weight.

Carbohydrate sensitivity is caused, in part, by a defect in blood sugar regulation. The cells become unresponsive or resistant to the action of insulin, making it difficult for glucose to enter the cells. This is called insulin resistance. Insulin resistance is the hallmark characteristic of type 2 diabetes—the most common form of diabetes. Because of insulin resistance, blood sugar levels in diabetics are always above normal.

Blood glucose levels can be measured by analyzing a blood sample. Since foods can dramatically influence glucose levels, samples are taken after a person has not eaten for at least eight hours. If you are an average, non-diabetic individual, when you wake up in the morning, your blood contains between 65 and 100 mg/dl (3.6-5.5 mmol/l) of glucose. This is known as the fasting blood glucose concentration. The ideal fasting blood sugar range is between 75-90 mg/dl (4.2-5.0 mmol/l).

When you don't eat and as your cells continue to draw glucose out of the blood, your glucose level gradually falls. Most people experience a feeling of hunger as blood glucose drops toward the low end of the normal range. The natural response to this sensation is to eat, which raises blood sugar. Normally, your blood sugar should not rise to more than 139 mg/dl (7.7 mmol/l) after eating a meal. This is called postprandial glucose level. Elevated fasting and postprandial glucose levels indicate insulin resistance.

Diabetes is officially diagnosed when fasting blood sugar is 126 mg/dl (7.0 mmol/l) or higher. This occurs when insulin resistance is severe. People with fasting blood sugar levels between 101 and 125 mg/dl (5.6-6.9 mmol/l) are considered to be in the early stages of diabetes, often referred to as "pre-diabetes." Fasting blood sugar levels over 90 mg/dl (5.0 mmol/l) indicate the beginning stages of insulin resistance. As insulin resistance increases, so do blood sugar levels. The greater the insulin resistance, the higher the blood sugar levels.

Insulin resistance is usually present in anyone who has a fasting blood sugar level over 90 mg/dl (5.0 mmol/l). Although fasting blood sugar levels up to 100 mg/dl (5.5 mmol/l) are generally considered to be normal, they are viewed this way only because so many people fit into this category. They are not "normal" for a healthy individual. Having insulin resistance, even if the condition is relatively mild, causes carbohydrate sensitivity. Whenever blood glucose levels are elevated, insulin will also be elevated, unless the pancreas has lost its ability to produce normal amounts of insulin. Remember, insulin is a fat storage hormone and if it is elevated, it is causing fat to be produced and stored. In insulin resistant individuals (those with fasting blood glucose over 90 mg/dl or 5.0 mmol/l), insulin levels are elevated 24 hours a day, promoting fat storage at every opportunity. An overweight diabetic person typically makes two to three times more insulin than a slender non-diabetic person. Whenever carbohydrate is consumed, the body will try to store it as fat no matter how much or how little is eaten. For these individuals, carbohydrate-based low-calorie diets, and particularly low-fat diets, do not work.

Empty Stomach Syndrome

One of the consequences of eating high-carbohydrate meals, particularly those loaded with simple and refined carbohydrates, is a condition I call *empty stomach syndrome* (carbohydrate induced hunger). Empty stomach syndrome is characterized by frequent or prolonged periods of hunger caused by eating carbohydrate-rich foods.

Hunger is the driving force that compels us to eat and to overeat. When you have an empty stomach, you feel miserable and want to eat. If there is nothing to compel you to not eat, you will tend to nibble and snack all day, along with eating your regular meals. Carbohydrate-rich foods don't satisfy hunger, they cause it. They may fill you up temporarily, but hunger will quickly return and constantly nag you. When you eat carbohydrates without adequate fat and protein, you will always be hungry.

When we eat carbohydrates, digestive enzymes break the links that hold the sugar molecules together. Individual sugars are then released. These sugars are absorbed into the bloodstream. Glucose is absorbed by our cells and used as fuel. Other sugars, such as fructose and lactose, are picked up by the liver and converted into glucose. All sugar molecules are eventually converted into glucose or fatty acids (fat).

Simple carbohydrates consist of only one or two molecules of sugar. They are instantly absorbed into the bloodstream. Starches and other complex carbohydrates take a little longer to break down into individual sugars. Small starches that may contain only 100 or so sugar molecules will digest more quickly than larger ones that may contain a 1000 or more. The more "complex" the carbohydrate, the longer it takes the body to convert it to sugar. Foods in their natural form, such as whole wheat, are composed of a higher percentage of large complex carbohydrates. Processed foods, such as white bread, are less complex and digest quickly.

When you eat carbohydrate-rich foods, they digest very quickly and pass in and out of the stomach in a short amount of time. As the stomach empties, feelings of hunger quickly return. This is why you will often feel hungry an hour or two after eating a high-carb, low-fat, low-protein meal.

The effect high-carb foods have on blood sugar levels makes matters even worse. When you eat a high-carb meal, especially one loaded with refined grains and sugar, blood sugar levels skyrocket. Since high blood sugar can be dangerous, the pancreas responds by frantically pumping out insulin as fast as it can. Blood insulin levels rise very rapidly. As insulin is being pumped into the bloodstream, blood glucose is rapidly shuttled into the cells.

Before long, blood levels of insulin become extraordinarily high and glucose levels abnormally low. Low glucose levels signal the brain the need for more glucose and initiates feelings of hunger to encourage eating to boost glucose levels. An empty stomach combined with low blood glucose levels brings on excruciating feelings of hunger. Typically, there are three responses: 1) you stick it out and suffer until the next meal, at which time you are so hungry that you overeat, 2) you break down and eat a snack, or 3) you suffer as long as possible, eat a snack anyway, and still overeat at the next meal. Any of these options sabotages your weight loss efforts.

Fat and protein digest much more slowly, so the stomach stays fuller longer. They also do not elicit the rapid insulin response that leads to the dramatic highs and lows caused by carbohydrates. As a result, hunger is forestalled for an extended period of time without the temptation to snack and when the next meal comes, you are not so famished that you overeat. At the end of the day you wind up consuming fewer total calories than if you had eaten carbohydrates. Eating fat in place of carbohydrate allows you to feel satisfied and consume fewer calories. Because we have been conditioned to be afraid of eating fat, it bears repeating again and again—fat does not make people fat, carbohydrates do.

Our Love Affair with Carbs

Carbohydrates, especially in the form of sugar, taste good. That's a problem. If they didn't taste good, people wouldn't eat them and we wouldn't have an obesity epidemic.

We just love that taste of sugar. We must, since we consume on average over 50 teaspoons of it a day. Some of our favorite foods are rich in simple and refined carbohydrates—candy, donuts, cake, cookies, chips, desserts, ice cream, chocolate, sweet breads, the list can go on and on. These foods are alluring and once you take a bite, you crave more, and before long you've eaten an entire box, whether you were hungry to begin with or not. Sweets especially have this effect. You know what I'm talking about. You eat one small bite of chocolate and you immediately want another. It's like a power that engulfs you, takes control over you, and won't go away until you've devoured at least 1,000 calories of the stuff. The pleasurable taste of carbohydrates drives us to overeat and consequently gain weight.

High-protein and fatty foods, on the other hand, don't have this mesmerizing power. Although they can taste terrific, you aren't compelled to keep eating and eating even when common sense tells you to stop. You stay in control and limit what you eat.

Catering to the concerns of weight-conscious customers, manufacturers have produced a variety of decadent foods made with low-calorie and zero-calorie sugar substitutes. Customers can have the same satisfaction with fewer calories. Despite the plethora of low-calorie foods now available, waistlines have not decreased an inch, but have expanded. Nor has caloric consumption declined. In fact, today we consume 600 more calories per day then we did in 1970.

Reduced calorie foods are as sweet and tasty as ever and continue to entice people to eat and overeat. To make matters worse, since these foods have fewer calories, people often have a tendency to eat more, thinking they aren't doing any harm. They end up eating more calories than if they ate the full calorie versions.

Avoiding sugar by using sugar substitutes doesn't solve the problem. In fact, it appears to have made matters worse. A number of studies have shown that zero-calorie sweeteners used as a means to aid in weight loss actually cause greater weight gain!

A University of Texas Health Science Center survey in 2005 found that people who drink diet soft drinks gain more weight than those who drink the full sugar versions. In that study, for every can of diet soda people consumed each day, there was a 41 percent increased risk of being overweight.

In a series of experiments conducted at Purdue University, researchers compared the effects of foods containing either zero-calorie saccharine or regular sugar. Animals fed with artificially sweetened yogurt over a two week period consumed more calories and gained more weight than animals eating yogurt sweetened with sugar.[1] This study was a continuation of work the Purdue group began four years earlier when they reported that animals consuming saccharin-sweetened liquids and snacks tended to eat more than animals fed high-calorie, sugar sweetened foods.

The researchers theorize that when the sweet taste of the artificial sweetener wasn't followed by the expected number of calories, it threw off the rats' normal physiological response to calories in general. Like Pavlov's dogs, trained to salivate at the sound of a bell, animals and humans are similarly trained to anticipate lots of calories when they taste something sweet — in nature, sweet foods are usually loaded with calories. As a result, they were compelled to eat more food to compensate for the phantom calories. This may explain why dieters find that after eating sugar-free food, they often compensate by indulging in other calorie-rich foods.

Artificial sweeteners not only cause the brain to crave calories and carbohydrates, driving people to eat more, but they also have a physiological effect. If total calorie consumption was held constant so that no extra food could be eaten, those people eating foods containing sugar substitutes would still gain more weight.

Studies have found that foods containing low-calorie sugar substitutes interfere with fundamental homeostatic processes of the body. For example, when we sit down and begin eating a meal, the body anticipating an influx of calories immediately prepares the digestive system to handle the load by revving up the metabolism. Metabolism will remain elevated for a couple of hours after eating as the food is being digested. This rise in metabolism can be measured by an increase in body temperature.

The same thing occurs in animals. Researchers at Purdue University demonstrated that sugar-fed rats, as expected, exhibited an uptick in core body temperature at mealtime, corresponding to a rise in metabolism in anticipation of processing the incoming calories. Animals given artificially sweetened foods, on the other hand, showed no such rise in body temperature.[2-3] The animals that received the artificial sweetener have a different anticipatory response. They don't anticipate getting as many calories. The net result is a more sluggish metabolism that stores, rather than burns, incoming excess calories. Many overweight people already have problems with a sluggish metabolism, they don't need to compound the problem by eating artificial sweeteners. It doesn't matter what type of zero-calorie sweetener is used— saccharine, aspartame, xylitol—the effects will be the same.

These studies help explain why, despite the enormous popularity of low-calorie foods and drinks, we are heavier than ever.

Sugar Addiction

White refined sugar is not really a food, but acts more like a drug. It is a pure chemical extracted from plant sources and in many ways resembles cocaine. Cocaine is extracted, refined, and purified from the leaves of the coca plant. Similarly, sugar is extracted from sugar beets or sugarcane and refined and purified. Like cocaine, you end up with a purified crystalline powder (sucrose) that is highly addictive.

Addiction involves more than just a preference for something because you like the taste. It can be defined as the persistent compulsive use of a substance that on cessation causes psychological or physical anxiety. Sugar cravings fit into this definition. Sugar can be just as addictive, and even more so, than cocaine. This may sound like an overstatement because a person can stop eating sugar without suffering from the severe physical withdrawal symptoms commonly associated with cocaine addiction. Nevertheless, sugar addiction can cause dependence, severe anxiety, and even physical symptoms upon withdrawal.

A study published by French researchers demonstrated just how addicting sugar can be. Given the choice between sugar or cocaine, they found that 94 percent of rats chose sugar. When exposed to both substances, their desire for sugar was stronger than the desire for cocaine. Even rats who were already addicted to cocaine quickly switched their preference to sugar as soon as they were offered a choice. The rats were also more willing to work for sugar than for cocaine.[4]

In addition, the researchers found that there is a cross-tolerance and a cross-dependence between sugar and addictive drugs. As an example, animals with a long history of sugar consumption actually became tolerant (desensitized) to the analgesic effects of morphine.

A study out of Yale University found that addictions to sugar and drugs result in similar activity in the brain. Test subjects filled out a questionnaire, based on established criteria for accessing drug addiction, to measure their addiction to certain foods. The questionnaire included statements such as, "I find that when I start eating certain foods, I end up eating much more than I had planned," and respondents rated how closely the statement matched their experiences.

Using magnetic resonant imaging (MRI), a brain imaging procedure, the researchers examined brain activity when the subjects saw, and then drank, a chocolate milkshake. What they found was that the brains of subjects who scored higher on the food addiction scale exhibited brain activity similar to that seen in drug addicts, with greater activity in brain regions responsible for cravings and less activity in the regions that curb urges.[5]

Like with drug addiction, cutting down on sugar and carbohydrate consumption all at once can cause withdrawal symptoms. Symptoms may include intense carbohydrate cravings, headache, lightheadedness, irritability, irrational behavior, fuzzy thinking, and a general overall feeling of tension or stress.

Everyone, almost without exception, who is significantly overweight or obese is addicted to carbohydrates. It is the overconsumption of carbohydrate that is the primary contributing factor to their weight problem. Eating sweetened low-carb foods isn't going to help them.

Zero- or low-calorie sweeteners do not help with weight loss or with overcoming sugar addiction. If you are trying to lose weight, *sugar substitutes are your enemies*. They give you a false sense of security while fueling the fire of sugar addition. Studies that showed sugar to be more addictive than cocaine also showed zero-calorie sweeteners were just as addictive.[4] Using sugar substitutes keeps sugar addictions, cravings, and bad habits alive.

This is why artificial sweeteners and sugar alcohols are not recommended. Even the use of stevia should be limited. This is also why many people fail when they go on low-carb diets. Low-calorie sweeteners are common in most low-carb diet programs. Atkins and other low-carb food manufacturers sell tons of low-carb candy bars, shakes, bakery goods, and desserts, all of which sabotage your weight loss efforts. The companies that make these products are catering to your sugar and carb additions by making similar tasting substitutes, keeping all of your addictions alive and active. Sooner or later your cravings will get the better of you and you will fail. Success requires you to conquer your sugar addition. It is possible.

When you can break your addiction to sweets, you will gain a tremendous advantage and gain control over yourself and your life. You will no longer become a slave to foods. Sweets may still entice you at times, but they will not control you like they had before. One of the major goals of the dietary program described in this book is to release you from sugar and carbohydrate addition. Fortunately, a high-fat diet helps curb sugar cravings and eases your separation from sugar addiction.

Leptin Resistance

Certain hormones can influence hunger and body composition. One of these is leptin. Leptin plays a key role in regulating energy intake and expenditure and works in tandem with insulin. Both insulin and leptin resistance are associated with obesity. While too much insulin can cause weight gain, too little leptin will do the same.

Leptin is a master regulator of our appetite. It reduces feelings of hunger. Leptin is produced by your fat cells. The amount in your blood is proportional to the amount of fat on your body. Leptin acts on receptors in the brain. In this manner, your fat cells communicate with your brain to let you know how much stored energy (fat) is available and what to do about it. When leptin signaling is working properly, if you are too thin and need to store more fat, your blood levels of leptin will be low. Low leptin levels cause hunger, leading to increased food consumption and, consequently, fat storage. As fat cells enlarge, more leptin is produced, signaling the brain to cut back on food consumption. In other words, not only do low leptin levels cause hunger, they also increases fat storage; high leptin levels depress hunger and reduce fat storage. In this manner, proper body weight is maintained.

Dieting lowers leptin levels, thus increasing feelings of hunger. This is why dieting can be so arduously difficult. To make matters worse, some people's leptin signaling system has gone awry. This is called leptin resistance. Although they may be overweight and may be producing a high amount of leptin, the leptin receptors in the brain are not picking them up. The brain interprets this as a leptin deficiency caused by a lack of body fat. In response, the brain turns on the hunger switch, and never completely turns it off. Going on a diet and reducing the amount of leptin produced, increases the feelings of hunger, making dieting sheer torture. Even if a dieter is capable of sticking it out long enough to lose a substantial amount of weight, leptin resistance persists, causing the person to gradually overeat and regain the weight.

How is leptin resistance caused? It's initiated by eating too much carbohydrate, particularly sugars and refined grains. After eating a high-carb meal, blood sugar surges, along with insulin, which triggers the conversion of sugar into fat and packs it away in storage. This added fat then produces a surge of leptin. Over time, constant exposure to excessive levels of leptin desensitizes the leptin receptors, leading to leptin resistance. It is very similar to the development of insulin resistance as a consequence to overexposure to high levels of insulin. If you are diabetic or insulin resistant, you are also very likely leptin resistant.

The way to reestablish proper leptin (as well as insulin) sensitivity is to prevent these surges. This is done by reducing carbohydrate intake, especially refined carbohydrates which exert more of an impact on blood sugar. A low-carb, coconut oil, ketogenic diet is the best treatment for leptin resistance.

Starch Is Just Another Form of Sugar

Refined sugar isn't the only problem. Starch can be nearly as bad. Starch is the carbohydrate found in grains, tubers, beans, and other starchy vegetables. Starch is sugar. It is composed of pure glucose. The only difference is that in starch, the glucose molecules are all linked together in a long chain. However, once we eat it, digestive enzymes break the links into individual sugar molecules. Like any other source of sugar, starch causes blood sugar levels to rise rapidly, increases insulin secretion and fat storage, depresses immune function, and has all the other detrimental effects associated with sugar. Eating a slice of white bread is essentially equivalent to eating 3 teaspoons of sugar. White bread begins to turn into sugar in our mouths as soon as we start chewing. Saliva contains digestive enzymes that immediately begin to transform the starch into sugar.

People who do not eat many sweets or use sugar may think they are immune to sugar's detrimental effects. Yet, if they eat white bread, white rice, white potatoes, and products made with white flour, they are getting just as much sugar as anyone else and maybe even more. White bread can cause weight gain, insulin resistance and diabetes, reduce resistance against cancer, and set the stage for Alzheimer's or Parkinson's disease.

White flour is made by refining whole wheat flour. During the refining process many nutrients are removed, along with most of the fiber. Manufacturers add back a few of the nutrients but not the fiber. Fiber plays an essential role in the digestion of starch. Fiber slows down the release of glucose into the bloodstream. This is very important because it slows down sugar absorption, moderating insulin secretion, making it more manageable.

Starch in and of itself is not necessarily bad. After all, the glucose in starch is used as a source of fuel for our cells. The problem is the overconsumption of starch or the disproportion of starch in the diet in comparison to fat, protein, and fiber. A moderate amount of starch and even sugar can be handled as long as adequate amounts of fat, protein, and fiber are also consumed.

A typical diet consisting of 2,400 calories per day includes about 350 grams of carbohydrate on average. This equates to 1400 calories of sugar and starch—that is almost 60 percent of the total daily calories consumed! It's no wonder obesity, diabetes, Alzheimer's, and other degenerative diseases are on the rise.

For all the reasons listed in this chapter thus far, you will gain more weight eating carbohydrates than you will by eating fat or protein. Again, fat does not make us fat, carbohydrates do.

OVERCOMING SUGAR ADDICTION

Our love affair for sweets has created a society of sugarholics. Sugar and artificial sweeteners are dangerously addicting, much like narcotics. Like cocaine and other drugs, they stimulate pleasure centers in the brain. The desire for this pleasurable sensation can become so intense that it controls our thoughts and actions, just like cocaine controls an addict. We can be going along fine and then all of the sudden we get a desire to eat something sweet. It can be a piece of chocolate, chewing gum, or a soda, anything just so long as we get a sugar fix. Because sugar stimulates feelings of pleasure, even when we are full, we often continue to eat sweet foods. How many times have you been full but just had to have dessert? Or you weren't feeling hungry but couldn't resist the temptation of a sweet treat that is placed in your view? Or you began eating something sweet, such as a cookie, thinking you'll only eat one or maybe two at most, but end up devouring nine or ten? No, you couldn't eat just one. The sweet taste often overpowers good intentions, sound reasoning, and the strongest willpower. If you can identify with any of these situations, you've become a slave to sugar.

Sweets have never been a major source of food in the human diet. In the past, fruit provided the majority of our sweets. Since fruit was only available during the summer, it was only eaten a few months out of the year. The lack of refrigeration prevented the storage of fruits for long periods of time. While refined sugar has been around for a couple of centuries, it never was a major part of the diet.

One of the big problems with both sugar and artificial sweeteners is that because they stimulate pleasure centers in our brain, we tend to overeat. Most sweetened foods are high in calories and low in nutrition. Therefore, we tend to fill up on nutritionally deficient, calorie-rich, artificially flavored foods, leaving little room for nutritionally dense, high-fiber, wholesome foods. When children grow up eating nutritionally poor foods, these are the foods they learn to like. Consequently, as they become adults they continue to eat these types of foods and suffer the consequences of poor health and obesity as a result. With each succeeding generation we eat more and more refined processed foods and fewer and fewer whole, natural foods. Kids nowadays, as well as adults, are fatter than ever before.

Another problem with eating a lot of sweetened foods is that they desensitize our taste receptors. As a consequence, sweets don't taste as sweet. Foods don't taste as good. You might wonder why taste receptors would become desensitized to sweets. I like to explain this using an analogy with another one of our senses—smell. It's like walking into a closed room that has a bad odor. When you first enter the room the smell may be overpowering. But if you remain in the room for any length of time the receptors in your nose become less sensitive and you no longer notice the smell. The smell in the room may not have gotten any weaker, but your ability to detect the smell has decreased. As long as you are exposed to the odor your nose remains desensitized. If you leave the room for a while and give your nose a break, it recovers and becomes resensitized, so that if you returned to the room with the offensive odor you will again notice the smell. In like manner, the sweet receptors in our mouths become dulled or desensitized when they are constantly bathed in sugary foods. Overstimulation causes them to become less sensitive to sweets. In response, we often increase the intensity of the sweets in our foods. This desensitizes the sweet receptors even more.

Like a drug addict that needs a larger and larger dose to achieve the same effect, we need more and more sugar in our foods in order to detect the same level of sweetness or get the same amount of pleasure. After a while, natural foods gradually become less appealing. This is one reason why sugar is often added to frozen fruit, and canned fruits are packed in syrup. Fresh fruit isn't sweet enough anymore.

Desensitizing taste receptors also makes vegetables and other natural foods less appealing. Kids nowadays don't like vegetables. In our great-grandparents' day kids ate their vegetables; they didn't turn up their noses to peas and broccoli like they do now. Nor did they get soda pop, candy, and sugar-coated breakfast cereal every day. Kids don't like vegetables because their taste buds are desensitized by eating too much sugar and artificial flavor enhancers. Many adults don't care much for vegetables for the same reason. If fresh, unsweetened fruits and vegetables aren't appealing to you, you're not going to eat them. Instead, you wind up eating less healthy foods which keep your sweet cravings alive.

One of the key ingredients to a successful weight loss program is gaining control over your sweet tooth. If you can harness your cravings for sweets, you will automatically eat less food. The only way to fight sweet cravings is to nip it in the bud—the taste bud, that is. If you remove the desire for sweets, they lose their power and control over you. This can be done. The key is abstinence, just like for any other drug addiction. Abstain from using sweeteners or eating sweet foods for a period of time. I recommend a period of at least six weeks. Six months is better. The longer you can go without eating any foods with added sweeteners, the more your taste receptors will recover and resensitize themselves. Abstaining from sweets is like leaving a smelly room and having your sense of smell restored. When you refrain from eating sweets, your taste receptors can recover.

When you do add a little sweetener back into your diet, you will find that you don't need as much as you did in the past. Not only will sweets taste sweeter, you will find that all foods taste better. You'll begin to appreciate the natural sweetness of peas, squash, and fresh fruits. You won't need as much sweetener as you did before in order to enjoy certain foods. In fact, commercially sweetened foods will taste too sweet. This fact was brought home to me some time ago. After not eating any sweetened foods (other than fruits occasionally) for several months, my wife and I decided to reward our good efforts by buying a pint of Haagen-Dazs ice cream and splitting it. We purchased vanilla with almonds because we thought it would not be as rich as

74

the other flavors. When we began eating we both noticed how overly sweet it tasted. We'd eaten this flavor many times before in the past, but now it seemed so sweet as to lose its appeal. Neither one of use could even finish the serving. We ended up throwing it away. Can you believe it, throwing away Haagen-Dazs ice cream? On occasion, we do eat homemade ice cream made with real cream, sweetened with a tiny bit of stevia, and topped with fresh fruit. It's not too sweet and tastes great.

I notice the same thing whenever I eat white bread, which isn't very often. Commercially made white bread, which almost always has added sugar, often tastes overly sweet. It's more like candy or sweet bread than just plain bread. All commercially made treats taste too sweet to me now, and they will to you too, once you break the sugar habit.

Artificial sweeteners should be completely avoided all the time. Natural sweeteners, such as raw honey and molasses, should be used in preference over the highly refined ones. As you resensitize your taste receptors, you will lose your desire for sweets. You will no longer have cravings. When you come face to face with sweet treats in the course of your day, you will not be drawn in by their beckoning call. You will have the will power to resist and not feel deprived because you have full control over your actions.

Sugar is the number one cause of weight gain because, like a drug, it creates addiction. If you are going to lose weight, and lose it permanently, you *must* conquer your sweet tooth. The only way to do that is through abstinence. Using so-called natural sweeteners in place of refined sugar won't do it. Switching to artificial sweeteners won't do it. Consumption of all sweets needs to be curtailed.

Once you've broken the grip sugar has over you, keep in mind that sugar addiction is like alcoholism. A recovered alcoholic can relapse with just a few drinks. Likewise, a sugarholic can relapse with just a few sweets. Even when you break the sugar habit, sweets may always retain some allure, but they won't control you as they once did. You will be able to resist them as long as you don't fall prey to their enticements.

Does this mean you can never eat sweets again? For some people, maybe so. Others may be able to handle a little sweetening or a treat now and then, but it is so easy to fall into the habit of eating sweetened foods that it is best to stay away from them as much as possible. Fruits or foods sweetened with a little whole fruit are okay, but not fruit juice. Fruit juice is too sweet and is not much different from Kool-Aid or soda. Fruit juice can easily jump-start sugar addiction. "Natural" sweeteners are not much better than any other sweetener. Sweet addictions can be kept alive and thriving on natural sweeteners just as well as any other. To keep sweet addictions away, you need to refrain from all added sweetening, with the possible exception of a little fresh fruit and occasionally a little stevia.

A LOW-SUGAR DIET

One of the primary reasons why most low-calorie, low-fat, and other reducing diets don't work is because they continue to allow sugar or other sweeteners. One of the biggest problems with most weight-reducing diets is that they focus too much on reducing calories instead of zeroing in on the main culprit—refined carbohydrates. Calorie reduction should not be a torturous affair filled with struggling and starvation. When you focus *only* on calorie reduction, you are setting yourself up for disappointment and failure. A better approach is to eliminate the *cause* for excess calorie consumption. If you eliminate the desire to overeat, you automatically eat fewer calories, feel satisfied, do not feel deprived, feel good about your dietary choices, and lose weight with much less effort and pain.

Most diets allow sweets in one form or another because we have become so addicted to them that many people would be turned off by a diet that didn't have them. But what do you want? Do you want to lose weight and lose it permanently, or do you want to keep both your sweets and your body fat? The choice is yours. If you conquer your sugar addictions, you will be far more successful in losing weight because you will be eating foods that are more filling and satisfying and that don't entice you to overeat. You end up eating less—by choice, not by restraint.

If your diet is going to be successful over the long run, you must gain control of your sweet tooth. I meet too many people so enslaved by sugar they won't or can't break away from it. Sugar controls their lives. They try diet after diet, but keep their sweet tooth and sugar addictions alive and their willpower at the mercy of sugar cravings.

A successful weight-loss program will be one that involves a low-sugar diet. When I say sugar, I include artificial sweeteners as well. You can't break sugar addictions by substituting one drug for another. A successful diet will also limit grains, especially white flour and white rice. All refined carbohydrates are addicting.

A good weight loss program, one that is healthy and can be maintained for life, will include foods with a mixture of complex carbohydrates, protein, and fat from a variety of wholesome, natural sources. These foods would be much like those typically eaten by our great-grandparents and their parents—whole milk, rich full-fat cream and butter, meat marbled with fat, fresh fruits and vegetables of all types. These are the foods that nourished our ancestors for thousands of years. These are the foods that nature, not some chemist or corporation, has provided for our nourishment.

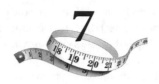

Not All Calories
Are Equal

CALORIES IN VERSUS CALORIES OUT

The causes of obesity and overweight are continually being debated. Some say it's a lack of exercise, others claim genetics or metabolism is to blame, while most people simply say it's because we eat too much. There is truth in all these statements. Many factors are involved. However, the one factor we hear most often is calories in versus calories out—if you eat more calories than your body burns off, the excess is tucked away into storage as fat, regardless of any other factors.

The food we eat is converted into energy to power metabolic functions and physical activity. Any excess energy is converted into fat and packed away into our fat cells, producing the cellulite on our legs, the spare tire around our middles, and the oversized seat cushions on our backsides. So, the more we eat, the bigger we get.

If that's all there is to it, the answer to being overweight seems obvious: eat less. This is not always a welcome answer or an easy one to implement. How many people have tried to diet by eating fewer calories? Probably everyone reading this book. If it worked, you wouldn't be here and I wouldn't have had to write it. In this chapter, you will learn why low-calorie dieting ultimately makes you *gain* more weight, why overweight people seem to gain weight more easily than thinner individuals, and why you need more than a simple low-calorie diet to lose weight permanently.

The energy we obtain from food is measured in calories. Everybody needs a certain amount of energy (calories) to keep basic metabolic processes functioning—the heart beating, lungs expanding and contracting, stomach digesting food, and every other cellular process that keeps the body alive.

The rate at which the body uses calories for these maintenance activities is called the basal metabolic rate (BMR). It is equivalent to the amount of calories a person would expend while lying down, completely inactive but awake. Any physical activity, no matter how simple, would require additional calories. At least two-thirds of the calories we use every day go towards fueling basic metabolic functions. Only one-third is used for physical or voluntary activity.

The BMR is different for each individual. Many factors determine our BMR and the amount of calories our bodies need and use. Younger people and physically active people require more calories. People who are fasting, starving, or even dieting use less calories than they ordinarily would. Overweight people use fewer calories than lean people. These last two are unwelcome news to people who are overweight and dieting. It means they have to eat even less to see a change.

On average, a person needs roughly 2,400 calories a day to maintain current weight, whether they are over- or underweight. This is the amount needed just to stay even. Out of this number, two-thirds or 1,600 calories are needed just to power basic metabolic processes. The remaining 800 calories are used for daily activities.

The theory behind all low-calorie diets is the idea that being overweight is caused by eating more calories than the body burns. For example, if your BMR and activity level requires you to consume 2,400 calories to maintain your weight, any excess calories over that amount will be converted into fat and stored in the body. In order to lose weight a person needs to eat fewer calories. In this case less than 2,400, because the body would need to take fat out of storage and burn it to meet energy needs. The fewer calories you consume, the more fat must be taken from the body and the more weight is lost. This process is commonly summed up as "calories in versus calories out." Body weight is determined by how many calories we eat versus how many we burn off.

Calories in > calories out = weight gain
Calories in < calories out = weight loss
Calories in = calories out = weight maintenance

While watching your calorie intake is important, losing weight successfully involves more than just limiting calorie consumption. Often, a dieter will reduce daily food consumption to less than 1,000 calories a day and still gain weight! Theoretically this can't happen. If you believe that weight loss is governed simply by the formula "calories in versus calories out," the average size person must have around 1,600 calories a day just to fuel basic metabolic functions. Any less than this should result in weight loss. I know people who have gained weight eating only 800 calories a day—half the amount needed to fuel basic metabolic functions!

It can be very frustrating when an overweight person eats nothing but lettuce and carrots and still gains weight. Friends, family, and even the doctor will often accuse the dieter of cheating, sneaking food when no one is looking, or failing to account for every bite eaten. Yet, this is very common. There are many overweight people who are gaining weight on starvation diets. Obviously, there is something very wrong with the calories in versus calories out formula. There is much more to successful weight management than simply counting calories.

DIETING MAKES YOU FAT

Someone once said, "Over the past several years I've lost 200 pounds. If I'd kept it all off, I would weigh a negative 20 pounds." I think many of us can relate to this statement.

Take Susan, for example. Susan was like many overweight people. She wanted to lose weight and worked hard at it. She tried one diet after another. Most of them seemed to work—at least at first. She would go on one diet and lose 10 or 12 pounds (4.5 or 5.5 kg), but before long the weight would come right back. She would try another diet and maybe lose 20 pounds (9 kg), but over time the weight would creep on back. Every diet she tried ended with the same results. After years of dieting, not only was she still overweight, but she weighed more than ever. All the dieting she did hadn't helped her lose a single pound. In fact, it seemed to make her even bigger. The truth is, dieting was part of her problem.

According to the Mayo Clinic, 95 percent of those people who go on weight-loss diets gain all their weight back within 5 years. Many add on more weight than they had before. Typical weight-loss diets not only don't work but often make matters worse. Yes, dieting can actually make you fat.

The problem with many weight-loss diets is that they focus only on calorie restriction. While paying attention to calorie consumption is important, it is not the only factor that influences body weight. The sad fact is that all low-calorie, low-fat diets are doomed from the start. No matter what type of food you eat, if the diet relies solely on calorie restriction, it is programmed to fail.

In addition to calories, you must consider other factors. One of these is metabolism. You can't ignore metabolism and expect to be successful. Let me explain why.

Your metabolic rate is affected by many things. One of the things is the amount of food you eat. Our bodies have a built-in mechanism that strives to maintain a balance between our metabolism and the environment. This mechanism was vital for our ancestors who relied on seasonal availability of foods for survival. When food was plentiful, metabolism ran at the height of efficiency. A higher metabolism has advantages in that it raises energy levels, keeps the brain alert, improves immune system function, and speeds healing, tissue growth, and repair. During winter or famine when food was less plentiful, metabolism slowed down. The advantage was that less energy (i.e. food) was needed to fuel metabolic processes. People were able to survive on fewer calories during times of scarcity.

Today with modern food preservation and delivery methods, getting enough to eat is no longer a problem for most people. Food is abundantly available all year around. However, our bodies still maintain the ability to adapt quickly to famine. If we suddenly start to eat less food, it signals to our bodies that there must be a famine and, as a means of self-preservation, our BMR decreases to conserve energy. The problem with this is that when we diet, we cut down on calorie consumption and the body thinks it's starving, so our metabolic rate slows down. Slower metabolism also means our bodies have less energy and we become fatigued more easily.

When you go on a calorie-restricted diet, your body reacts as if it were experiencing a famine. For the first few days, while your metabolism is still running at normal, the restriction in calories works and you lose weight. Weight loss is always greatest for the first few weeks. After a while as your body adjusts to lower calorie intake, metabolism gradually slows down. Now the calories you consume are balanced with the calories you burn. Weight loss stops. You hit a plateau.

In order to lose more weight you must cut your calorie intake even further. If you do, you will lose a few more pounds until your body adapts and your metabolism again slows down. As long as you continue to restrict calories your metabolism will drop to balance calorie intake with calorie output. Dieting becomes very restrictive and uncomfortable (some would say painful). This is why some people can decrease their total daily intake to less than 1,000 calories and not lose any weight.

When you decide to end the diet, even if you still eat less than you did when you started, the extra calories start to add on weight because your metabolism is depressed. It still thinks you're in a famine. Now when you increase calorie intake, the excess calories are packed on as fat, even though you may be eating fewer calories than you did before you started the diet. By the time your metabolism has figured out that the famine is over, you've added back the weight you've lost. In addition, your body tends to add on more fat to protect itself in case of another famine. So after dieting, you gradually gain back all the weight you lost and a few extra pounds for good measure. In the end, you weigh more than when you started. This whole cycle may take only a few months or drag out for several years. The end result is the same.

The next weight-loss diet you attempt has the same outcome, as does the next and the next. Each time you diet, you end up weighing more than you did before. This process is termed "dieting-induced obesity" or the "yo-yo effect."

Most weight-loss diets are considered temporary dietary restrictions and as soon as the weight is lost, old eating habits are resumed. It's these habits that caused the weight problem in the first place. Consequently, weight comes back on. You can never stay slim by eating the way you used to. In order to lose weight permanently, you must make a permanent change. This, however, is undesirable for most people. Who in their right mind would want to remain on a weight-loss diet forever? These diets are just too restrictive and, in many cases, unhealthy. In order for any diet to work, it needs to be something you can feel comfortable with, something you can do for the rest of your life. You've got to make it a permanent part of your life. So the diet you choose must be one that is satisfying, filling, and healthy. If a diet isn't satisfying, it won't last long.

Notice that I said that for a diet to be successful, it must also be healthy. A diet which is lacking in nutrition, as are most all low-calorie, low-fat diets, has a negative effect on metabolism and encourages overeating as a means to prevent starvation and malnutrition. Metabolism is discussed in more detail in Chapter 13.

ALL CALORIES ARE NOT ALIKE

Calories are units by which energy is measured. Technically, a calorie is the amount of energy needed to raise the temperature of 1 gram of water 1 degree C. In our bodies, carbohydrate, protein, and fat are metabolized to produce energy, which is measured in calories.

Scientists have determined that a gram of carbohydrate produces 4 calories, a gram of protein also produces 4 calories, but a gram of fat delivers 9 calories—more than twice that of the other two. A person can eat over twice as much carbohydrate or protein to equal the same amount of calories they get from fat. If you are cutting down on calories as a means to lose weight, but still want to eat enough so you don't feel hungry, it would seem logical to cut out as much fat as possible and replace it with carbohydrate or protein. This is the basic reasoning behind all low-calorie and low-fat diets.

According to this model of weight loss, all calories are assumed to be equal regardless of their source. This has led to the saying that "a calorie is a calorie is a calorie" whether it comes from fat, carbohydrate, or protein. This assumption, however, is wrong and is why low-calorie and low-fat diets don't work. Since a calorie is a unit of measurement like centimeters or degrees, it would seem logical to say a calorie is a calorie just as it is to say a centimeter is a centimeter regardless of what you are measuring. However, centimeters and degrees are direct measurements. You can determine the exact height of a person in centimeters using a measuring tape or a person's temperature in degrees using a thermometer. Calories are not direct measurements. There is no device that can measure calories inside our bodies, so there is no way to actually measure the energy released in our bodies from the foods we eat. We can only make a calculated guess.

Calories are calculated using a machine known as a bomb calorimeter. Food is placed in a sealed container surrounded by water and completely burned. The resulting rise in water temperature is measured. From this process the number of calories in carbohydrate, protein, and fat is determined. Knowing this, the number of calories in a food with a mixture of each of these three nutrients can be calculated. If our bodies *always* functioned *exactly* like a bomb calorimeter regardless of the types of food eaten, then maybe a calorie would be a calorie. However, many other biological factors can influence the net calorie effect of our foods. For example, some hormones and enzymes promote fat burning over carbohydrate, and certain fats boost the metabolic rate. These variables are not taken into account in bomb calorimeter measurements. The measurements obtained from a machine when it burns calories, is not necessarily the same as when the human body burns calories. The source of the calories is very important. This is why one person can eat like a horse and be as thin as a rail, while another can eat like a rabbit and yet still pack on weight.

Innumerable books have been published on low-calorie, low-fat diets promoting the "calorie is a calorie" principle. An entire weight-loss industry has been built around this concept. Millions of people have read these books, cut fat out of their diets, counted their calories, and yet have grown fatter and fatter. The calorie theory is, in a sense, quite cruel. If you gain weight while limiting your calories, something is clearly wrong. It couldn't be the theory, most people would agree. So, if it isn't the theory, it has to be you! You must be cheating, sneaking food when no one is looking and lying about it. Nobody could gain weight eating fat-free salads and steamed veggies—right? When you deny it, they just wink or grin, signaling they'll keep your little secret.

Most of the fat in our bodies does not come from the fat in our diets, it comes from the carbohydrates we eat. All of the carbohydrate in our diet, which is not used immediately for energy, is converted into fat and stored in our fat cells. That spare tire around your middle was once the stack of pancakes you ate for breakfast, the donut you had as a snack, and the large order of fries you wolfed down at lunch. The vast majority of food we eat comes from carbohydrates. On average, we consume about 60 percent of our daily calories in the form of carbohydrate, only 40 percent comes from protein and fat. Most of the protein and fat we consume is used as structural materials to build and maintain muscles, bones, and other tissues. Only a tiny fraction of the protein and fat we eat is used to produce energy or is stored as fat. The body does not need to use protein and fat for energy because there is so much carbohydrate available, even an excess. This excess carbohydrate is what ends up as body fat.

Studies have shown that a carbohydrate-rich diet, like we normally eat, increases the synthesis of fat and cholesterol. When some of the carbohydrate is replaced by fat, fat and cholesterol production in the body decreases![1-2] These studies disprove the theory that all calories are equal. Therefore, replacing most of the carbohydrates in the diet with fat will lead to less fat production and lower body weight (and cholesterol levels improve too). It is really that simple.

Not only are the calories from carbohydrate different from those of fats, but even the type of carbohydrate can have varying effects. Sugars, for example, are not all alike when it comes to calories. Studies have demonstrated that sugars can have different effects on bodyweight, even though their calorie content may be the identical.

You will gain more weight eating foods sweetened with fructose than you will with foods sweetened with sucrose or glucose. Researchers can cause rats to become obese by feeding them high fructose corn syrup, yet rats do not become obese consuming the same amount of calories in the form of sucrose.[3]

While fructose contains the same amount of calories as sucrose, the effects on metabolism are different. Studies have shown that fructose increases plasma free fatty acids that get stored as body fat, increases the effects of the hormone ghrelin, which signals hunger to the brain, and interferes with the normal transport and signaling of the hormone leptin, which helps to produce the feeling of satiety.[4-6] All of these promote weight gain and fat storage. Essentially, fructose is metabolized to produce fat, while glucose is largely being processed for energy or stored as glycogen in the liver and muscles.

DO THE MATH

Scientists have calculated that eating 3,500 calories over what we burn, causes a weight gain of 1 pound (0.45 kg) of fat. Some people eat far more than the typical 2,400 calories a day—1,000 to 3,000 calories more, without compensating for it by burning off those calories from additional physical activity. According to the "all calories are equal" theory, they must be eating far more than normal in order to be overweight. One cup (236 ml) or about 2 scoops of vanilla ice cream contains 500 calories, which is the same number of calories you would get from eating 3 ounces (85 g) of potato chips or a couple of candy bars. Eating 500 extra calories than you burn, will cause you to gain 1/7 pound (0.065 kg). Doesn't seem like much, however, if you snacked on 500 extra calories every day for a year, you would gain 52 pounds! In ten years, you would balloon to 520 pounds (235 kg), over and above your starting weight! Now what if you ate 1,000 extra calories a day? It would be a very easy thing to do just by eating junk foods, snacks, or soda between meals. You would gain 104 pounds (47 kg) the first year and a staggering 1,040 pounds (472 kg) in ten years! If you weighed 150 pounds (68 kg) when you started, in ten years you would weigh nearly 1,200 pounds (544 kg).

Here is the problem. How many people eat a few snacks during the day which amount to 1,000 or more added calories but don't come anywhere near weighting 1,200 pounds? If all calories were equal there would be a lot more 1,200 pound people walking around, or perhaps they wouldn't be mobile enough to walk around, but there would be far more of them. According to Wikipedia's list of the world's heaviest people, there have been only three people in all recorded history who have weighed more than 1,200 pounds. I'm sure they didn't all get this heavy only from snacking on a few candy bars and potato chips between meals. This fact alone should tell you there is something wrong with the theory.

A case in point is Water Hudson (1944-1991), who holds the Guinness World Record for the largest waist—119 inches (300 cm). Hudson is the fourth largest person in medical history. At his heaviest, he weighed 1,197 pounds. His daily diet consisted of two boxes of sausages, 1 pound (0.45 kg) of bacon, 12 eggs, a loaf of bread, four hamburgers and four double cheeseburgers, eight large portions of fries, three ham steaks or two chickens, four baked potatoes, four sweet potatoes, four heads of broccoli, and a large cake, which was washed down with an average of 18 quarts (17 liters) of soda.[7] His total daily caloric intake amounted to over 30,000 calories a day! This was just from his meals. On top of all of this, he ate a variety of snacks. Now, according to the calorie in verses calories out concept, it was only from eating the snacks that accounted for all of his excess weight!

Let's look at the formula again and actually calculate how much weight he would gain eating 30,000 calories a day; we'll ignore the snacks for this calculation. According to the theory, Hudson should have gained 8.6 pounds (3.9 kg) each day! In one year he would gain 3,139 pounds (1,424 kg) for a total weight of 4,336 pounds (1,966 kg). In just ten years he would weigh over 43,360 pounds (19,660 kg)! Can you see how ridiculous the calorie theory becomes?

The opposite is also true. If you cut out 1,000 calories from your diet (say down from 3,500 to 2,500), you would be expected to lose 104 pounds in a year. If you cut out 2,000 calories, down to about 1,500 a day, as many low-fat dieters actually do, you should lose over 200 pounds a year, assuming you could lose that much. Very few people successfully lose this amount of weight in that time frame. Again, something must be wrong with the theory.

Looking at the evidence, the outdated concept that "a calorie is a calorie" is totally blown out of the water. The source of the calories is important—very important! In the following chapter you will learn more about the differences between fat calories and carbohydrate calories and how adding fat into your diet can help you lose excess weight.

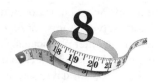

Eat Fat and Grow Slim

FAT IS NOT THE PROBLEM, IT IS THE SOLUTION

Herman Taller, MD, had been chubby all his life. As an adult he stood 5 feet 10½ inches (179 cm) and weighed 265 pounds (120 kg). There didn't seem to be anything he could do about his weight.

When Taller entered medical school at the University of Pavia in Italy, he studied medical papers on nutrition and asked physicians about weight reducing diets. There were theories and diets by the dozen. He tried them all, but none of them worked for him. One of these diets had him eating nothing but fresh fruit. He lost a few pounds that way, but when he came off the diet, he gained back what he had lost and then some. He couldn't maintain this type of diet forever because it made him weak and nervous. Fruit alone was not enough to sustain him.

He tried limiting his food to just milk and vegetables. For an entire month, that was all he ate. At the end of the month, he found he had gained three pounds. He tried an all protein diet, concentrating on meats and fish. This turned out to be just one more way for him to gain weight. The entire time he was in medical school he was on one diet after another and was constantly hungry. By the time he graduated, he weighed 35 pounds (16 kg) more than he had when he started.

He graduated shortly before the outbreak of the Second World War. Fearing the impending conflict in Europe, he accepted a medical position in Chile and departed for South America. Eventually, he moved to the United States and began working as an obstetrician and gynecologist in New York.

As a young doctor, his weight continued to grow. He discussed weight control with other physicians and his failure with the various diets. Some of them hinted that he must have "cheated," eating on the sly, admitting to no one, perhaps not even to himself, what he had been doing. Other physicians who had weight problems themselves simply shrugged their shoulders.

Taller proposed to one of the other physicians, who seemed particularly convinced that he was cheating, that they conduct an experiment. They would go away on a vacation together for ten days, stay in each other's company continually, eat and drink the same foods, and then evaluate the results. His colleague accepted and they went off to a resort. Taller followed the accepted method of weight control: a low-calorie, low-fat diet. He concentrated on eating salads and avoided all fats and fatty foods, and since this was a vacation, he drank a cocktail each night before dinner. His physician friend, who was slim, did the same. At the end of the vacation, his friend had lost a pound or two but Taller gained nine pounds! His friend couldn't explain it and simply brushed it off as an anomaly.

It's not that semistarvation diets didn't help him lose weight, at least initially. Whenever he tried one, he lost some weight, but afterward he invariably gained back more than he had lost. In addition, there were unpleasant side effects to these crash diets, specifically fatigue, irritability, and constant nagging hunger.

In 1955 doctors were becoming interested in cholesterol and its relationship to coronary disease. At the time, there seemed to be some connection between obesity and cholesterol, and so, being heavy, Taller had his cholesterol measured. It was 350 mg/dl, far above the 225 mg/dl which was considered normal at the time. So now he had something else to worry about.

The physician who tested his blood told Taller he wanted him to try something to help lower his cholesterol. Taller asked him what it was. The physician didn't want to tell him yet and told Taller to trust him. To show Taller it was safe, he drank some of the oily substance and told him to take it every day.

Because of his high cholesterol, Taller was willing to experiment, so he began drinking 3 ounces of the mystery substance daily. He was to report for blood cholesterol tests every two weeks.

As the physician had anticipated, Taller's cholesterol level began to drop. Surprisingly, so did his weight. Although his diet remained unchanged, his weight began to melt off. Within two or three weeks he noticed that he was fastening his belt on a tighter notch. This mystery substance was not only reducing his cholesterol but taking off pounds as well. What was this miracle substance? It was nothing more than vegetable oil, basically the same kind you would buy in the grocery store. Taller was dumbfounded. In addition to his regular meals, he was consuming 3 ounces of oil, which amounted to 6 tablespoons (89 ml) of added fat into his daily diet. He was consuming some 5,000 calories a day—and losing weight! The average daily calorie consumption for a normal sized adult is between 2,000 to 3,000. He was consuming nearly twice that amount.

The drop in weight was steady and dramatic. He was feeling better. Chronic sinus congestion that had troubled him for years was clearing up. His complexion was improving. After eight months he had lost a total of 65 pounds (29 kg)—all without dieting. At 200 pounds (91 kg) he was still not a thin man, but he was far thinner and far happier than he had been in years.

All these years Taller tried to eliminate fat from his diet because he believed it promoted weight gain. Now that he was eating fat, as well as more calories, he was losing weight. For decades he had read that in order to lose weight you had to cut calories. This was considered an unshakable rule. Yet, by increasing his caloric intake by adding more fat, he was losing weight. He began thinking that perhaps all calories are not alike when it comes to weight management.

Taller began spending all his spare time in the medical library looking up everything he could find on obesity and metabolism. In his research be came across the work of Dr. Alfred W. Pennington. Pennington wrote an article in the April 1951 issue of the *Journal of the Medical Society of Delaware* titled "The Use of Fat in A Weight-Reducing Diet."

In the article Dr. Pennington stated, "Contrary to the claims of the low-calorie school of thought, low-calorie diets have failed under the most rigid experimental conditions. Low-calorie diets, based on the principle of caloric requirements, are crudely devised in the service of simplicity. There are fat people, plenty of them, who are actually starving."

Then he encountered a key sentence of explanation: "The ability of tissues to oxidize fat is, in contrast to carbohydrates, unlimited." The word "oxidize" in this case means to burn up or convert into energy. Just as you car burns gasoline to produce the energy to power the engine. Your body burns up food to create the energy you need to move and function. Dr. Pennington was making an interesting point. The body, he was maintaining, can burn up an unlimited amount of fat, can transform an unlimited amount of fat into energy. If you burn all the fat you eat, there is not going to be any fat left. Fat, then, is not going to make you gain weight, provided you have sufficient exercise.

What about carbohydrate? Here, Dr. Pennington believed, the chemistry of the body was limited. The body could burn only a certain quantity of carbohydrates, the exact quantity varying with the individual. What happens to the carbohydrate that isn't burned? The body stores it as fat. In men, the body concentrates excess fat about the stomach, as "middle-age spread," and at the back of the neck; and in women, it concentrates excess fat on the buttocks, the upper arms, the upper legs and the breasts, as well as the abdomen.

Dr. Pennington discovered that in the body all calories are not the same. With his discovery, it became evident that it was not the quantity of food a person ate, as much as the types of food he ate that mattered. To say that a specific number of calories will make you fat is as silly as saying that a certain number of microbes will make you sick. What kind of calories? What kind of microbes?

After the end of the Second World War the incidence of heart disease quickly rose and by 1950, it had become the number one cause of death in America. Obesity was also on the rise. Back in those days, large companies often had their own medical staffs to look after their employees. In 1948 officials at E.I. DuPont company in Wilmington, Delaware, were becoming increasingly concerned about the rising obesity and heart disease rates among their employees. Low-calorie diets had already failed to stem the problem. DuPont physician, Dr. Alfred Pennington, decided to take a different approach. He became convinced that obesity was not caused by overeating, but instead by an inability to completely metabolize carbohydrates. Eating too many carbohydrates was making the employees fat, as well as promoting heart disease.

To test his theory, he placed 20 overweight DuPont executives on a high-fat, low-carbohydrate, unrestricted-calorie diet. They immediately began to lose weight, averaging nearly 2 pounds per week. "Notable was a lack of hunger between meals," Pennington wrote, and "increased physical energy and sense of well-being." In three and a half months the executives lost an average of 22 pounds each. They lost weight on a diet that did not restrict calories; they ate 18 ounces (510 g) of meat with 6 ounces (170 g) of fat (primarily saturated fat) divided over three meals, averaging over 3,000 calories a day. Carbohydrates were restricted to no more than 80 calories (20 g) per meal. "In a few cases," Pennington reported, "even this much carbohydrate prevented weight loss, though an ad-libitum (unrestricted) intake of protein and fat was successful."

Pennington considered low-calorie diets a form of starvation and as such were nutritionally poor and unhealthy—which they are. He believed that the safest and most effective method of weight reduction was to eliminate carbohydrate from the diet completely and to allow unrestricted intake of protein and fat. He recommended eating fresh meat with all the fat. Most of the meat sold at the stores, he said, did not contain enough fat, so he advised adding extra meat or kidney fat. The proportions he prescribed were 9 ounces (255 g) of lean meat to 3 ounces (85 g) of fat, cooked weight, at each of the three meals of the day, with the patient at liberty to take more, if he chose, in that proportion—three parts of lean to one of fat. The total quantity of food eaten was not important, but the three-to-one ratio needed to be maintained because any decrease in the fat would reduce the rate of weight loss. "The entire success of the diet depends on eating enough fat," he states. "Otherwise, the patient would be on a mere low calorie diet, with all the disadvantages such a diet entails." He claimed that a loss of weight of 12 pounds a month was usually accomplished on such a regimen. When normal weight is reached, the weight loss stops.

One of the chief advantages of this diet is that it maintains energy production. The body is never tricked into thinking it is experiencing a famine and starving, so metabolism remains steady. Calories are burned off at a normal rate. This eliminates the constant need to lower calorie consumption to keep pace with declining metabolism that happens on a calorie restricted diet.

Word of Pennington's low-carbohydrate, high-fat approach to weight loss spread, and by the early 1950s, it became popularly known as the DuPont Diet. By the end of the decade, however, fat, especially saturated fat, was being accused of elevating blood cholesterol levels and contributing to heart disease. Out of fear, people started cutting fat out of their diets. The DuPont Diet, which was high in saturated fat, eventually faded away and was forgotten.

Using what he learned from Pennington's work, Dr. Taller began recommending a low-carb, high-fat diet to all of his overweight patients. Also fearful of saturated fat, Taller replaced saturated fat with vegetable oil, specifically safflower oil because it was high in polyunsaturated fat. He recommended that his patients consume 3 ounces (90 ml) of oil and 2 ounces (60 ml) of margarine a day. One ounce (2 tablespoons/30 ml) of liquid vegetable oil was consumed before each meal and 2 ounces of margarine was used in meal preparation. It worked. His overweight patients shed pounds easily, without reducing their calorie intake. In 1961 he wrote a book titled *Calories Don't Count*. While using safflower oil and margarine rather than saturated fat was still effective in promoting weight loss, the high linoleic acid content of the safflower oil and trans fatty acids of the margarine would eventually cause greater harm in the long run, as you learned in Chapter 3. Taller's diet gained popularity initially, but the general fear of fat, eventually spelled its doom and it, too, fell into by the wayside.

USE FAT TO LOSE FAT

Taller and Pennington weren't the only investigators to discover that fat is needed for successful weight loss. As early as 1928, researchers at the Russell Sage Institute in Troy, New York discovered the same thing. During calorimetric testing, a male subject lost excess weight while eating a diet of fatty meat containing between 2,000 and 3,000 calories daily. As 80 percent of the calories in his diet were derived from fat, it was apparent that his body was able to burn more food on this diet than on an ordinary low-calorie diet.[1]

One of the first researchers to draw the connection between fat and carbohydrate consumption and body weight was famed thyroid expert Broda Barnes, MD, PhD. When he was fresh out of medical school in 1938 he began working with Dr. Robert W. Keeton at the University of Illinois. Because of Barnes' background (he had a PhD in endocrinology—the study of the thyroid and other glands), Dr. Keeton assigned him to study the relationship between the endocrine system and obesity.

He assembled a group of obese volunteers and for three months every morsel of food they ate was carefully recorded. When he analyzed the types of foods they were eating he discovered something totally unexpected. While the diets of the volunteers all varied, the one factor that they all had in common was a high consumption of carbohydrates. Their protein intake was moderate, but they avoided fat like the plague. Butter and fatty foods were avoided and all fat was carefully trimmed off meat. It became obvious to Dr. Barnes that the low-fat, high-carbohydrate diet was the cause of their obesity.

At this time, one of Barnes' colleagues was studying the effects of high-fat diets in rats. He found that overweight rats lost excess weight when given a high-fat diet. He suggested to Barnes to try a similar diet on human volunteers.

Dr. Barnes designed a moderate-protein, low-carbohydrate, high-fat diet. The diet consisted of 50 grams of carbohydrate, 70 grams of protein, and 90 grams of fat, adding up to about 1,300 total calories a day. The average number of calories normally consumed ranges from 2,000 to 2,800 per day, so this was also a low-calorie diet. The fat supplied 63 percent of the total calories consumed.

For breakfast they typically ate two eggs with bacon, ham, or sausage; two ounces of fruit juice; and a beverage with cream if they desired; but no sugar or toast. Lunch and dinner consisted of fatty meat, a vegetable topped with butter, a salad with a generous amount of oil-based salad dressing, a glass of raw whole milk, and a small serving of fresh fruit for dessert.

The vegetables and fruits most often used were relatively low in carbohydrate. On occasion, a smaller quantity of higher carbohydrate vegetables were served. All bread and cereals were eliminated.

The volunteers were kept under observation in the hospital. During this time, they steadily lost weight, averaging 10 pounds per month. Even more astonishing: although the diet contained fewer calories than normal, they enjoyed the food and didn't feel hungry. Every one of the volunteers was comfortable and did not suffer with hunger pangs. At times, they even left food unfinished.

At the beginning of the study all the volunteers, with one exception, weighed over 300 pounds. The smallest of the bunch weighed only 295, but was included because she was only 18 years old. She had been fat all of her life and was very embarrassed about it. Whenever company would drop by to visit, she would hide under her bed and stay until they left. She was brought into the outpatient department because she had grown so large that she could no longer squeeze under the bed.

She remained at the hospital for 13 months. In that time, she lost 110 pounds. Her abdomen and hips showed the most remarkable loss. Dr. Barnes noted that her face was not drawn and haggard as so often is the case with people who lose this much weight.

Knowing what to eat, she continued with the diet when she went back home, where she lost an additional 48 pounds. Eleven months later she weighed 137 pounds. Within just two years she had lost a total of 158 pounds!

For the next 35 years Dr. Barnes prescribed this high-fat diet for his overweight patients. In that time, all of his patients who stayed on the diet reported successful weight loss.

In the 1950s two British scientists, Alan Kekwick and Gaston L. S. Pawan, discovered that all calories are not alike and that the source of the calories plays a significant role in weight management. Kekwick and Pawan set out to study the relative effects of fat, protein, and carbohydrate on weight loss in a low-calorie diet. They put 14 obese patients on four different diets in succession over a period of time. Each of the diets provided 1,000 calories per day, but differed in the amount of fat, protein, and carbohydrate. One diet had 90 percent fat, the next 90 percent protein, the next 90 percent carbohydrate, and the last was a normal mixed diet. The patients rotated through each of the diets. The subjects stayed in a hospital so they could be kept under constant observation to insure strict dietary compliance.

If all calories are equal, as most scientists believed at the time, the 1,000 calorie diet should have produced the same amount of weight loss in each of the subjects. But that is not what happened. The 90 percent fat diet (high-fat, low-carb) produced the greatest weight loss, followed closely by the 90 percent protein diet. Next, came the mixed diet. Last of all was the very low-fat 90 percent carbohydrate diet.[2] In essence, the higher the carbohydrate content, the lower the weight loss; the higher the fat content, the greater the weight loss.

In a follow-up study, Kekwick and Pawan compared the weight loss of obese subjects on a high-carbohydrate diet with a high-fat diet, eating twice as many calories as in the previous study. Subjects on a high-carbohydrate 2,000-calorie diet failed to lose any weight. The same subjects on a high-fat diet not only lost weight at 2,000 calories, but lost weight even when calorie consumption increased to 2,600![3] A typical example of the subjects in this study was BJ. After eight days on the high-carbohydrate, 2,000-calorie diet, BJ didn't lose an ounce, but lost 9 pounds in 3 weeks on the 2,600-calorie, high-fat diet.

Kekwick and Pawan discovered a hormonal substance in the urine referred to as "fat-mobilizing substance" (FMS). This substance apparently stimulates the breakdown and burning of body fat, resulting in increased weight loss. FMS increases with the consumption of dietary fat. Thus, adding fat into the diet stimulates the burning of body fat. Eating fat, it turns out, increases the body's utilization of stored fat, leading to weight loss. This provided the reason why eating fat caused greater weight loss than eating carbohydrate or protein. It also demonstrated why all calories are not alike.

91

Eating a high-fat diet is even more effective than not eating at all. In the 1960s Dr. Frederick Benoit and colleagues at the US Naval Medical Research Institute compared two groups of overweight subjects; one group ate a high-fat diet, while the other group consumed no food at all. The subjects' weight loss over time was measured. The high-fat group consumed 1,000 calories a day, 90 percent of which came from fat. The remaining calories came from approximately 15 grams of protein and 10 grams of carbohydrate. The other group consumed no calories at all, only water. After ten days the fasting group lost 21 pounds on average, but most of that was from lean body tissue and water; only 7.5 pounds was body fat. In comparison, the high-fat diet group lost on average 14.5 pounds, 14 of which was from body fat.[4] The group that ate 1,000 calories, mostly from fat, lost twice as much fat as the group that ate nothing! Plus, they lost very little water and lean muscle. A reduced calorie diet with ample fat and limited carbohydrate will produce much greater weight loss than any low-fat diet, regardless of the number of calories consumed—even if this number is zero! Therefore, including an ample amount of fat in the diet is essential for greatest weight loss. This is a very important concept to remember for anyone trying to lose weight. You need to eat fat to lose fat. The discoveries of Kekwick, Pawan, and Benoit disproved the common belief that a calorie is a calorie. The source of the calories is important.

Based on the work of these and other researchers, Robert Atkins, MD, developed a very successful method of weight loss which he described in his book *Dr. Atkins' Diet Revolution*, which was first published in the 1970s. It was this book that really introduced the concept of low-carb dieting to the public. Dr. Atkins updated the book in 1992 and republished it as *Dr. Atkins' New Diet Revolution*. The book became an international bestseller.

One of the major criticisms with low-carbohydrate diets is the higher percentage of fat, which is really the key ingredient that makes the diet so effective. With a reduction of carbohydrates, protein and fat consumption increases. Due to the fear of consuming too much fat, critics claimed that low-carb diets will raise blood cholesterol levels and increase risk of heart disease. However, Dr. Atkins found, after working with over 25,000 patients, that just the opposite happens. Blood cholesterol levels improve on the low-carb, high-fat diet. What was even more aggravating to the critics was that there was no restriction on saturated fats. Animal fats were freely eaten without showing any harmful effects. The high-saturated fat, low-carb diet had beneficial effects on blood cholesterol levels and also improved blood sugar levels in diabetics. People not only lost excess weight, but their health in general greatly improved.

Kevin Vigilante, MD, co-author of *Low-Fat Lies*, says, "Low-fat diets as commonly conceived do not work, can be medically harmful, and do not represent the best diet for many people—especially if they want to lose weight and keep it off."

Dr. Vigilante confesses that physicians in general know very little about nutrition. "So like most Americans I was a low-fat fanatic for years," he says. "I preached it to my overweight patients, and I tried to practice it myself. But I had a hard time sticking to the program. Either I hated the food or I was hungry all the time." Nevertheless, he kept exhorting his patients to avoid fat.

He then had an experience that changed the way he looked at diets. He went on vacation to Italy. While there, he lifted his barrier to fatty foods and ate for the sheer enjoyment of it without regard to fat. "Everything I ate was awash in olive oil," he said. All foods were full of fats—cheese, cream, sauces—nothing was made with low-fat ingredients. Judging by the foods he was eating he expected an increase in his waistline, but when he returned home, "I felt my clothes were looser. Then I got on the scale. I had lost almost five pounds!"

He mentioned this unusual experience to a nutritionist friend, Dr. Mary Flynn. She wasn't surprised. "Sure, a little fat helps you lose weight."

He was shocked. "It seemed too good to be true," he said. "I just couldn't accept the notion that you could lose weight without immense suffering."

"I don't believe in low-fat diets," Dr. Flynn said. "They just don't work. Fat makes food taste good, and it makes you feel full. Without a little fat you're always going to be hungry."

The key she said was to eat the right kind of fat in the right amounts. Dr. Vigilante was so impressed with this information that in 1999 he teamed up with Dr. Flynn and wrote a book exposing the low-fat myth titled *Low-Fat Lies*.[5]

SATISFY HUNGER

The problem with most low-fat diets is that they lack satiety. What is satiety? It's the feeling of fullness or satisfaction at the end of a meal, the feeling that you are no longer hungry. The longer you can maintain this feeling, the longer you can go without eating and without overeating at the next meal. Some foods provide greater and longer lasting satiety than others. A T-bone steak provides greater satiety than a slice of watermelon. A ham and cheese omelet offers more satiety than a bowl of lettuce and tomatoes. Satiety is one of the ingredients for successful weight reduction.

When the volume of food we eat is not adequate enough to achieve satiety, or if the food digests rapidly, we become hungry again long before the next meal. This encourages snacking and feelings of hunger that make dieting a challenge.

It is true that consuming too many calories promotes weight gain. Unfortunately, calorie intake is all that most weight-loss diets focus on. High-calorie foods (i.e., those that contain the most fat) are restricted so you can eat more low-calorie foods. In theory, if you cut out high-calorie foods, you will be able to eat a larger volume of low-calorie foods and feel satisfied on fewer calories. While this idea may sound logical, in real life it doesn't work. The problem with this approach is that most low-calorie foods aren't very satisfying. For instance, after eating a lettuce and tomato salad, how long can you go without feeling hungry again? If you are like most people, hunger returns within a couple of hours. These low-calorie foods digest very quickly, leaving your stomach empty and complaining. You have to eat again to satisfy your hunger or you must suffer until the next meal. Most of us can only take so much suffering before we call it quits and go back to eating the way we did before.

A diet that allows you to eat until you are satisfied and keeps you from getting hungry until the next meal is a much better way to control total calorie intake. When your stomach is full you don't think about eating, you don't spend time dreaming about foods, you don't suffer, and you don't feel the need to cheat in order to satisfy hunger pangs.

You can control calorie intake easier if the food you eat gives you a feeling of lasting fullness. What you need is a diet that allows you to eat a satisfying volume of food while balancing calorie consumption with energy needs. However, the foods that are the most satisfying are generally the highest in calories.

Fortunately, we don't eat foods based on calories, we eat based on satiety, which is determined by volume, not calorie content. When the stomach is full, hunger is satisfied. It's that simple. And the longer food remains in the stomach, the longer we can go between meals without feeling hungry and without eating. So even though the foods you eat may contain more calories, if they satisfy your hunger and keep you from overeating, your total calorie intake will be less and you will lose weight.

There are certain foods that satisfy hunger and keep us feeling full for several hours. There are other foods that digest quickly and cause us to be hungry sooner. Each of these are discussed below.

Dietary Fiber

If you had your choice between two nearly identical pieces of cake with one having half as many calories as the other, which one would you choose? If you are concerned about your weight you would choose the one with fewer calories.

If the foods you ate had fewer calories, you could eat just as much as you normally do and still lose weight without going hungry. One way to lower the calorie content of your food, without lowering the volume, is to eat foods which are high in fiber. Fiber contains no calories, but does provide bulk and can help with feelings of satiety. High-fiber foods are also good sources of nutrients.

Foods that are high in fiber are generally low in calories and provide bulk, so they are more likely to fill you up, not out. A slice of whole wheat bread, for example, is five times more filling than a slice of white bread. Whole wheat bread also contains fewer calories than white. The same volume of whole wheat bread provides less starch (calorie producing carbohydrate) and more fiber (non-calorie carbohydrate) than white bread. Ounce for ounce, the whole wheat bread supplies fewer calories because it contains more fiber (as well as vitamins and minerals).

Fiber not only provides bulk with fewer calories, but it also delays hunger. Fiber tends to linger in the stomach, delaying gastric emptying. Fiber also delays the absorption of carbohydrates and fats in the small intestine. This provides a feeling of fullness and satiety. Increasing your fiber intake will help make your stomach and brain think you are full, even when you are taking in fewer calories.

During a meal it takes about 20 minutes to get the feeling of fullness that prompts us to stop. Whether you eat quickly or slowly, it still takes the same amount of time. In today's fast-paced world many people don't take the time to eat. They gulp down a meal and off they go. Studies show that when people eat meals at a rapid rate, they became hungry again more quickly than when they eat exactly the same volume of food at a slower rate.[6] So the rate at which you eat not only influences how much you eat at a meal, but also influences the length of time a person can go without eating between meals. Fast eaters, therefore, tend to eat more than slow eaters. Several studies have shown that overweight people usually eat more rapidly than slim people. Fiber is helpful here, too. Since fiber is chewy, it takes more time to eat high-fiber foods. Eating is slowed down, so we end up eating less.

Eating high fiber food is an important step in any permanent weight-loss program. In summary, high-fiber meals provide low-calorie bulk, keeps your stomach full longer, slows down digestion of other carbohydrates, and slows down eating time so you take in less food. Even a small increase in fiber can make a difference. A study in England discovered that lean adults averaged 19 grams of fiber a day, while obese ones consumed only 13. This is a difference of only 6 grams a day. Fresh fruits, vegetables, and nuts are among the best sources of fiber.

Protein

An adequate amount of protein in the diet can help you lose weight because protein satisfies hunger longer than carbohydrates. It takes the stomach longer to digest protein than carbohydrate. Consequently, food remains in the stomach longer, extending the feeling of satiety.

If you eat a breakfast of ham and eggs (high-protein foods), it will easily hold you over until lunch. A low-protein breakfast, such as a slice of toast, glass of juice, and a half grapefruit won't last long. By lunchtime you will be so hungry that you will overeat (if you didn't snack on donuts or candy). The calories you didn't get at breakfast are added on at lunchtime. You will eat faster and your sense of satiety won't kick in until you've loaded up on more calories than you otherwise would. If you also eat a low-protein lunch, the same thing will happen at dinner. You either end up consuming more total calories on the diet or feel miserable all day long.

Studies have shown that eating a high-protein meal is associated with a decrease in hunger afterwards and ultimately eating fewer total calories during the day. Volunteers in these studies were able to wait longer between meals before eating and ate less during the meals. In a study performed in Canada, men were given either high-protein or moderate-protein meals for 6 days and could eat as much as they liked: those eating more protein took in fewer calories each day. Observations such as this support the idea that a very high-protein diet may reduce total calorie consumption, which has increased the popularity of high-protein weight-loss diets.

Fat

For years now fat has been labeled as the primary cause, or at least a major contributor, to obesity and overweight. It is ostracized from all weight-loss diets. Even many high-protein diets limit fat consumption. Indeed, no self-respecting weight-loss diet would be caught dead recommending fat. That is, until now.

Like protein, fat also slows down the digestion of food, allowing the stomach to feel full longer and quenching the pangs of hunger. Fat stimulates the release of hormones that slow down the rate at which food leaves the stomach, allowing you to feel full longer. The small intestine also has fat receptors that act in much the same way. When you eat fatty foods you feel satisfied longer and don't sense a need to snack or to overeat at the next meal. For this reason, adding fat to your diet can help you lose weight!

After years of exclusion, fat can now be welcomed back into the diet with open arms. No longer do you need to buy lean cuts of meat or trim off every speck of fat. No longer are you required to eat tasteless non-fat milk and low-fat cheese. You can now add a pat of butter to your vegetables and cook with oil without fear. Adding fat to your foods and eating full-fat foods will help you to eat less and lose weight.

In one study, volunteers were given either a high-fat or a low-fat breakfast containing the same number of calories. Those who ate the high-fat breakfast felt full longer and delayed the time of their next meal, thus avoiding between meal snacks.[5]

Research has shown that when people get hungry soon after a meal, they tend to overeat at the next. Thus, a high-fat breakfast helps to prevent both between meal snacking and overeating. The end result is the consumption of fewer total calories. When used properly, fat can be an important aid in helping you lose weight and keeping it off.

Without fat, food is less filling, and we tend to overeat to get the same feeling of satiety. Also, low-fat foods are not necessarily low-calorie foods. Fat gives food flavor. If you take the fat out, it becomes bland and less desirable, so manufacturers add in more sugar to improve the taste. You end up with a low-fat food that has just as many calories as the full-fat version. However, without the fat, the food is less satisfying and digests more quickly, making you hungry sooner. For this reason, many so-called low-fat and non-fat foods actually promote snacking, overeating, and, ultimately, weight gain!

In another study, a group of women were given a mid-morning yogurt snack and then later served lunch and dinner. There were two choices of yogurt. One was regular full-fat and the other was low-fat. Each was labeled, but there was no mention of total calorie content. Each, however, contained the same number of calories. The only difference was the fat content. Participants were allowed to choose whichever one they wanted. When the women were later served lunch, those who had the high-fat yogurt ate less than those who ate the low-fat variety. The extra fat in the yogurt snack satisfied their hunger longer and encouraged them to eat less at lunch.

Researchers also wanted to learn if those who ate less at lunch would eventually make up for it at dinner. But at dinner the ones who ate the high-fat yogurt and less food at lunch didn't eat any more than the others. They weren't any hungrier for eating less at lunch. So at the end of the day those women who ate the high-fat yogurt ended up consuming fewer total calories than those who ate the low-fat snack.[7]

Some fats exert a greater degree of satiety than other fats. Coconut oil is at the top of the list on the satiety scale. This has been demonstrated in both human and animal studies. For example, in a study conducted in Japan, rats were given diets containing either MCT-based oil (derived from coconut oil) or vegetable oil. The amount of food eaten was determined every hour. As early as one hour after feeding, total food intake significantly decreased in the MCT-fed animals. Rats were then given a choice between the two foods to confirm if palatability of the diets had any influence. There was no difference in food intake between the two diets.[8] This study showed that the oil composed of MCTs was more satisfying than other oils, at least in rats.

The effect in humans is the same. In a study with human subjects, women were given a drink which contained either MCT based oil or vegetable oil. Thirty minutes later they were offered lunch in which they could choose and eat as much as they wanted. The women who had the MCT oil before the meal ate less food, and as the authors of the study stated, "significantly decreased caloric intake in the lunch."[9]

Another study was divided into three phases. In each phase the subjects had free access to high-fat foods for 14 days. The phases differed in the amount of both MCTs (from coconut oil) and LCTs in the foods. The first phase contained 20 percent MCTs and 40 percent LCTs of total energy. The second contained equal amounts of MCTs and LCTs. The third had 40 percent MCTs and 20 percent LCTs. Researchers recorded the total amount of food each subject consumed. It was found that as MCT content increased, total food consumption decreased.[10]

In another study, normal-weight men were given breakfasts differing only in the type of fat used. Food intakes at lunch and dinner were measured. Those eating breakfasts containing MCTs ate less at lunchtime. At dinner there was no difference. This study showed that when MCTs are eaten at one meal, hunger is forestalled for longer and less food is eaten at the next. Also important was that even though subjects ate less at lunch, they did not make up for it by eating more at dinner. Total daily food and calorie intake decreased.[11] Studies show that test subjects consume on average 62.5 fewer calories per day when their meals contain MCT in place of LCTs.[12]

These and other studies suggest that eating coconut oil in place of other oils can provide longer satisfaction and hold off hunger longer, resulting in lower total-calorie consumption. For this, and other reasons, coconut oil is known as a low-calorie fat. The idea that any fat could be considered low-calorie is strange indeed, but it is an accurate description.

Another reason why coconut oil is called a low-calorie fat is because it actually has fewer calories than other fats. Fat in general supplies 9 calories per gram. Coconut oil, because of its smaller molecular size, supplies 8.6 calories per gram. That is 0.4 calories per gram less. This may not seem like a lot, but when you consider the total amount of fat in the diet, this could add up. For example, take a typical daily consumption of 2,400 total calories with 30 percent of those calories coming from fat. We can assume that half of the fat comes from added sources such as cooking oils, salad dressings, and such. If all the added fat were replaced with coconut oil, it would reduce the total number of calories consumed by 16 calories a day. This deficiency of 16 calories can be combined with the 62.5 reduction in calories caused by the satiety effect (as seen above) for a total reduction of 78.5 calories per day. In a month, that would amount to 2,355 fewer calories consumed. Now that will make a difference!

LOW-FAT DIETS PROMOTE FAT PRODUCTION

The body needs fat. If it is not supplied in the diet, it will make its own (except for the essential fatty acids). If you don't eat enough fat, the body, sensing fat deprivation, increases the production of fat-making enzymes. People on very-low-fat diets manufacture fat at a dramatically increased rate. So eating less fat actually can cause your body to make and store more fat.

Researchers at the University of Colorado found that when people go on low-fat diets, a fat-storage enzyme called lipoprotein lipase becomes more active, causing the small amount of fat you eat to be stored more easily, thus increasing fat storage in the body.[5] It's ironic that we avoid eating fat to lose weight, but end up producing more body fat in the process.

The less fat you eat, the more fat your body tries to make and pack away into storage; no wonder low-fat dieting doesn't work! A recent study clearly demonstrated this fact. Researchers at Brigham and Women's Hospital and Harvard Medical School showed that subjects on a moderate-fat diet lost weight more effectively than those on a low-fat diet, even though they consumed the same number of calories. Those on the low-fat diet consumed no more than 20 percent of their daily calories as fat. The moderate-fat diet included 35 percent of daily calories as fat. Keep in mind that the current recommendations for fat consumption by The American Heart Association and others are no more than 30 percent of calories and many recommend no more than 20 percent, so the 35 percent fat diet used in this study could even be considered a high-fat diet in comparison. Those subjects on the high-fat diet lost an average of nine pounds, while the low-fat diet participants gained an average of 6.3 pounds![13] Both groups ate the same number of calories, yet the high-fat group lost weight while the low-fat group gained. It appears that if you want to pack on extra weight, you should reduce the amount of fat you eat! It's no wonder we've been getting fatter over the past few decades in our fat phobic society.

In recent years a number of other studies have confirmed the fact that low-carb, high-fat diets produce greater weight loss and produce more favorable changes in blood cholesterol and glucose control than low-fat diets. For instance, the prestigious *Journal of the American Medical Association* published a yearlong head-to-head study between the Atkins diet and the Zone, Ornish, and LEARN diets. The LEARN (Lifestyle, Exercise, Attitudes, Relationships, and Nutrition) diet follows the American government's recommendations for a diet low in fat and high in carbohydrate. The Ornish diet also involves several lifestyle changes as well as calorie restriction and very low-fat intake. At the end of the yearlong study the Atkins diet came out the clear winner in both weight loss and overall improvement in measurable health parameters, such as cholesterol and blood glucose levels. Subjects on the Atkins diet lost more than twice as much weight as any of the other diets with no signs of undesirable side-effects. Those in the Atkins group achieved greater reductions in weight, body fat, triglycerides, and blood pressures, and a greater increase in HDL (good) cholesterol—all signs of improved cardiovascular and overall health.[14]

Any way you look at it the Atkins diet performed better than all these other popular diets. "This is the best study so far to compare popular diets," said Walter Willett, chair of the department of nutrition of the Harvard School of Public Health. The findings confirm, he said, that reducing carbohydrates, "especially those with refined starch and sugar like that found in the US diet, has metabolic benefits." It also shows that replacing carbohydrates with fat "can improve blood cholesterol fractions and blood pressure."

Many other studies have also confirmed that low-carb, high-fat diets produce greater weight loss, better blood cholesterol and triglyceride levels, better blood sugar control, and lower markers for inflammation than low-fat diets.[15-17] The scientific community in general now recognizes low-carbohydrate diets as superior to low-fat diets. However, despite the evidence, many medical professionals, organizations, and businesses continue to support and promote low-fat dieting for philosophical (e.g. vegetarianism) or monetary reasons.

You can lose weight on a low-fat diet, but it's a struggle. You feel deprived and miserable the whole time. However, by replacing carbohydrate with fat, you can enjoy the food more, feel satisfied, and lose more weight! On a low-carb diet with adequate fat you can lose weight eating the same number of calories that you used to gain weight on. The bottom line is that calorie for calorie, you can lose more weight on a low-carb diet that allows ample fat than you can on any other type of diet. In addition to the weight loss, you will also experience an improvement in your blood chemistry and in your overall health.

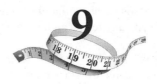

Dietary Ketosis

WEIGHT LOSS WITHOUT PAIN

If you lived in Europe during the Middle Ages and were brought before authorities and charged with a misdeed, you might have ended up in the torture chamber. Here you would be shackled to a rack and stretched until your limbs nearly pop out of their sockets, or your flesh might be seared with a red hot iron. Nowadays we're more civilized. We don't send people to the torture chamber for mistakes in judgment; we put them on low-fat diets. The suffering can be just as intense.

Most weight-loss diets are basically the same. To reduce calorie consumption you are limited to tiny portions of food that have had all traces of fat removed. Fat gives food flavor and improves taste. When it is removed, you end up with a small portion of some tasteless gruel. Perhaps the reason for this is that if it tastes bad enough, you won't even want to eat it and you will consume fewer calories. My vision of a satisfying meal is not a grilled tofu patty resting on a bed of raw bean sprouts. If I have to eat this way, I'd rather be fat.

Most weight-loss diets ultimately fail because they make you hungry. The low-calorie foods you are allowed to eat are not satisfying. Honestly, how long is a bowl of shredded lettuce and a slice of cucumber going to sustain you? Low-fat diets are inherently doomed to failure because of the mistaken assumption that in order to reduce calories, you must cut out as much fat as possible.

But you say you've lost 50 pounds on one of these low-fat diets or know someone who has. Let me ask you this question: are those pounds still gone? If you gained them back, then the diet didn't do you a bit of good. It didn't work. If a weight-loss diet cannot keep the lost weight off permanently, it is useless. In fact, it may be worse than useless because yo-yo dieting encourages weight gain. Statistics show that 95 percent of those people who go on weight-loss diets eventually regain all their weight. That's an incredible 95 percent failure rate!

Why do these low-fat diets fail? Because they are torture! Following such diets is nothing more than slow starvation—literally. You feel hungry and miserable all the time. You rarely feel satisfied. You think about food constantly. When you're trying to stop from eating, continually being reminded of food by a groaning stomach is agony.

An ideal diet is one which lets you eat until you're satisfied and keeps you from being hungry until the next meal. In addition, the food you're allowed to eat should be flavorful and delicious. Impossible, you say? Yes, if you follow the mistaken idea that eating a low-fat diet is the only way to lose weight. But if you add fat into your diet while avoiding the real troublemakers, you can eat until you are content, feel satisfied, and still lose weight. Since you can eat satisfying meals and aren't constantly hungry (or, in other words, miserable), you can easily maintain this diet indefinitely and, consequently, keep the excess pounds off permanently.

Energy Metabolism

Glucose is the primary source of energy used by all the cells in the body. We get glucose mostly from the carbohydrates in our foods. When food is not eaten for a time, such as between meals, during sleep, or when fasting, blood glucose levels decline, limiting the amount available for energy production. However, our cells demand a continual supply of energy 24 hours a day. To maintain energy levels, body fat is mobilized and fatty acids are released from fat cells. In this manner, the body always has access to either glucose or fatty acids to fuel its constant need for energy.

While this process works well for the body, it does not work for the brain. The brain cannot use fatty acids to satisfy its energy needs, so it requires an alternative source of energy. This alternative fuel source comes in the form of ketone bodies or ketones. Ketones are a special type of high-energy fuel produced in the liver from fatty acids. All the cells in the body, except for liver and red blood cells, can burn ketones to produce energy, but they are made specifically to feed the brain and nervous system. Between meals, when blood glucose levels fall, the liver starts converting fatty acids into ketones and blood ketone levels increase. After eating a meal containing carbohydrate, blood glucose levels go up, signaling the liver to stop producing ketones, and blood ketone level gradually declines. This way the brain has a continual supply of energy from either glucose or ketones to rely on.

The adult human brain uses approximately 100 to150 g of glucose per day. If the brain relied on glucose only, in a state of total starvation in which only water is consumed, the brain would have to get glucose by cannibalizing body protein. Making 100 to 150 g of glucose per day available to the brain would require the breakdown of some 172 to 259 g of body protein each day.

At this unsustainable rate of protein breakdown, death would occur within 2 weeks. Yet people have fasted, consuming nothing but water, for more than two months. How can this happen? The reason they can fast this long is that a portion of the fatty acids released from storage are converted into ketones, which satisfies the brain's energy requirements and, therefore, spares lean body tissue.[1]

If the diet is lacking in fat, more lean tissue is broken down because ketones are made from fat. Much of the weight loss people experience when they go on low-fat diets is due to the breakdown of muscle. On a low-carb, high-fat diet, lean muscle tissue is conserved. Weight loss occurs primarily from reduction of body fat.

There are three ketone bodies derived from fatty acids: beta-hydroxybutyric acid (BHB), acetoacetic acid (AcAc), and acetone. Like glucose, ketones are present in the blood at all times.

A healthy adult liver can produce as much as 185 g of ketone bodies per day. Ketones supply 2 to 6 percent of the body's energy needs after an overnight fast and 30 to 40 percent after a three-day fast. A person is said to be in ketosis when the body shifts from burning glucose to burning fatty acids and ketones.

Ketone production begins to increase within a few hours after a meal is skipped. The level of ketones normally present in the blood after an overnight fast is usually around 0.1 to 0.2 mM/L but can be as high as 0.5 mM/L. As fasting (or carbohydrate restriction) continues, ketone production increases. After two days of fasting, ketones rise to about 1.0 to 2.5 mM/L. Ketosis associated with a water only fast does not become substantial until 3 to 5 days have elapsed. After a week or more of fasting, nondiabetic individuals have ketone levels of about 5 to 7 mM/L. Once it reaches this level during a fast, ketone levels remain fairly constant. Ketone levels do not rise any higher regardless of the length of the fast.

You can't go into ketosis unless your carbohydrate consumption is very low. For most people this means below about 40 grams a day. To put this into perspective, most people consume about 300 grams of carbohydrate a day and some eat much more. When you are fasting, you are eating no carbohydrate at all, so you shift from burning primarily glucose to mostly fat. You go into ketosis within just two or three days. When you are on a low-carb diet, it takes a little longer, usually 5 to 7 days or more depending on how much carbohydrate and how much total food you eat.

The maximum amount of carbohydrate a person can consume and still be in ketosis varies from person to person. Some people are more carbohydrate sensitive than others, and they must reduce their carbohydrate intake more than average in order to get into ketosis. Most people could go into a mild state of ketosis by limiting their carbohydrate intake to 40 or 50 grams per day. Carbohydrate sensitive people, which includes most overweight individuals, would need to reduce their carb intake to 20 or 30 grams for the same effect.

103

The Ketogenic Diet

Ketosis induced by dietary means is referred to as dietary ketosis or nutritional ketosis. Dr. Robert Atkins called it benign dietary ketosis. He added the word "benign" to distinguish it from diabetic ketoacidosis, which is a serious complication associated with type 1 diabetes. When you are in dietary ketosis it is a sign that your body is mobilizing its stored fat and using it to satisfy your body's energy needs. In other words, your body is burning off its fat and you are losing weight.

A ketogenic diet is one that puts a person into ketosis—a state of fat burning. For a diet to be ketogenic, it must be very low in carbohydrate, high in fat, with moderate but not too much protein.

Ketogenic diets are nothing new, they have been used therapeutically for over 90 years. The first scientifically formulated ketogenic diet was developed in the 1920s as a means to treat epilepsy. Back then doctors often used fasting therapy to treat difficult health problems such as cancer, arthritis, gastritis, and neurological problems. One of the conditions that responded very well to fasting therapy was epilepsy. Fasting for a period of 20 to 30 days, consuming noting but water, could significantly reduce epileptic seizures with long lasting results. It was observed that a high level of ketones produced on a continual basis had a very pronounced therapeutic effect, especially on the brain and nervous system.

Doctors discovered that the longer the patients could remain on the fast, the better the outcome. Obviously there was a limit to how long a person could remain on a fast, so doctors devised a diet that mimicked the metabolic effects of fasting while providing all the nutrients needed to maintain good health. The result was the ketogenic diet. The ketogenic diet proved to be very successful, even against very severe drug-resistant forms of epilepsy.

Since the ketogenic diet proved to be useful in correcting the brain defects associated with epilepsy, researchers began to test it on other brain and nerve disorders. Initial studies with neurodegenerative disorders such as Alzheimer's disease, Parkinson's disease, ALS, Huntington's disease, traumatic brain injury, and stroke all responded very favorably to the ketogenic diet.[2-5]

Not only are brain and nerve disorders improved but so are many of the parameters by which we measure a person's overall state of health, such as blood lipids (cholesterol, triglycerides), blood pressure, blood sugar and insulin levels, C-reactive protein levels (a measure of inflammation throughout the body), and body fat.[6-9] The ketogenic diet has proven to have an overall therapeutic effect on the body.

With the classic ketogenic diet, carbohydrate intake is kept to around 2 percent of total calories. This is done in order to produce therapeutic levels of ketones. Carbohydrate ordinarily accounts for about 60 percent of our daily calories. When this is dropped to only 2 percent, the void must be filled by another energy producing nutrient. In the ketogenic diet, fat is used to replace the carbohydrate, fat supplies the needed building blocks for ketone production, comprising up to 90 percent of total calories. Protein provides the remaining 8 percent.

This is the type of diet used to treat severe disorders such as epilepsy, however, weight loss can be accomplished with a much less strict diet that allows more protein and carbohydrate and less fat. Limiting total carbohydrate to about 40 grams or less per day can still induce ketosis.

In the treatment of epilepsy and other disorders the patient, usually a child, is given enough calories for normal growth and development. In a weight loss regimen, however, the modified ketogenic diet restricts total calorie consumption. But this is not a problem because a modified ketogenic diet, with its meat, eggs, cheese, and cream, is much more satisfying than any other type of diet. You can fill up on less food and still consume fewer calories.

Is A High-Protein Diet Ketogenic?

There are a lot of low-carbohydrate diets around, but not all of them are ketogenic. This is particularly true of diets that allow unrestricted meat and other protein-rich foods. Back in the late 1920s researchers discovered that Canadian Eskimos subsisting on their traditional diet of meat and fat with virtually no carbohydrate had low ketones levels similar to those people eating typical carbohydrate-based diets. When game was abundant, the Eskimos ate their fill of meat. The glucose derived from the breakdown of ingested meat protein was sufficient to prevent ketosis.[10]

Similar results were found in a clinical study where subjects ate a carbohydrate-free diet high in meat (an Eskimo-type diet) for many months while under close observation in a metabolic ward at a hospital.[11] The investigators' findings led them to conclude that, in persons subsisting on diets very low in carbohydrate, ketosis varies inversely with the quantity of protein eaten. This occurs because approximately 48 to 58 percent of the amino acids in most dietary proteins can be converted into glucose. For every 2 grams of protein consumed in a carbohydrate-free diet, somewhere between 1.0 and 1.2 grams are potentially convertible to glucose. Therefore, in order to successfully lose weight on a low-carb, ketogenic diet, protein-rich foods cannot be eaten without limit. This is important to understand because many people who go on low-carbohydrate diets assume meat and other high-protein foods have little or no effect on their ability to lose weight. They stuff themselves full with protein-rich foods and wonder why they aren't losing weight like they expected or why they may even be gaining weight. They then complain that low-carbohydrate dieting didn't work for them.

An all meat diet may be low-carb, but it is not a ketogenic diet. A ketogenic diet can be defined as one that is very low in carbohydrate and high in fat with adequate, but not excessive, protein. Fat comprises 60 percent or more of total calories consumed.

105

The Problem with Lean Protein

Everywhere you go you hear people tell you to eat lean protein, cut off the fat, discard the skin, eat only the lean white meat, choose chicken and fish over red meat because it has less fat, eat low-fat cheese and milk, etc., etc., ad nauseam. Why all the emphasis on lean protein? Apparently it's a holdover from the anti-fat hysteria we've experienced over the past few decades. Even many low-carb and Paleo adherents repeat the mantra—choose lean meat. Many authors of low-carb dieting books, even those that praise the virtues of eating fat, will instruct readers to choose lean cuts of meat. That makes no sense. Fat is not the enemy! Fat—the right type of fat—is your friend. The natural fats in dairy and meats, including red meats, are good for you! You should not be discarding the fat or avoiding meat marbled in fat. Fat makes meat taste better. You should never feel guilty about eating fat.

The ketogenic diet, including the Coconut Ketogenic Diet, is not a high-protein diet. It is a high fat diet, with adequate, but not excessive, amounts of protein. Fat, not protein, is the secret to the success of this diet. In fact, protein consumption needs to be limited for optimal success, not only for weight loss but for better overall health.

Eating lean meat without adequate fat can actually be detrimental to your health! An excellent example of this occurred in the 1970s with a liquid protein craze called the "protein-sparing modified fast." The idea behind the diet was based on the fact that cutting down on calories causes not only fat loss but also lean tissue loss. If the dieter consumed an adequate amount of protein on a low-carb, low-calorie diet, muscle protein would be spared from being broken down. Theoretically, the dieter would lose only body fat without any lean tissue loss. It was believed that the best way to consume the protein was to drink it. Almost overnight the craze caught on and stores were stocked full of liquid protein diet beverages.

The source of the protein in these shakes came from gelatin, a purified protein product made from the tendons, cartilage, and skin of cattle. While gelatin is a good source of protein, its mixture of amino acids is of lower quality, that is, not as balanced as the amino acids you get from real foods such as eggs, milk, meat, and fish. But that was not the main problem with the diet. A much more serious issue was the complete absence of fat. Without fat, protein (amino acids) cannot be properly metabolized—regardless of the quality. Fat is essential for complete protein metabolization. As a consequence, people following this diet for any length of time became malnourished and sick, many of them died from heart failure even though they had no signs of heart disease. Taking vitamin supplements and even supplementing the diet with a small portion of lean meat did not help, people still died, at least 60 in all, thousands more became ill. Popularity of the diet quickly faded, although liquid protein shakes and meals are still available.

The sickness that occurs from eating lean protein without an adequate source of fat is called "protein poisoning," also referred to as "rabbit starvation." Symptoms can include diarrhea, headache, fatigue, low blood pressure, slow or erratic heart rate, and general feelings of discomfort. Without adequate fat, protein can actually become toxic. This fact has been known and documented for centuries. In ages past, our hunter-gatherer ancestors didn't eat lean meat—they avoided it when possible. They went for the fattiest meat possible and relished fatty organ meats and bone marrow. They would not eat lean meat because they knew that without an adequate source of fat, it could be harmful, even deadly. The Eskimos of northern Canada and Alaska were familiar with protein poisoning. Traditionally, their diet consisted almost entirely of meat, yet they knew the importance of getting an adequate amount of fat. They always carried seal oil or other fats with them to supplement their meals. All meat was dipped into a bowl of seal oil, like a dipping sauce, before being eaten. In addition to fish and seals, they hunted caribou, moose, fox, bear, geese, ptarmigan, and other game, but they generally avoided rabbit. Arctic rabbits are very lean and they would not hunt them unless they had plenty of fat available for dipping. They had learned that eating too much rabbit would make them sick. Even if they could eat enough rabbit meat to fill them up, including the organ meats, which provided a complete high-quality source of protein, without added fat they would become sick. You could live longer consuming only water with no other source of food than you could on a diet of water and all the rabbit meat you could eat. Among the Eskimos and Canadian Indians it was known that eating rabbit brought on death from "starvation" quicker than a complete abstinence of food, thus the term "rabbit starvation." The same would happen if they ate too much of any source of lean meat, including caribou that had lost their reservoir of summer fat and were exceedingly thin.

Arctic explorer and anthropologist Vilhjalmur Stefensson (1879-1962) wrote extensively about his years living off the land in the Canadian Arctic, just as the primitive Eskimo. He describes how at one point he and his companions were forced to hunt and eat lean caribou because of a lack of other food. He was aware of the Eskimo's reluctance to eat lean meat, but the lack of food compelled them to eat it anyway. Within a couple of weeks they all became deathly ill. Only when they got a source of fat did they recover. At other times when food was scarce and they had seal oil available, they would survive by just eating the seal oil. Unlike lean meat, eating just the oil did not cause them any harm.

When Stefensson wrote about living off of meat and fat without any vegetable foods and maintaining good health, he was criticized by the doctors of his day. They claimed it was impossible, he would get scurvy or some other deficiency disease. To prove them wrong Stefensson and one of his arctic companions, Karsen Anderson, agreed to live on nothing but meat and fat for one year under the observation of a medical team at Bellevue hospital in New York City. The year was 1928. Both men completed the year-long experiment without any deficiency diseases and ended the experiment in excellent health. Although this story is often told to illustrate the safety of eating meat, it really demonstrates the safety of eating fat. While they ate different cuts and types of meat, none of it was lean, and 79 percent of their calories came from fat—mostly saturated fat.[12]

Curious about what Stefansson wrote regarding eating lean meat, Dr. Eugene DuBois, who headed the experiment, wanted to see what effect a lean meat diet would have. Reluctantly, Stefansson agreed to temporarily restrict his diet to lean cuts of meat, while Anderson would eat whatever mix of fat and meat he wanted. This sub-experiment was conducted at the very beginning of the study, but it didn't last long. It only took two days for symptoms of protein poisoning to kick in. Stefansson explains, "The symptoms brought on at Bellevue by an incomplete meat diet (lean without fat) were exactly the same as in the Arctic, except that they came on faster—diarrhea and a feeling of general baffling discomfort. Up north the Eskimos and I had been cured immediately when we got some fat. Dr. DuBois now cured me the same way, by giving me fat sirloin steaks, brains fried in bacon fat, and things of that sort. In two or three days I was all right, but I had lost considerable weight."

Anderson, on the other hand, eating a mixed meat and fat diet experienced no problems. It only took a couple of days at Bellevue for symptoms of protein poisoning to appear. In the Arctic it took 2 to 3 weeks. Stefensson speculated that the reason for the difference in time was that when they ate lean caribou in the arctic, they got a little fat from behind the eyeballs and from the bone marrow, which must have slowed down the advent of the disease. In the hospital, he had no source of fat so symptoms came on much faster.

When primitive humans went looking for game, they didn't hunt for lean animals, they went for the fattest they could find. They relished in the fat and ate every bit they could get. Primitive humans knew the dangers of eating lean meat. Low-carb and Paleo diets that advocate eating lean meats, trimming off the fat, and low-fat dairy and other low-fat foods are harmful. High-protein diets are not the key to successful, healthy weight loss, fat is.

THE SECRET TO SUPER SUCCESSFUL WEIGHT LOSS
Reduced Hunger
Consuming too many calories, regardless of their source, can contribute to weight gain. Whether the calories come from carbohydrate, protein, or fat, consuming more calories than what is needed immediately by the body is converted into body fat. While eating fat has a metabolic advantage, if you consume fat along with excessive amounts of carbohydrate, you lose that advantage. Even eating too much fat in excess of daily caloric needs can sabotage weight loss efforts. The one thing all weight loss diets have in common is the reduction in total calorie consumption. Even the ketogenic weight loss diet is most effective when total calorie consumption is limited.

108

What is the biggest stumbling block to successful weight loss? What aspect about dieting causes more pain and contributes to the failure of the diet more than any other? The answer is *hunger*. Constant nagging hunger makes dieting tortuous and doomed to failure. If the pangs of hunger could be eliminated, dieting would be much easier and far more successful.

The ketogenic diet offers the solution. Ketosis has an appetite suppressing effect.[13] If you can conquer the endless feelings of hunger that accompanies most diets, you won't be tempted to snack or overeat at mealtime and may even skip meals without missing them. The appetite suppressing effect of the ketogenic diet is the secret weapon of super successful weight loss. When you go into ketosis, hunger is greatly diminished even when you consume fewer calories. You can cut down on your total calorie consumption and lose excess weight without suffering from hunger, lack of energy, nervousness, irritability, or any of the common symptoms associated with low-calorie dieting, and which ultimately sabotages most diets. At the same time, you can enjoy eating meats, eggs, cheese, cream, gravies, and other rich, fatty foods to your satisfaction. The food tastes so good and is so satisfying that you can eat this way for a lifetime.

The effects of the ketogenic diet on appetite suppression was clearly demonstrated in a study by researchers at Kraft Foods and published in the *American Journal of Clinical Nutrition*.[14] In this study subjects were divided into two groups. One group ate a typical low-fat, calorie-restricted diet. Total calorie intake was cut by 500-800 calories per day. The second group ate a low-carb, high-fat diet without any restriction on the total number of calories consumed per day. The low-carb group was instructed to eat three meals per day, plus snacks and to eat until hunger was satisfied, without overeating. In essence, only one group was actually "dieting," the other group simply modified the types of foods they ate, eating their heart's content of fat, meat, and low-carb vegetables, without regard to calories. After 12 weeks, the low-fat group on average lost 5.5 pounds (2.5 kg) and the low-carb group lost 10.8 pounds (4.9 kg)—twice the amount of the low-fat group. The low-carb group also had nearly twice the reduction in waist circumference, losing 1.7 inches (4.3 cm) compared to 1.1 inches (2.8 cm).

Despite the fact that the low-carb group was allowed to eat all they wanted, their hunger was satisfied with less food, and consequently, they consumed fewer calories than the low-fat group. At the start of the study, the average calorie intake of the low-carb and low-fat groups respectively was 2,050 and 1,961. After 12 weeks, the low-carb group was taking in on average 1,343 calories, compared to 1,500 calories in the low-fat group. The low-carb diet satisfied the participants' hunger without forcing them to cut calories, they did it naturally by choice. This is a natural method of weight loss, not a forced one accompanied by constant hunger and discomfort.

Several studies have shown that ketosis depresses hunger and reduces calorie intake. In one study, the caloric intake of subjects on a ketogenic diet was reduced by 1,000 calories below that being eaten by subjects on a low-fat diet in order to produce the same level of hunger.[15] Another study, which assessed hunger and cognitive restraint, found that after a week on a low-carb diet, hunger was reduced by 50 percent in comparison to those on a low-fat diet.[16]

Some researchers have suggested that part of the reason for the reduced appetite associated with low-carb dieting may be due to lower blood insulin concentrations. Insulin seems to promote hunger. Studies have found that foods with high insulin responses are less satiating, and elevated insulin levels increase food intake. Suppressing insulin secretion with the use of certain drugs, has also shown to dampen hunger and promote weight loss.[17]

When you are in ketosis, that means fat is coming out of your fat cells and is being burned to produce energy. Blood insulin remains low, but normal, which means there is no excess insulin in your blood that would be shoveling fat into your fat cells. Your body transforms from a metabolic state in which you burn sugar and store fat, into one that pulls fat out of storage and burns it. Weight loss is the result.

Ketones provide your body with a high quality source of fuel that produces significantly more energy than glucose. It's like the difference you get when you burn coal as compared to paper. With coal the fire burns hotter and longer. Even when total calorie consumption is decreased, the body does not sense it is starving. As a consequence, energy levels and metabolism remain normal or may even be elevated. You can diet for extended periods of time without suffering from a drop in metabolism that accompanies other calorie restricted diets. Since your metabolism and energy levels remain normal, you can lose more body fat on a ketogenic diet then you can on a complete water fast.

When you go on a ketogenic diet, you can tell when you are in ketosis by the absence of hunger. This may take about 5 to 7 days. As strange as it may seem, if you are hungry on a ketogenic weight loss diet, that means you are eating too much! Reducing the amount of food you eat will put you deeper into ketosis and actually relieve hunger.

Let me share with you experiences of some of those who have followed the guidelines outlined in this book:

"I weighed 179 pounds, not too heavy, but still a good 20 pounds overweight for my height. My wife often commented about my pot belly. That's where most of my excess weight seems to settle. I'd tried to lose the weight but constant hunger pangs eventually foiled every attempt. I would go on a diet, cut out fattening foods, eat more salads, and reduce my calorie intake. I'd lose a few pounds at first, but then it became harder and harder to take the weight off. I had to cut back more on my calories. After several weeks of starving myself, I would conclude it just wasn't worth the discomfort and go back to my old way of eating.

"When I learned about the Coconut Ketogenic Diet I was excited. Here was a diet that promised me weight loss, without the discomfort and constant feelings of hunger. It lived up to its promise. I switched to a very low-carbohydrate, high-fat ketogenic diet initially eating three meals a day. The fat satisfied my hunger and I didn't feel the need to eat as much as I had before. My meals became smaller but still satisfying. After about a week or so my hunger had diminished so much that I began skipping meals. I would eat breakfast, which usually consisted of a couple of eggs and 1 or 2 ounces of meat (bacon or sausage), with lots of fat. I would cook the eggs in three tablespoons of coconut oil and pour the oil over the eggs before eating. Occasionally, I would include a cup of whole milk with a little added cream, to increase the fat content. This high-fat meal was so satisfying that when lunchtime came around I was rarely hungry. I would either skip lunch completely or have just a light snack. The snack usually consisted of two tablespoons of coconut oil mixed into two tablespoons of cottage cheese. Most of the time I would just skip lunch. I wouldn't be hungry or even tempted to eat until dinnertime. At dinner I would eat about 6 ounces of fatty meat and some vegetables, again with lots of added fat—coconut oil, butter, red palm oil, bacon drippings, etc. The meals were delicious! The amount I ate was far less than I would normally eat. The ketogenic diet really suppressed my appetite. I never felt the hunger I had experienced with other weight reducing diets. In comparison, this diet was a breeze.

"For my body type and activity level I should eat about 2500 calories a day just to maintain my weight. Even though I was eating huge amounts of fat, I was getting about 1700 calories a day, 1300 just from the fat. Except for the first week, my energy levels were soaring. I was able to exercise three days a week as I normally do without any drop in strength or energy. In fact, my energy levels seemed to improve. After three months, I lost a total of 24 pounds—an average of 2 pounds a week. I had reached my goal weight of 155 pounds. My weight hadn't been this low in years."

"I have been on a low-carb, ketogenic diet for 2 years now and it's the best thing that's happened in my life. I am 55 years old and all my life I have always had a problem with weight control. I reached my limit when I weighed over 525 pounds. In just less than 2 years I have lost over 125 pounds and sill losing. I am never hungry and my energy level is higher and my blood work constantly improves."
Brian C.

"I've been on a low-carb diet for four years and plan to stay on it for the rest of my life (I'm 72). I started when I was diagnosed as diabetic. My blood glucose is very well controlled with only diet and herbs. All my health indicators are excellent and I feel wonderful. My carb intake averages about 25 grams a day, mostly low glycemic index. I eat all the veggies I want, except the starchy. I get lots of fiber from the veggies and flaxseed freshly ground in my coffee grinder. I don't count calories and am never hungry. I no longer am losing weight but maintain a very healthy 165 pounds, down about 50 pounds from my highest."

Roy H.

Motivation to Stick with the Diet

Hearing success stories helps keep up enthusiasm and maintain motivation to stick with the diet. But there is another motivating factor. The ketosis-hunger connection can work as a fantastic motivational tool to keep you from cheating. It takes three days on a water fast to get into ketosis to a level where hunger is noticeably depressed. It takes twice as long on a ketogenic diet to achieve the same level of ketosis. This requires strict adherence to a very low-carb, high-fat, moderate protein diet to achieve and maintain.

It only takes one meal or high carb snack (a piece of cake, candy bar, soda, fruit juice, etc.) to kick you out of ketosis and you must start all over again. You need several days of low carbing with hunger pangs before you get back into a hunger suppressed level of ketosis.

Oftentimes we are tempted at a friend's house, walking by a restaurant and smelling the foods, at a party, and so on. We try to justify cheating by saying "Oh, just this one little piece won't hurt." Big mistake! It will hurt. Just that one little piece of pie can throw you out of ketosis (and may even make you gain weight), and you have to start all over again. Once you are out of ketosis your hunger pangs will come back! You will feel hungry and be tempted to eat more. Even if you don't eat any additional high carb foods, you will be so hungry you will over-eat allowed foods—meats and vegetables. And consequently, consume excess calories that will stop your weight loss progress.

Any time you are tempted to consume any high carb food or drink, stop and think of the consequences. If you eat this stuff, you will lose all the work you put into getting into ketosis and you will have to do it over again. (Remember, it takes 3-7 days to get back into ketosis). Eating it will also make you hungry and crave more food. These thoughts alone should be enough to keep you motivated to keep with the program and not cheat—even a little.

IS A HIGH-FAT DIET SAFE?

Some people have criticized ketogenic diets because of the high amount of fat, especially saturated fat, that is consumed. They fear that eating this much fat could be harmful and promote atherosclerosis (hardening of the arteries), heart attacks, strokes, and other health problems. They claim that overweight people, who are already at an increased risk of heart disease, would increase their risk by adding more fat into the diet.

As we have seen in previous chapters, dietary fat does not cause heart disease. That theory has been soundly disproven and researchers are now recognizing this fact. Most people would be better off if they added more fat into their diets. The ketogenic diet has been studied and tested and proven useful for nearly a century without any harmful effects being noted. Epileptic patients remain on the diet for two or more years. Thousands of people have been following the ketogenic way of eating for years, with saturated fat being their primary source of fat, without suffering from heart attacks or strokes as a consequence.

In the biggest analytical study on the safety and efficacy of the classic ketogenic diet to date, investigators failed to find any harm being done over time, even though up to 90 percent of the patients' calories came from fat; the effects were all positive. "We have always suspected that the ketogenic diet is relatively safe long term, and we now have proof," says Eric Kossoff, MD, a neurologist at Johns Hopkins University who participated in the study. "Our study should help put to rest some of the nagging doubts about the long-term safety of the ketogenic diet."[18] The effects of the ketogenic diet have been overwhelmingly positive, whether it has been to treat a brain disorder, correct a metabolic problem, or to lose unwanted weight.

Not only is a high-fat, ketogenic diet safe, but it brings about better overall health in comparison to lower-fat diets. For example, researchers at the University of Connecticut compared cardiovascular risk factors of two groups of overweight men, one following a very low-carb, high-fat diet and the other following a low-fat diet. Blood tests were performed at the beginning of the study and at its conclusion 6 weeks later. Both diets showed improvements in total blood cholesterol levels, blood insulin levels, and insulin resistance, but the differences in these parameters between the two groups were not significant, which shows that the high-fat diet is just as good as a low-fat diet. However, only the low-carb group had significantly lower fasting triglycerides, triglyceride/HDL ratio, and blood glucose levels, which showed the superiority of the low-carb diet.

The low-carb group also had better LDL cholesterol readings. LDL cholesterol is often referred to as the bad cholesterol because it is believed to be the primary type of cholesterol that leaves deposits in the arteries. However, there are two types of LDL cholesterol: one large and fluffy and the other small and dense. The large and fluffy LDL is harmless, in fact, it is actually beneficial because it is the type of cholesterol that is incorporated into cell membranes to give them strength and is also used to produce many of our hormones; it is the small dense LDL cholesterol that is associated with increased risk of heart disease. Blood tests generally do not separate the two and only give a single value for the total. The number for total LDL is thus completely useless. In this study, the two types of LDL were measured

113

separately. Total LDL cholesterol was significantly reduced by the low-fat diet but not by the low-carb diet. On the surface this may appear to show an advantage to the low-fat diet, but that is not the case. While the total LDL did not change much in the low-carb diet, the type of LDL did, decreasing the undesirable small LDL and increasing the beneficial large LDL. Although the low-fat diet decreased total LDL, it did not significantly improve the percentage of the good LDL.[19]

In addition to the better blood lipid and sugar levels, the low-carb dieters also lost significantly more weight, 13.5 pounds (6.1 kg) versus 8.6 pounds (3.9 kg). All these changes indicate a much greater reduction in the risk of heart disease and diabetes in comparison to a low-fat diet.

Researchers at Duke University performed a similar study.[20] One hundred and twenty overweight, hyperlipidemic (i.e. those with high cholesterol) men and women volunteered for the study. Half of the subjects ate a low-carbohydrate, ketogenic diet (less than 20 grams of carbohydrate per day) with no calorie limit; they could eat as much meat, fat, and eggs as they wanted. The other half ate a low-fat, low-cholesterol, calorie-restricted diet (reduced by 500-1000 calories per day).

After 24 weeks, the low-fat group lost 10.6 pounds (4.8 kg) of body fat while the ketogenic group lost 20.7 pounds (9.4 kg), twice as much as the low-fat group. For weight loss, this study clearly demonstrates the advantage of the ketogenic diet. Blood pressure, which had been slightly elevated in the test subjects, decreased in both groups. In the low-fat group, systolic (top number) and diastolic (bottom number) blood pressure decreased by 7.5 and 5.2 mm Hg respectively. In the ketogenic group, systolic and diastolic blood pressure decreased by 9.6 and 6.0 mm Hg respectively. The higher your blood pressure is, the greater your risk of heart disease. Even a small increase in blood pressure increases risk. The advantage again goes to the ketogenic group.

Blood triglycerides are considered an independent and separate risk factor from cholesterol for heart disease. The higher the triglyceride value, the greater the risk. Blood triglyceride levels dropped by 27.9 mg/dl in the low-fat group and fell by a whopping 74.2 mg/dl in the ketogenic group, more than 2.5 times as much as the low-fat group. HDL cholesterol is considered the "good" cholesterol and is believed to help protect against heart disease; the higher this number the better. HDL cholesterol decreased by 1.6 mg/dl in the low-fat group but increased by 5.5 mg/dl in the ketogenic group.

The cholesterol ratio (total cholesterol/HDL) is considered far more accurate as an indicator of heart disease risk in comparison to total cholesterol or LDL values. The lower the ratio, the lower the risk. The cholesterol ratio dropped by 0.3 in the low-fat group and by 0.6 in the ketogenic group, twice that of the low-fat group.

Another independent risk factor is the triglyceride/HDL ratio. The smaller the ratio, the better. The low-fat group saw a drop of 0.6 while the ketogenic group fell by 1.6, or nearly three times as much. The triglyceride/ HDL ratio is considered one of the most accurate indicators of heart disease risk. A ratio of 6 or more indicates very high risk, a ratio of 4 or more signals high risk, and a ratio of 2 or less is ideal, or low risk. At the end of the study, the low-fat group's ratio averaged 3.4 or moderate risk, while the ketogenic group averaged 1.6, signifying a very low risk of heart disease. With each risk factor measured, the ketogenic diet proved superior to the low-fat diet, collaborating the results of the previously mentioned study.

Both of these studies were published in 2004. Since that time, study after study have confirmed these results. Low-carb, high-fat, ketogenic diets, in comparison to low-fat, calorie-restricted diets, show better results on weight loss, body fat loss, blood pressure, HDL cholesterol, triglycerides, cholesterol ratio, triglyceride/HDL ratio, LDL particle size, blood sugar, insulin levels, and insulin sensitivity.[21-26]

Even in long-term studies lasting up to 2 years, the results have been the same.[27] High-fat, ketogenic diets have proven to be not only safe, but more protective against heart disease and diabetes than low-fat diets.

KETOACIDOSIS

There is widespread confusion among both physicians and lay people about the ketogenic diet and ketosis. Many doctors have voiced concerns about the use of dietary ketosis, believing it can lead to acidosis—excessively low blood pH (too acidic). This belief is based on observations of a life-threatening condition sometimes seen in untreated type 1 diabetics called ketoacidosis. Ketones are slightly acidic. The presence of too many ketones can make the blood acidic, causing ketoacidosis, which can throw a person into a diabetic coma. Doctors learn about ketoacidosis in school but don't learn much about dietary ketosis or the ketogenic diet. For this reason, they tend to view any level of ketosis as a warning sign of keotacidosis and often caution patients about ketogenic dieting.

Regardless of what you may hear from your doctor or read on the Internet, following a ketogenic diet will not cause ketoacidosis. Dietary ketosis is not the same as, nor is it even similar to, diabetic ketoacidosis. The former is a normal metabolic condition of the body that can be manipulated by diet. The latter is a disease state that only occurs in type 1 diabetics and cannot be influenced by the diet.

Insulin is required in order to transport glucose from the blood into the cells. Type 1 diabetics are unable to produce an adequate amount of insulin. For this reason, they require regular insulin injections. Ketoacidosis can occur after eating a high-carbohydrate meal. Without an injection of insulin, glucose cannot enter the cells and blood glucose levels can rise dangerously high. Not only is the high glucose level toxic, but without glucose, the cells in the body literally begin to starve to death. This is a life-threatening situation that affects the brain, heart, lungs and all other organs. To prevent imminent death, the body shifts into crisis mode and begins frantically pumping ketones into the bloodstream to provide the cells the fuel they need to survive. Cells can absorb ketones without the aid of insulin. Since none of the cells are able to access the glucose, ketones are continually being pumped into the bloodstream as an alternative fuel source. Ketone levels rise so high, they cause the blood to become acidic, creating a state of acidosis.

Ketoacidosis occurs only in untreated type 1 diabetics and in very rare occasions in severe cases of alcoholism. It cannot be triggered by diet alone. Low-carb ketogenic diets produce ketone levels in the blood of about 1 to 2 mM/L. Extended periods of complete fasting raises ketone levels to 5 to 7 mM/L. This is as high as it gets from dietary manipulation because the body carefully regulates ketone production. In ketoacidosis, however, ketone levels may exceed 23 mM/L. The body is fully capable of buffering the effects of ketones at fasting levels, but when they rise above 20 mM/L, it is beyond the body's ability to handle.

KETONE TEST STRIPS

A simple way to tell when you are in ketosis is by using a urine ketosis test strip, also known as a lipolysis test strip. The strips are made of thin strips of chemically treated paper. One end of the test strip is dipped into a fresh specimen of urine. The strip changes color depending on the ketone concentration in the urine. Using the test strip, a person can tell if their blood ketone level is "none," "trace," "small," "moderate" or "large." The test is helpful in that it indicates that the dietary changes you are making are producing ketones and to what degree.

Another method of testing ketone levels is a blood meter. This method requires you to prick your finger with a needle and take a blood sample. It is much more accurate than the urine test because it tests the blood directly. The readings are given numerically in mM/L so you get a precise number. The cost, however, is substantially greater.

When a person is in dietary ketosis it means body fat is being dissolved and burned for energy. In a sense, it is a measure of how much body fat is being burned away. Testing can be useful in that it can tell you when you are in ketosis and approximately to what degree. You can also see how changes in your diet affect your ketone levels. If you add more carbohydrate into your diet, ketone levels will drop. To increase ketosis you can reduce carbohydrate consumption. This can be helpful in making sure you are not eating too much carbohydrate.

Ketone test strips sound like a great tool, and some low-carb diet programs recommend using them, however, they are not very accurate, nor are they very useful in a weight loss program. They were designed to test for ketoacidosis, not dietary ketosis.

Dietary ketosis can be influenced by several factors that can affect the readings. For example, ketone levels will vary depending on the time of day and your level of physical activity. After waking in the morning or when you are sedentary, readings are lower than when you are active or after exercising. The amount of water you drink will also affect the reading on urine test strips. If you drink a lot of water, it will dilute your urine and the ketones in it, giving a lower than actual reading.

Readings will also be influenced by the amount and type of fat in your diet. When a person is in ketosis, much of the fat that is eaten is transformed directly into ketones, which raises blood ketone levels. If you eat a lot of fat, your blood ketones will be elevated from the diet (this happens only when the body is already in ketosis or has been fasting). Also, MCTs are converted directly into ketones, so if you eat coconut oil, it will raise blood ketone levels as well. MCTs produce ketones regardless of the other foods in your diet. For example, you could eat a typical carbohydrate based diet and after eating coconut oil, test positive for ketosis. You would be in a temporary MCT- or diet-induced ketosis, not a metabolic ketosis. The ketones are from the fats in the diet and not from dissolved body fat. A diet high in fat and MCTs can give a much higher reading on urine and blood ketone tests, making the readings meaningless as an indicator of weight/fat loss.

As a means of evaluating the degree of body fat being consumed, ketone test strips are only accurate if you are fasting, consuming nothing but water. Even then the amount of water you drink will affect the readings on the urine test strips. If you eat any type of food, the readings will reflect your diet and not the amount of fat you are burning. This is one of the reasons why the readings in the morning, after an 8 to 12 hour fast, are generally lower than during the day when you are active and eating.

Ketone test strips are useful in letting you know when you are in ketosis and, to a limited extent, the degree of ketosis—mild, medium, large. However, test strips are not necessary, you can also tell when you are in ketosis when your hunger decreases, and the less hungry you are, the deeper you are into ketosis. If you do want to use the strips, the cheap urine test strips are all you would ever need. Buying expensive blood testing equipment is totally unnecessary and provides no additional useful information.

HIT THE REST BUTTON

Have you ever been working on the computer when it locked up on you, or became trapped in a program that wouldn't allow you to exit? To get out of the situation you hit the rest button or reboot the computer to close it down and restart afresh. When the computer comes back on, the trouble is gone and everything is working properly.

Our bodies can be like that computer, they get locked up and won't respond properly. These glitches manifest themselves as symptoms like high blood pressure, high blood sugar, insulin resistance, leptin resistance, high triglycerides, low HDL cholesterol, indigestion, poor immune function, aches and pains, stiff and sore joints, inflammation, low thyroid function, chronic headaches, constipation, low energy, insomnia, obesity, and any number of other conditions. Drugs usually don't help matters. Most drugs are designed to ease symptoms, not fix a problem. They mask the symptoms rather than correct the underlying cause.

Symptoms are not in themselves diseases, but indications that something is wrong. It's like the low oil warning light on your car. The light can be annoying and putting a piece of tape over it or removing the light bulb from the dashboard won't correct the problem. The symptom—the bright red light—may be removed, but the underlying problem—low oil—still exists. If you ignore the warning light, eventually your engine will overheat, burn out, and die. The same thing happens to our bodies when we ignore the warning signs and mask them with drugs.

Often, once you start taking a drug to ease one symptom, it causes another. The doctor will prescribe a second drug to counter the side effects of the first, but this second drug may cause other side effects, which will lead to another drug, and on and on. Before long, you are taking a handful of drugs to treat all the symptoms and still feel miserable because the underlying problem has not been corrected. It's like a computer that has so many programs running that it locks up. Trying to install or run a new program won't fix the problem and will probably make things worse.

Wouldn't it be nice to have a reset button for our bodies that clears away all of the symptoms and allows us to start over with our body chemistry back in balance? We, in fact, do have a reset button that can do just that. The way to activate this reset button is through the Coconut Ketogenic Diet.

The ketogenic diet was originally developed to treat epilepsy, which it does very successfully. It reboots the brain, so to speak, allowing the body to rewire neurological circuits and correct the underlying problem.[28] The ketogenic diet has also showed promise in treating Alzheimer's disease, Parkinson's disease, ALS, Huntington's disease, autism, multiple sclerosis, traumatic brain injuries, stroke, and other brain disorders.[29-36] In every instance, the ketogenic diet has brought about remarkable improvement. Even in otherwise healthy people who are not afflicted by neurodegenerative disorders, it improves mental alertness and clarity.

The ketogenic diet has also been found to be a tremendous benefit to diabetics. It lowers high blood sugar and insulin levels, and reverses diabetic symptoms, such as neuropathy and nephropathy, that were once considered irreversible.[37-41]

It helps restore reproductive health. Improves sperm vitality and motility, important for successful fertilizaition.[42-43] It boosts immune function and protects against cancer.[44-45]

It enhances heart function by improving its efficiency and strength while utilizing less oxygen. The heart thrives on ketones and prefers ketones over glucose as a source of fuel. With ketones available, the hydraulic efficiency of the heart is increased by 25 percent in comparison to glucose.[6, 46] Ketones calm inflammation. Inflammation is associated with almost every type of disease, including heart disease, diabetes, and atherosclerosis. Calming runaway inflammation could be helpful in alleviating the detrimental effects of a multitude of health problems.[6, 9, 47]

The ketogenic diet reduces the formation of destructive free radicals formed in the body. [48-49] Like, inflammation, free radicals are associated with most diseases and contribute to the damage and pain they cause.

The ketogenic diet helps balance body chemistry. It resets or resensitizes hormone receptors, reversing leptin and insulin resistance and brings about better appetite control. It improves thyroid gland and system function, improves blood lipid levels, balances blood sugar, normalizes blood pressure, and brings about greater weight loss than other diets.

Some of the changes you can expect to see after going on the Coconut Ketogenic Diet:

Weight/fat loss
Reduced waste circumference
Reduced hunger, better appetite control
More energy
No more mid-afternoon energy crashes
More control over foods, less cravings, end addictions
Improved blood sugar levels
Reduced blood pressure, if high (will not affect normal blood pressure)
Higher HDL
Lower triglycerides
Lower cholesterol ratio
Reduced systemic inflammation (lower C-reactive protein readings)
Better sleep at night
Improved digestion
Sharper mind, more alert
Fewer aches and pains
Improved symptoms associated with low thyroid function (see list on
    pages 156-157)
Improved feelings of well-being

There are no harmful side effects associated with the Coconut Ketogenic Diet. Most people are fat starved and overloaded with carbohydrate. Replacing carbohydrate calories with fat calories can have a dramatic positive effect on weight and overall health. Below are some comments from people who have increased their daily fat consumption by adding coconut oil or virgin coconut oil (VCO) into their low-carb diets.

"I have low thyroid, even on Synthroid it was borderline before starting the VCO. That was about 6 months ago. It is in the middle of the normal range, more than double what it was 6 months ago. I had my blood work done last week, my cholesterol was ok, but good cholesterol was wonderful making my ratio of bad to good 2.7. The triglycerides had reduced by 50 points. I feel better knowing all of this and will continue…and no signs of fatty liver."
Pat

"There is something to this VCO stuff, let me tell you. My blood pressure went from 210/142 to 134/77, and this after actually decreasing my blood pressure medication!"
Alice

"Once I started to read your book, I started taking the coconut oil. Within two weeks I had my blood tested. My TSH levels greatly improved as did my HDL/LDL cholesterol ratio. This ratio improved so drastically, that my doctor's office said they never saw anything like it. On top of that, I feel a lot better than I had been for years. I can only attribute these improvements to the coconut oil. I am so grateful for having stumbled across your book.'
Margaret

"I have diabetes and now that I'm using VCO daily with meals, I no longer need to take any diabetes medication. Unless of course, I get foolish and have something nice like an ice cream cone, then I would have to take a pill. Otherwise the VCO totally controls my blood sugar."
Bonnie

"I take 3 tablespoons daily at different times before meals and my low thyroid is improved greatly, my blood work I just had done is better than it has ever been. This means my cholesterol, HDL, and triglycerides have all improved since I started on the VCO. I had the blood work done before I started and it has been about 6 months or so and just had more blood work done and the numbers are great. My Dr. told me to just keep doing whatever I was doing. The only thing I have done differently is the coconut oil. I feel better, have energy I did not have and cannot say enough about how it has helped my sense of well-being…I had aches and pains and felt tired all the time."
Patricia

"My cholesterol is stable and healthy. Glucose is stable which means I have not had to sustain those nasty insulin spikes. Diabetes runs high in my family and by keeping my blood glucose under control, I probably will avoid diabetes, or at least prolong its onset. My itchy skin has vanished along with my migraines. I just ran in a 5K run back in November to wave goodbye to my 49th birthday. I will run it again this coming November to welcome my fifties. Thanks to low carb, I learned about the health benefits of coconut oil. I wonder when the other "more healthy" diets will catch on. Women at my age generally expect to get osteoporosis. I had to have a bone x-ray [a couple of years ago] which revealed healthy bone mass. This struck the doc by surprise. I wasn't surprised because I practice a healthy low-carb diet. I have never been so unworried about my health."

Mary

"I am 33 pounds down and feel like I'm in my 30's again even though I'm pushing 65. No longer taking pain medicine and have more energy than I ever dreamed possible. Blood pressure is down and my work friends are amazed at how good I'm looking and feeling—no more complaining because I hurt! I always feel great and without taking pills!"

Wendy

"I have lost 56 pounds so far and have another 20 to 50 pounds to go. I know I'll get there. I have added coconut oil to a low-carb diet that I've been on for 11 months. I am now off all prescription medications for high blood pressure, asthma, and allergies. My cholesterol levels have improved greatly—triglycerides were 940, and in three months have gone down to 247. I have energy again and can exercise. A year ago I could not walk around the mall without stopping to rest. Now I go day hiking with my hubby. The coconut oil fits perfectly with this way of eating. I have my life back!"

Dabs

"My cholesterol dropped from 270 to 200, while my HDL soared from 30 to 56 in three months. My hypothyroidism has disappeared. The doctors are scratching their heads. They can't understand how I have normal thyroid levels without medication."

Edie

Simply adding coconut oil into your diet can bring about beneficial changes in your health. When you combine coconut oil with a low-carb, ketogenic eating plan, the changes can have a remarkable effect. This is the basis for the Coconut Ketogenic Diet.

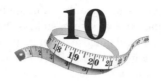

10

Is Your Thyroid Making You Fat?

We face a serious problem. A plague of gigantic proportions is sweeping across the civilized world, claiming millions of victims. You could be one of them. Unlike the plagues of the past which strike quickly, this new plague is more deceptive. It creeps up on its victims very slowly and often goes undetected for years. By the time you begin to suspect something is wrong, symptoms are far advanced. What is this insidious new plague? It's not an infectious disease. It's a spectrum of metabolic disorders that affect thyroid function. They include hypothyroidism, hyperthyroidism, goiter, Graves' disease, Hashimoto's disease, and others. The most common being hypothyroidism, or low thyroid function.

An estimated 20 million Americans have some form of thyroid disease. Up to 60 percent of these people are unaware of their condition. Women are five to eight times more likely than men to have thyroid problems. At least one in eight women will be diagnosed with a thyroid disorder during her lifetime, many others will go undiagnosed. Levothyroxine (e.g., Synthroid), a synthetic thyroid hormone, is the 4th highest selling drug in the US. Thirteen of the top 50 selling drugs in the US are either directly or indirectly related to hypothyroidism. Each year the number of people affected by thyroid disorders continues to rise.

Your thyroid is a butterfly-shaped gland located in your neck, just below the Adams' apple. The thyroid gland produces two important hormones, triiodothyronine (T3) and thyroxin (T4). Every organ and cell in our body requires an adequate amount of thyroid hormone for proper functioning. These hormones regulate body temperature, metabolic rate, reproduction, growth, the making of blood cells, nerve and muscle function, the use of calcium in the body, and more. They affect your cells' ability to utilize blood sugar and insulin and determine the rate at which calories are metabolized, thus having a dramatic effect on body weight.

Your pituitary gland and hypothalamus control the rate at which the thyroid hormones are produced and released. The process begins when the hypothalamus—a gland at the base of your brain that acts as a thermostat for your whole system—signals your pituitary gland to make a hormone known as thyroid-stimulating hormone (TSH). Your pituitary gland—also located at the base of your brain—releases a certain amount of TSH, depending on how much T3 and T4 are in your blood. Your thyroid gland, in turn, regulates its production of hormones based on the amount of TSH it receives from the pituitary gland. If the thyroid does not produce an adequate amount of thyroid hormone, a low thyroid state exists called hypothyroidism. Sensitivity to cold, lack of energy, and weight gain are common symptoms. If the thyroid gland produces too much hormone, it creates a hyperactive state called hyperthyroidism. Symptoms include rapid or irregular heart rate, irritability, nervousness, muscle weakness, unexplained weight loss, sleep disturbances, and vision problems.

Thyroid function can be influenced by many factors—genetics, diet, chemical exposure, radiation, infection, and others. Under certain conditions the thyroid gland can come under attack by the body's own immune system causing inflammation and swelling (goiter), this is called autoimmune thyroiditis. Although relatively rare, Graves' disease and Hashimoto's disease are the two most common autoimmune thyroid disorders. In the case of Graves' disease, antibodies produced by the immune system attack the thyroid gland, causing it to produce excess thyroid hormone (hyperthyroidism). This overstimulation causes the thyroid to swell. With Hashimoto's disease, the attack by antibodies damages the thyroid gland causing it to become underactive, producing hypothyroidism.

Doctors don't fully understand why the immune system would attack our own bodies leading to autoimmune disease. There are many theories. According to David M. Derry, MD, PhD, noted thyroid researcher and author of the book *Breast Cancer and Iodine*, "In the course of a minor illness, damaged thyroid cells dump their contents into the bloodstream. Several proteins coming from the dead cells are foreign to the body's immune system. The immune system having made antibodies to these proteins now attack normal thyroid tissue causing inflammation and further death of thyroid gland cells. This mechanism is responsible for the initiation of Hashimoto's and Graves' disease."[1]

HYPOTHYROIDISM

When people say they have low metabolism or low thyroid function, what they are generally referring to is hypothyroidism. How can you tell if you have an underactive thyroid? Symptoms of hypothyroidism include overweight, sensitivity to cold, lack of energy, muscle weakness, slow heart rate, dry and flaky skin, hair loss, constipation, irritability, mental depression, slowness or slurring of speech, drooping and swollen eyes, swollen face, recurrent infections, allergies, headaches, calcium metabolism problems, and female problems such as heavy menstrual flow and cramping. Hair loss is frequently associated with thyroid problems. One peculiar characteristic or tell-tale sign of a thyroid problem is the thinning of the eyebrows, and in particular the outer edge, which may even disappear. Hair loss of the outer edge of the eyebrows is one of the very unique signs that point specifically to an underactive thyroid. If thyroid problems are resolved, the brows often grow back. If hypothyroidism occurs in childhood and remains untreated, it may retard growth, delay sexual maturation, and inhibit normal development of the brain.

If you are hypothyroid, you may not experience all or even most of above symptoms. Severity of the symptoms depends on the degree of thyroid hormone deficiency. Mild deficiency may cause no observable symptoms; severe deficiency may produce many of the above conditions.

Thyroid hormones regulate metabolism. Metabolism controls the rate at which the body uses energy to power the processes within living cells. As cells consume energy, heat is produced. The heat produced from metabolic processes is fairly constant, normally fluctuating less than a degree or so throughout the day. It is lowest when we are at rest (when energy needs are low) and increases with physical activity (when energy needs are greater). Vigorous physical activity can raise body temperature by as much as two or three degrees.

Normal body temperature is 98.6° F (37° C). During the day body temperature can vary up or down by a full degree (or half a degree C). A temperature of 97.6° F (36.4° C) could be considered normal depending on the conditions in which the reading was taken. If metabolism is low due to insufficient secretion of thyroid hormone, body temperature would be chronically lower than normal. Obvious symptoms would be sensitivity to cold. Being easily chilled and frequently experiencing cold hands and feet are typical signs of hypothyroidism.

Another consequence of low metabolism is being overweight. When metabolism is slowed down, less energy is used. If your body doesn't use all the energy supplied in the foods you eat, it converts it into fat. So the lower your metabolism, the more likely you will store fat and gain weight. For this reason, calorie consumption alone is not the cause of overweight. A person with low thyroid function could eat a normal amount of food and still gain weight.

There are many factors that can contribute to the development of hypothyroidism including heredity, lifestyle, diet, and environment. In most

124

cases, low thyroid function can be corrected either with medication or with diet and lifestyle changes. The following sections discuss some of common contributing factors and offers help in overcoming this condition.

MALNUTRITION
Overweight but Undernourished

Believe it or not, the reason you may be overweight is because you are malnourished. Yes, you read that correctly. You may be overweight because of malnutrition. When I say this, I'm not suggesting that you run out and eat more food. What you need to do is learn how to make wise food choices.

Malnutrition is one of the major underlying causes of obesity. How could someone who overeats be malnourished? The amount of food you eat doesn't determine your nutrient status. You could stuff yourself with 10 pounds of donuts every day and still be malnourished. Donuts are not a good source of nutrients. They provide lots of calories but little in the way of vitamins and minerals.

Most of the foods we eat nowadays are nutrient deficient. Processing and refining remove and destroy many nutrients. Sugar, for example, has a total of zero vitamins and minerals. But it does contain fattening calories. White flour, likewise, has been stripped of its vitamin and mineral rich bran and germ, leaving almost pure starch. Starch is nothing more than sugar. White rice is the same. The vitamin-rich bran is removed leaving the white starchy portion behind. Potatoes are almost all starch. The skins contain most all of the nutrients, but how many people always eat the skins with their potatoes?

Most all of the foods we typically eat are made from sugar, white flour, white rice, and potatoes. These foods supply roughly 60 percent of the daily calories of most people. Another 20–30 percent comes from fats and oils. That in itself wouldn't be bad except the most popular oils are margarine, shortening, and processed vegetable oils like soybean and corn oils. Oils are often hidden in our foods. All packaged, convenience, and restaurant foods contain loads of poor quality fats, including a high percentage of hydrogenated fats. Ugh!

For the most part, our typical diet consists of foods which are mostly empty calories—starch, sugar, processed vegetable oils. Few of us eat fruits and vegetables. When we do, it's generally as condiments—pickles and lettuce on a sandwich, tomato sauce and onions on a pizza. Our food is loaded with calories, but nutritionally deficient. We consume lots of calories and few nutrients. The consequence is that you can eat and eat and eat until you are overweight, yet be malnourished.

The US Department of Agriculture states that most all of us don't get enough (100 percent of the RDA) of at least 10 essential nutrients. Only 12

125

percent of the population obtains 100 percent of seven essential nutrients. Less than 10 percent of us get the recommended daily servings of fruit and vegetables. Forty percent of us eat no fruit and 20 percent no vegetables. And most of the vegetables we do get are fried potatoes (cooked in hydrogenated vegetable oil).

The Journal of the American Dietetic Association reported a study of 1,800 second- and fifth-graders in New York State and found that on the day they were surveyed, 40 percent of the children did not eat any vegetables, except potatoes or tomato sauce; 20 percent ate no fruit, and 36 percent ate at least four different types of high-calorie, nutritionally poor snack foods. It's no wonder kids nowadays are getting fat.[2]

It's bad enough that most of the foods we eat are nutritionally poor, but the problem is compounded even further by the fact that these same foods also destroy the nutrients we get from other foods. Sugar, for example, has no nutrients, but it does use up nutrients when it is metabolized. Eating sugary and starchy foods can drain the body of chromium, a mineral vital to making insulin. Without insulin, you develop blood sugar problems like a diabetic. The more processed our food is, the more nutrients we need in order to metabolize it. Polyunsaturated oils, another source of empty calories, eat up vitamins E and A, and zinc; certain food additives burn up vitamin C. A diet loaded with white-flour products, sugar, and vegetable oil quickly depletes nutrient reserves, pushing us further toward malnutrition. Healthy thyroid function requires good nutrition, without it thyroid function suffers.

Consuming excessive amounts of carbohydrate also promotes insulin resistance. Thyroid function is intrinsically liked to insulin function. If you have low thyroid function, you likely have some level of insulin resistance as well.[3] Even when thyroid hormone production is on the low end of normal, risk of insulin resistance is significantly increased.[4]

Vitamin C Deficiency

If you eat more than 200 mg of carbohydrate in a day (300 mg is typical), mostly from refined grains and sugar, and do not eat much fresh fruit or vegetables, I can just about guarantee that you are vitamin C deficient. This is important because vitamin C is essential for the production of thyroid hormones.

When you eat large amounts of refined carbohydrate you can create a vitamin C deficiency even when you are consuming the recommended dietary allowance (RDA) of vitamin C (in the US it is 60 mg/day). If you are diabetic or prediabetic the risks are even greater.

Glucose and vitamin C molecules are very similar in structure. Most animals can make their own vitamin C from glucose derived from the carbohydrates in their diets. It is a very simple process. Humans, however, cannot. We do not have the enzymes that can make this conversion, so we must get our vitamin C directly from the foods we eat. The similarity between glucose and vitamin C extends beyond the molecular structure but also includes the way they are attracted to, and enter, cells. Both molecules require help from insulin before they can penetrate cell membranes.

Glucose and vitamin C compete with each other for entry into our cells. But this competition is not equal. Our bodies favor glucose entry at the expense of vitamin C. When blood glucose levels are elevated, vitamin C absorption into the cells is severely restricted. Whenever you eat a meal that contains carbohydrate, it will be converted into glucose, which will interfere with vitamin C absorption. The more carbohydrate you eat, the higher your blood glucose goes, and the less vitamin C your body utilizes. It is ironic that you can drink sweetened orange juice or sugary breakfast cereals that are fortified with extra vitamin C, yet the sugar in these products almost completely blocks the absorption of the vitamin. A high-carbohydrate diet can lead to vitamin C deficiency. If a person is diabetic or is insulin resistant (even a little), blood glucose is elevated for extended periods of time, blocking vitamin C absorption even more.

For this reason, diets high in carbohydrate can cause vitamin C deficiency and, consequently, low thyroid function. The effect of carbohydrate on blocking the absorption of vitamin C is highly significant, yet generally unrecognized by the medical profession. It is possible to develop severe vitamin deficiency even when the diet contains what we might consider ample sources of vitamin C.

Severe vitamin C deficiency leads to scurvy, which may include any of the following symptoms: anemia, depression, frequent infections, bleeding gums, loosened teeth, muscle degeneration and pain, joint pain, slow healing of wounds and injuries, and the development of atherosclerosis (hardening of the arteries), which can lead to heart attacks and strokes. The disease eventually leads to death. It is far more likely for you to suffer a heart attack or stroke from eating a vitamin C robbing, high-carbohydrate diet than by eating a high-fat diet.

Scurvy was a common disease prior to the 20th century before the cause was discovered. Sailors were among the most prone to get the illness. During long voyages, the fresh produce would be consumed first, leaving little more than salted meat and hardtack for the remainder of their journey. Hardtack is a dry biscuit made from flour, salt, and water. This was the mainstay for most sailors. Since flour and meat are poor sources of vitamin C, scurvy often resulted. On a vitamin C deficient diet, scurvy can surface anywhere from 1 to 3 months, depending on the person's vitamin reserves prior to the restricted diet.

When it was discovered that fresh produce could prevent the disease, lemons and limes were added to sailor's diet. The British navy was the first to supply their crews with citrus fruits and for this reason, British sailors were often referred to as limeys.

In the late 1800s and early 1900s many explorers traveled in search of the Northwest Passage through the Canadian arctic or to be the first to reach the North Pole. To prevent scurvy, they added fruits and vegetables to their standard supplies of flour, sugar, coffee, and salted meat. Time after time, expeditions ended in tragedy due to scurvy. Their supply of produce did not protect them.

In the early 1900s anthropologist Vilhjalmur Stefansson traveled to the Canadian Arctic to study the Eskimo way of life. He was particularly interested in the primitive Eskimo and lived among them for several years. During his explorations he would bring only enough food to last a month or two. As his supplies ran out he and his companions would live completely off the land, as the Eskimos did. The Eskimos, he reported, ate no plant food at all, but subsisted totally on wild game. He ate the same way for several years. He never experienced scurvy, nor did any of the natives he lived with. Later, when he wrote about his experiences he was met with strong criticism to his claim. It was believed that an all meat diet was vitamin deficient and would surly cause scurvy. To quiet his critics, Stefansson and a colleague lived on an all meat and fat diet for an entire year without coming down with scurvy.

The reason why Stefansson and the Eskimos didn't suffer from scurvy is because they did not eat any carbohydrate. Even though their meat diet was very low in vitamin C, what vitamin C they did get was absorbed because it did not have to compete with glucose. However, when bread or flour are added, scurvy quickly follows. Stefansson reported that others in his exploration team who ate flour and sugar soon developed scurvy and were healed only when they resumed their no-carb, high-fat and meat diet.

Most people who eat a high-carbohydrate diet do not develop the symptoms of full-blown scurvy, but they can still be vitamin C deficient and suffer from mild or subclinical scurvy. This deficiency disease can be more insidious than full-blown scurvy because the signs and symptoms are not easy to recognize and diagnose. Health declines slowly, giving little warning that anything is wrong until it is too late. Over time, dental health declines, aches and pains arise, atherosclerosis develops, and thyroid function declines. This is another good reason to reduce your carbohydrate intake.

Subclinical Malnutrition

Advanced stages of malnutrition can exhibit themselves as a number of characteristic diseases such as scurvy (vitamin C deficiency), beriberi (thiamin deficiency), and pellagra (niacin deficiency). Such conditions leave the body vulnerable to infections, depress immunity, slow down healing, disrupt normal growth and development, and promote tissue and organ degeneration. If left untreated, all are lethal.

According to the World Health Organization, 70–80 percent of people in developed nations die from lifestyle- or diet-caused diseases. The majority of cancers are caused by what we put into our bodies. Heart disease, stroke, and atherosclerosis, the biggest killers in industrialized nations, are dietary diseases. Diabetes is a diet related disease. Numerous studies have shown that vitamins, minerals, and other nutrients in foods protect us from these diseases of modern civilization.

When we think of malnutrition, we usually think of emaciated drought victims in Africa or starving people in India. In more affluent countries, the problem is more subtle. Symptoms of malnutrition are not as evident. Overweight people don't look malnourished and methods of diagnosing deficiency diseases require malnutrition to be in an advanced stage before they can be detected.

When a variety of food is available, few people develop obvious symptoms of malnutrition, even when their diets are nutritionally poor. Instead, they suffer from subclinical malnutrition. Subclinical malnutrition is a condition where a person consumes just enough essential nutrients to prevent full-blown symptoms of severe malnutrition, but the body is still nutrient deficient and prone to slow, premature degeneration. This condition can go on unnoticed indefinitely. In Western countries the problem of subclinical malnutrition is epidemic. Our foods are sadly depleted of nutrients. We eat, and even overeat, but may still be malnourished because our foods do not contain all the essential nutrients our bodies need to function optimally. As a result, the immune system is chronically depressed, the body cannot fight off infections well, and tissues and cells starving for nutrients slowly degenerate. The body, sensing a lack of nutrition, may shift into low gear, slowing down metabolism to conserve the nutrients it is receiving.

When the body is starved for nutrients, the stage is set for developing low thyroid function and weight gain. In order for the thyroid gland and its hormones to function properly you need adequate amounts of vitamins A, B_{12}, C, D, and E; minerals iodine, selenium, zinc, copper; and amino acids (the basic building blocks for protein). A deficiency in any one can cause low thyroid function. For example, in order to make the thyroid hormone thyroxin, the thyroid gland needs iodine and the amino acid tyrosine. A diet lacking in tyrosine containing protein or iodine will depress thyroid function. Because of the great importance iodine has on thyroid function, the following chapter will cover it in more detail. Meat and other animal products are important because they not only supply protein but also vitamins A and B_{12}. Vitamin A can be produced from beta-carotene found in plant foods, but some people have difficulty making the conversion. Vitamin B_{12} is only available in animal products and cannot be synthesized from other nutrients. Vitamin and mineral supplementation may be necessary to assure complete nutrition.

Food Additives

I have already discussed the effects of sugar, artificial sweeteners, and high fructose corn syrup and how they affect your weight. Many other food additives also contribute to the battle of the bulge.

If you want to get fat, one surefire way is to eat foods containing monosodium glutamate (MSG). MSG is a flavor enhancer as well as a belly fat enhancer. When researchers want to do obesity studies with mice they first need to create obese mice. There is no strain of rat or mice that is naturally obese, so the scientists inject them with MSG when they are first born. MSG triples the amount of insulin the pancreas creates, causing the rats to become obese.[5] When we eat foods containing MSG, the same thing happens to us.

MSG may be one of the primary culprits fueling our obesity epidemic. It is found in everything from canned soup and lunch meats to potato chips and salad dressings. It's found in thousands of packaged, canned, boxed, and frozen foods. If MSG is not listed in the ingredient label that doesn't mean it is not there. Manufacturers use a variety of ingredients that contain MSG without actually having to specifically list it as an ingredient. Other ingredients that contain MSG include hydrolyzed vegetable protein, bouillon, glutamic acid, glutamate, calcium glutamate, autolyzed yeast, yeast extract, textured protein, soy protein, whey protein isolate, and natural flavoring, among others. The list can go on and on and you could never remember all the different names.

All these food additives are used in packaged, prepared foods. The safest way to avoid MSG and other harmful additives is to simply not eat these types of foods. Instead, eat fresh produce, meats, eggs, and dairy—real foods. These are the foods that supply the best nutrition with the least additives. Whenever you read an ingredient label and see MSG, think of it as a fat enhancer that will convert whatever you eat with it into body fat.

Fats and oils are common food additives. When vegetable oils are hydrogenated, the chemical process transforms natural fatty acids into strange creatures called trans fatty acids. When consumed, these toxic artificial fats are incorporated into our cells and organs just like natural fats. However, they don't function like normal fats and can disrupt normal cellular processes. These fats can wreak havoc on the thyroid, pituitary, and other glands involved in governing and controlling metabolism and body weight. Partially hydrogenated vegetable oil is a common food additive. If you see it listed on the ingredient label, don't eat it. Your thyroid will be happy.

Non-hydrogenated vegetables oils can be a problem as well, especially when they are used in packaged, prepared foods or in deep frying (e.g, in french fries, potato and corn chips, onion rings, fried fish, chicken nuggets, donuts, etc.). While we need some polyunsaturated fats in our diet, the overconsumption of these fats can potentially promote weight gain. For instance, they can depress thyroid activity, thus lowering metabolic rate. Any polyunsaturated vegetable oil that is added to a packaged, processed food has been damaged. The reason vegetable oils can be a problem is because they oxidize quickly and become rancid. Oxidized oils block thyroid hormone secretion, its movement in the circulatory system, and the response of tissues to the hormone.[6]

As you learned in Chapter 3, polyunsaturated vegetable oils are highly vulnerable to oxidation. Exposure to heat, even low cooking temperatures, accelerates oxidation and free-radical generation. Since free radicals are toxic, our bodies have a built-in defense mechanism—antioxidant enzymes. Antioxidants neutralize free radicals. We get the building blocks for antioxidant enzymes from our foods. Nutrients such as vitamins A, C, and E and minerals selenium, copper, and zinc are essential in synthesizing our defensive antioxidant enzymes. For example, zinc and copper are needed to form superoxide dismutase, one of our most potent antioxidant enzymes. In addition to vitamins and minerals, plants contain a variety of phytochemicals with potent antioxidant properties, such as beta-carotene, lutein, lycopene, anthocyanins, and others.

The overconsumption of polyunsaturated oils, particularly those that have been damaged by excessive heat, can produce such a large number of free radicals that our body's antioxidant reserves can quickly become exhausted. This leads to a deficiency in essential antioxidant nutrients. These nutrients are not only used to form antioxidant enzymes but are used in thousands of other enzymes necessary for the proper regulation and function of our bodies.

Vitamins C and E, selenium and other antioxidant nutrients are essential for the production and utilization of thyroid hormones. When these nutrients are deficient, due to either eating a nutritionally poor diet or consuming excessive polyunsaturated oils, thyroid function suffers. Studies have shown that excessive use of polyunsaturated oils can interfere with thyroid gland and system function, leading to hypothyroidism.[7-8]

Selenium is crucial for both the production of T4 in the thyroid gland and essential for the conversion of T4 to T3.[9] A diet high in polyunsaturated oils also interferes with the conversion of T4 to T3, probably because it drains selenium reserves.[10] A deficiency in any number of antioxidant nutrients can lead to thyroid dysfunction. Free radicals themselves can also interfere directly with T4 to T3 conversion. Reducing the amount of polyunsaturated oils in the diet and adding antioxidant nutrients can improve thyroid function.[11-13]

Oxidized polyunsaturated vegetable oils are not the only source of free radicals that attack our bodies; free radicals can also be generated by chemical food additives, alcohol, tobacco smoke, toxic metals (e.g., mercury, lead, aluminum), polluted air, and other environmental toxins. Even if you avoided all sources of polyunsaturated fat, you are still exposed to free radicals.

Consuming good sources of antioxidants is essential for maintaining good thyroid function. Some antioxidants complement or revitalize others, so getting a variety of antioxidants provides the best protection. While taking antioxidant dietary supplements can be helpful, studies consistently show that antioxidants are more effective when they are obtained from whole foods, containing dozens of antioxidants, rather than from a tablet that supplies only a few.

When vegetable oils oxidize and go rancid they set in motion chemical reactions that affect flavor and shorten shelf life. In an attempt to extend shelf life as long as possible, food manufacturers add antioxidants as preservatives. Vitamin E is often used as a natural antioxidant preservative, but the most common are the synthetic antioxidants butylated hydroxytoluene (BHT), butylhydroxyanisol (BHA), and tert-butylhydroquinone (TBHQ). Nearly every cold breakfast cereal contains one or more of these synthetic antioxidants. You will also find them in pastry, cakes, breads, cookies, salad dressings, and chewing gum, as well as lipsticks, moisturizers, and other cosmetics. Almost any packaged food that contains fat will likely be preserved with one of these antioxidants. They are added to these products specifically to retard the oxidation of polyunsaturated fats and sometimes are even added to processed vegetables oils and margarines.

While these synthetic antioxidants may slow down fat oxidation and extend the expiration date on packaged foods, they introduce some problems of their own. Studies have shown that long term use (90 days or more) can be toxic to the liver, lungs, kidneys, bladder, and thyroid gland and promote cancer—one of the areas of major concern to researchers.[14] To make matters worse, these chemicals tend to accumulate in the body. While the amount of these chemicals in a single serving of breakfast cereal may not cause much harm, when eaten regularly over time they can accumulate and have potentially devastating effects.

There are many additional food additives—dyes, emulsifiers, artificial flavorings, preservatives, and such. Some like vitamin E, citric acid, sea salt, or non-aluminum containing baking powder are relatively benign. But many others, particularly those with long, hard to pronounce chemical sounding names, have raised concerns because of their potential adverse effects. It is best to avoid any packaged food that contains ingredients with which you are not familiar.

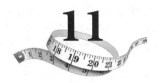

Iodine and Your Health

AN ESSENTIAL NUTRIENT

Iodine is an essential nutrient that is contained in and utilized by every cell in our bodies. The thyroid gland contains a higher concentration than any other organ or tissue. This gland takes up as much as 6 mg of iodide from circulation daily to use in the production of the thyroid hormones. Three iodine molecules are needed to make T3 (triiodothyronine) and four for T4 (thyroxine), the two key hormones produced in the thyroid gland. These hormones are synthesized and then stored and released from the thyroid as they are needed. Ideally, there should always be an adequate amount of thyroid hormone available to meet the body's daily needs even when daily consumption of iodine varies. However, when daily iodine intake cannot maintain the storage capacity of the thyroid gland or meet the body's daily needs, then a deficiency can occur, leading to low thyroid function or hypothyroidism.

A common misconception about iodine is that its only function in the body is for the production of thyroid hormones. The thyroid gland is not the only organ to concentrate and use iodine. The majority of the iodine in the body is not used for thyroid hormone synthesis, but is located in tissues outside the thyroid gland. Large amounts of iodine are found in the salivary glands, cerebrospinal fluid, brain, breasts, ovaries, kidneys, joints, arteries, bones, and the ciliary body of the eye.

Iodine is essential to every cell in the human body. It is needed for maintaining the function and structure of the mammary glands, it functions as a protective antioxidant, displays antitumor properties, acts as a detoxification agent, supports immune function, and protects against pathogenic bacteria.

Iodine deficiency causes a spectrum of disorders including goiter, hypothyroidism, mental retardation, cretinism, and varying degrees of other growth and developmental abnormalities in children. It is the world's leading cause of preventable brain damage. The World Health Organization (WHO) estimates that iodine deficiency disease affects 740 million people worldwide and that nearly 35 percent, about 2 billion, of the world's population are iodine deficient.[1] In addition, iodine deficiency increases the risk of thyroid, breast, endometrial, ovarian, and prostate cancers and possibly infant death syndrome (SIDS), multiple sclerosis, and other disorders.[2-4]

Next to the thyroid gland, the breasts are the body's main storage and utilization sites for iodine. Iodine is essential for development and maintenance of normal breast structure and function, especially in females. Milk from lactating breasts contains four times more iodine than the amount taken up by the thyroid gland.[5] The only source of iodine for breastfeeding infants comes from mother's milk. Iodine deficiency in breast tissue can lead to breast cancer and fibrocystic breast disease. In an iodine deficient condition, the thyroid gland and the breasts will compete for what little iodine is available. As a consequence, both tissues will be lacking.

Iodine functions as a protective antioxidant, preventing the formation of destructive free radicals derived from polyunsaturated and monounsaturated fatty acids. Iodine binds to the double and triple bonds of unsaturated fats, protecting these delicate fatty acids from oxidation as they are being transported to sites in the brain, eyes, and other organs of the body.[6]

Lipids (fats) make up the cell membranes throughout our bodies. Iodine incorporates itself into the lipids that make up the cell membrane. These substances are known as iodolipids. Iodine helps stabilize the membrane and participates in regulating the normal life cycle of the cell.

Normal cells have a distinct life cycle, and after a period of time they die and are replaced by new cells. For example, cells lining the digestive tract live 3 to 4 days, red blood cells live for 4 months, and skin cells live for 2 to 3 weeks. This process of programmed cellular death is known as apoptosis. Cancer cells, unlike normal cells, do not have a normal life cycle; the program for apoptosis has been turned off, allowing them to keep dividing over and over and never die. As a result, they grow unrestrained and eventually encompass and take over the surrounding tissue.

One of the functions of iodine in cell membranes is to monitor the cell's life cycle and induce apoptosis at the proper time. Tissues that are properly saturated with iodine have a greatly reduced risk of becoming cancerous. When breast cancer is present, increasing iodine intake has shown to restore normal breast tissue.[7] Populations with a high iodine intake, like the Japanese, have low breast cancer rates, as well as fewer thyroid problems.

Women are up to eight times more likely than men to develop thyroid problems.[8] Why are women more susceptible to hypothyroidism than men? One reason is that women require more iodine than men. It has been estimated that if adequate iodine is available, the thyroid gland will absorb 6 mg a day. In a 110 pound (50 kg) woman, the breasts absorb approximately 5 mg

134

per day. A larger women or a woman with larger breasts would absorb even more iodine. Other tissues and organs absorb another 3 mg. All these tissues compete for the available iodine. Since men have much smaller breasts than women, they have a lower iodine requirement. Consequently, an iodine deficient diet will become evident in a woman before it is noticeable in a man.

IODINE DEFICIENCY

As important as iodine is to our health, it is not present in adequate amounts in most foods. Plants absorb iodine from the soil. We get iodine from eating these plants and from the animals that feed on these plants. The amount in the diet is variable and generally reflects the amount present in the soil. While iodine is widespread in the earth's crust, it is not very abundant. It is grouped in the bottom third of the elements in terms of abundance.

The ocean contains the highest proportion of iodine. Land masses that have at one time been under the ocean, are overlain by sedimentary rocks and soils rich in iodine. Soils derived from igneous and volcanic rocks are very poor sources. Decades of continuous farming have depleted the iodine in most inland soils. Coastal soils are replenished by ocean spray. Even then, crops grown on these soils have low iodine levels. Livestock feeding on crops grown on iodine-containing soils concentrate iodine in their tissues. As in humans, iodine is concentrated in the mammary glands of livestock and enriches their milk with the nutrient. Whole milk, cream, butter, and other full-fat dairy products are good sources of iodine, provided the animals' diet contained the nutrient. Low-fat milk and dairy products are completely devoid of it, as is margarine and vegetable oils. The yolks of chicken eggs are also a good source. Animal fat supplies some iodine, if they were fortunate enough to be fed crops grown on iodine-containing soils or were given supplemental iodine. The most abundant source of iodine comes from seafood—ocean fish, shellfish, and seaweed. Seaweed is a particularly rich source of iodine. It captures iodine from the surrounding water and concentrates it to about 20,000 times that of ocean.

Iodine deficiency occurs most commonly in areas of the world where the soil and water are deficient in this nutrient. In severe cases of iodine deficiency, the cells of the thyroid gland begin to enlarge so as to trap as many atoms of iodine as possible. If the gland swells until it is visible, the condition is called simple goiter. In extreme cases, the gland can grow as large as a grapefruit. Goiter afflicts about 200 million people throughout the world, most of them in Africa. In 96 percent of these cases the cause is iodine deficiency.

Some areas are iodine deficient because they are covered by volcanic rock and soil, such as in the inland valleys of Oregon and Idaho, or have been stripped of iodine-containing soils by glaciers during the ice ages, like in the Great Lakes area of the United States and central Canada.

135

For many years, farmers living in iodine poor areas routinely gave their livestock blocks of rock salt. The salt, which was mined from ancient seabeds, supplied iodine to the cattle. Iodine from salt blocks and from trace amounts in the feed was concentrated in their milk fat. Butter made from the milk fat of these cows provided people with enough iodine to prevent goiter. As long as people ate an adequate amount of butter, goiter wasn't a problem.

During the Great Depression money was scarce, so people began using the cheaper margarine in place of butter. For many people butter had been their primary source of iodine. Although goiter was already a problem in some areas, when people switched to margarine, it suddenly became an epidemic. In an effort to prevent goiter, iodine was added to table salt.

Iodine is a very effective disinfectant and when combined with certain organic elements can become highly toxic. Iodine has been recognized as an essential nutrient since the 1800s, but due to fears that too much could become harmful, iodine supplementation was set as conservative as possible. The lowest daily dose of iodine needed to prevent goiter has become the standard. The US Recommended Dietary Allowance (RDA) of iodine for adults is 150 mcg (0.15 mg) per day. Because needs are greater during pregnancy and lactation the recommended amount in these cases is 220 mcg and 290 mcg per day, respectively. Most countries have adopted similar guidelines. While these amounts are enough to prevent goiter, the optimal intake of iodine has never been established.

Iodized salt wasn't the only added source of iodine in the diet. Sometime after the introduction of iodized salt, bakeries began using potassium iodide in their products as a dough conditioner. Potassium iodide increases the elasticity of the dough, allowing more air bubbles to be trapped, thus giving the bread a lighter texture. A single slice of bread supplied 150 mcg of iodine—the government's daily recommended dose. Since the iodization of table salt and the addition of iodine to baked goods, the incidence of simple goiter was nearly eliminated in the US and Canada.

In 1965 the National Institutes of Health reported that the average iodine intake from bakery products was 726 mcg per day. In the 1970s it climbed to over 800 mcg a day. Fearful that people eating a lot of salt and bread may be getting too much iodine, the government put a stop to the use of potassium iodide in baked goods. In the early 1980s bakeries discontinued the practice of using iodine in baked goods, substituting potassium bromide for the potassium iodide.

At about this same time, criticism was being directed toward salt as a contributor to the increasing rate of high blood pressure. Doctors began telling their heart disease patients to avoid salt and prescribed salt-restricted diets. Others, fearing high blood pressure and heart disease, cut down on salt consumption as well. Food manufacturers began making products with reduced or no added salt. Over the past 30 plus years salt consumption has declined by 65 percent. As a result of the removal of iodine from baked goods and the reduction in salt consumption, iodine intake has declined dramatically over the past 30 years. To make matters worse, our exposure to a number of goitrogenic substances that interfere with iodine absorption has increased, enhancing the risk of iodine deficiency.

With the widescale use of iodized salt, iodine deficiency was thought to be a thing of the past. While goiter is still uncommon where iodized salt is used, iodine deficiency is occurring at near epidemic rates. David Brownstein, MD, author of the book *Iodine: Why You Need It, Why You Can't Live Without It*, says, "Iodine deficiency is rampant." After testing 4,000 patients with various health problems, Brownstein says over 95 percent showed deficiency on laboratory testing for inorganic iodine. A study conducted by investigators at the CDC found that between 1971 and 1994 iodine levels in the US population had declined by 50 percent.[9] Iodine intake is likely even lower today. Over the past three decades the incidence of hypothyroidism has been steadily increasing.

Low iodine levels depress thyroid function. Severe iodine deficiency leads to goiter and serious hypothyroidism. Moderate iodine deficiency may not show any signs of goiter but can exhibit marked hypothyroidism. Mild iodine deficiency can lead to subclinical hypothyroidism—displaying some of the symptoms of hypothyroidism while thyroid hormone levels remain within the generally recognized range considered normal. Depressed metabolism and easy weight gain are common features of hypothyroidism, including subclinical hypothyroidism.

THE HALOGENS

Is your tap water making you fat? As bizarre as it may sound, drinking tap water may contribute to your weight gain. How, you ask? Water contains no nutrients, no fat, and no calories, so how can it contribute to weight gain? It's not actually the water that is at fault, it's what's in the water that's the problem—halogens. Halogens are a group of related elements that include fluorine, chlorine, bromine, and iodine.

When people talk about these elements you will often see them referred to in two different ways, for example, fluorine and fluoride. Fluorine (ending with –ine) refers to the element. Fluoride (ending in –ide) refers to the fluorine ion generally combined with other elements; for example, when sodium and fluorine combine, they form sodium fluoride. Although there are differences, the element and ion names (fluorine/fluoride, chlorine/chloride, bromine/bromide, iodine/iodide) are often used interchangeably. All of the halogens in pure form are toxic, but when combined with other elements can become less toxic or even benign, and in the case of chloride and iodide, become essential nutrients. Even when combined with other elements fluoride and bromide can be highly toxic. For this reason, these toxic halogens are often used as disinfectants and as the active ingredients in insecticides, fungicides, and rat poisons.

The halogens all have a similar structure and somewhat similar chemical properties. In the body, fluorine and bromine compete for the same receptors that capture iodine. In the synthesis of the thyroid hormones, for example, these toxic halogens can be used in place of iodine. When they are, the hormone becomes dysfunctional—useless. Iodine absorption decreases and its excretion by the kidneys increases. As a consequence, fluorine and bromine intake can lead to iodine deficiency, hypothyroidism, and even goiter.[10]

We are exposed to both fluorine and bromine in tap water. Bromine is sometimes added as a disinfectant and fluorine is added to supposedly reduce the risk of tooth decay. Both can contaminate water in areas where they are found naturally in the soils or as a consequence of industrial waste. Consuming and bathing in water containing these halogens on a daily basis can contribute to low thyroid function, and consequently, promote weight gain. So, in this manner, drinking tap water can be a contributing factor to your weight problem.

Of all the halogens, fluoride is perhaps the most troublesome because it has the greatest affinity to iodine bonding sites in the body and will easily displace iodine if present. In fact, fluoride has been used as a drug to treat hyperthyroidism—an overactive thyroid—because it is highly effective in blocking thyroid hormone production.

Fluoride is marketed as a means to prevent tooth decay because it is absorbed into teeth (as well as bone and other tissues) and hardens the enamel. While fluoride may harden the teeth, it has never been shown to actually prevent cavities, in fact, some studies show that it increases the incidence of cavities. In quantities typically added to drinking water it has been shown to cause a multitude of health problems including osteoarthritis, fluorosis (discoloration of the teeth), memory impairment, delayed brain development in children, and psychiatric disorders, among others, in addition to hypothyroidism.[11-12]

Even if you don't live in a community that adds fluoride to its water supply, you can still be exposed to fluoridated water. Commercially produced soda, fruit juice, sports drinks, beer, and other beverages are typically processed using fluoridated water. Any canned or bottled product that is processed using water can have fluoride; this includes canned vegetables and fruits. Since commercial products do not disclose the type of water used, you have no idea which contain fluoride and which do not.

Tea is a major source of fluoride even if the water is fluoride-free. Most black and green tea contains fluoride. The tea plant readily absorbs fluoride from the soil and concentrates it in the leaves. As a result, tea leaves contain high levels of fluoride. Herbal teas are a safer option.

138

Fluoride is added to toothpaste, mouthwash, gum, and many other products. You need to read ingredient labels, and choose products without fluoride.

Teflon used on non-stick cookware is made with chloroform and hydrogen fluoride. When food is cooked, some of the fluoride is released into the food and the air. You might think this may be a small amount, but it can give unfluoridated water twice as much fluoride as fluoridated water and triple the concentration of fluoride in fluoridated water. The fluoride released in the air from Teflon coated pans, especially if they are overheated, can be high enough to kill pet birds in the house, who are more sensitive to toxins than humans. The DuPont company claims that its coating remains securely intact at temperatures up to 500° F (260° C), however, pet owners have reported deaths with cooking temperatures as low as 325° F (160° C).

Because of their toxicity, both fluorine and bromine are commonly used in pesticides to kill insects and rodents. Fruits and vegetables almost always contain pesticide residue and should be thoroughly washed. Since some produce absorbs the pesticides, eating organically grown produce would be an even better option.

Bromine can be found in a number of places. Along with chlorine, bromine is used in hot tub and swimming pool treatments. It is added to some toothpastes and mouthwashes, where it is used as an antiseptic and astringent. Brominated vegetable oil is used in making soft drinks, such as Mountain Dew, Squirt, Sun Drop, and Fresca, and in some citrus flavored sports drinks, such as lemon lime and orange flavored Gatorade. Brominated vegetable oil is added to citrus drinks to help suspend the flavoring in the liquid.

Since the 1980s bakeries have replaced potassium iodide with potassium bromate. In the 1970s a single slice of bread contained 150 mcg of iodide, which supplied recommended dietary requirement for this nutrient. Today bread contains roughly the same amount of bromine, which means that if you eat several slices of bread a day, you are consuming huge amounts of bromine. If you eat commercially made sandwich bread, hamburger buns, donuts and other baked goods, or bread at restaurants, your thyroid may be screaming, "No more bromine!"

Chlorine gas (Cl_2), like iodine gas (I_2), is highly toxic. In pure form, both chlorine and iodine are used as disinfectants. However, when they are combined with potassium, sodium, or other metallic elements they form salts that are harmless and even beneficial. Table salt is composed of sodium chloride ($NaCl$). Like iodide (I^-), chloride (Cl^-) is an essential nutrient. Chloride is necessary for all known species of life. Along with sodium, it is the fifth most abundant mineral in the human body. Unlike fluoride and bromide, chloride generally does not interfere with iodine absorption or utilization in the body.

When combined with hydrogen and/or oxygen, chlorine can become a strong oxidizer and produce some very toxic compounds. One of these is perchlorate—a common environmental pollutant found in surface and groundwater and, unfortunately, tap water. Perchlorate consists of one chlorine atom surrounded by four oxygen atoms. In the form of perchlorate, chlorine can displace iodine in our bodies. Contamination of our water supply from perchlorate is widespread and is increasing.

Much of our exposure to the toxic halogens comes from baked goods and tainted tap water. High-carbohydrate foods and beverages such as sodas, juices, breads, and other baked goods can be sources of thyroid strangling halogens. Going on a low-carb or ketogenic diet would eliminate these troublemakers. Drinking filtered water would remove fluorine, bromine, and perchlorate. Washing your fruits and vegetables or eating organically grown produce would help to eliminate halogen-containing pesticide residue.

DIETARY GOITROGENS

Some of the foods we eat each day depress thyroid activity and promote hypothyroidism. These foods contain antithyroid substances called goitrogens. Goitrogens interfere with the uptake of iodine and the production and function of thyroid hormones and can even induce goiter formation. Goiter caused by toxins in foods is called toxic goiter.

Ironically, what some people consider to be health foods, contain the most goitrogens. All cruciferous vegetables (the cabbage family) contain goitrogens. This would include cabbage, cauliflower, brussels sprouts, mustard greens, broccoli, bok choy, turnips, kohlrabi, kale, collard greens, radishes, and horseradish. Eight million people worldwide, mostly in Africa, have toxic goiter because of the overconsumption of cruciferous vegetables. Legumes also contain goitrogens. This includes soybeans, peas, lentils, kidney beans, etc. Two more products that are commonly sold in health food stores are goitrogenic—rapeseed (canola) and flaxseed. Canola oil is found as an ingredient in many products, especially baked goods. Flaxseed is not only used as a dietary supplement, but in numerous products.

Does this mean that you should avoid all these foods? Fortunately, most goitrogens are heat sensitive and are neutralized when cooked. Fermentation also reduces goitrogenic activity. When these foods are cooked or fermented the goitrogenic toxins can be significantly reduced or eliminated, making the foods safer to eat.

For most people, who are getting an adequate amount of iodine, eating small amounts of these vegetables raw is not harmful. If you suspect you have a thyroid problem, however, it is best that you stay away from them unless they are cooked or fermented.

Of all the goitrogenous foods, soybeans pose the greatest threat. The antithyroid substances in soy are not destroyed by cooking. Soy products such as tofu and texturized vegetable protein have gained a great deal of popularity, particularly as meat extenders or replacements. But you say you don't eat soy? Think again. If you eat like most people, you're consuming soy in one form or another every single day whether you know it or not. Since soy is used in a wide assortment of foods, exposure can come from many sources. Soy byproducts have found their way into an incredible number of everyday foods. Soy is often used as a replacement for meat and dairy. It is disguised as everything from cheese, milk, burgers, and hot dogs to ice cream, yogurt, and protein drinks. It's even in baby formula. At least 60 percent of the foods on America's grocery shelves contain soy derivatives—soy flour, texturized vegetable protein, vegetable oil, partially hydrogenated oil, soy protein isolate, etc. Almost every packaged, prepared food you pick up now contains soy in one form or another. It makes me wonder if part of the reason why we are experiencing a growing problem with hypothyroidism and overweight is due to the increasing amount of soy in our food supply.

Many soy containing foods are marketed as low-fat, dairy-free, or high-protein meat substitutes which are eaten by people conscious about their weight. Little do they know that by eating these "low-fat" diet foods they are ruining their metabolism, and setting the stage for obesity.

We have been bombarded with the supposed benefits of soy for so long that many people find it hard to believe that soy promotes weight gain by interfering with thyroid function. However, there exists a significant body of research that demonstrates goitrogenic and even carcinogenic effects of soy products.[13] There are many reports of goitrogenic effects on children resulting from the use of soy-based infant formula.[14-15] Even healthy adults can develop thyroid problems when they begin eating soy.[16] Researchers have clearly shown that soy protein (isoflavones) inhibits the thyroid's ability to produce hormones.[17] Soy protein has even been linked to autoimmune thyroid disease—another mechanism that causes hypothyroidism.[18]

Soy protein isn't the only villain. Soybean oil also attacks the thyroid. The oil doesn't necessarily cause goiter but is equally as toxic, because it interferes with the production and utilization of thyroid hormones. Approximately 80 percent of the oils in our diet come from soy: soybean oil, partially hydrogenated soybean oil, margarine, and shortening. Look at ingredients labels for soybean oil of one type or another. If you see anything that contains soy, don't touch it. The only exception would be soy products that have undergone a long period of fermentation. The microbial action in fermentation neutralizes most of the toxins. Fermented soy products include miso, soy sauce, and tempeh. Small amounts of these items may be okay on occasion. All other soy products should be avoided, this includes tofu.

Don't be taken in by the argument that soy products must be safe because the Asians have been eating them for centuries. Contrary to what the soy industry would like you to believe, soy has never been a staple in Asia. A study of the history of soy use in Asia shows that the poor used it during times of extreme food shortage, and then the soybeans were carefully prepared using fermentation to destroy the toxins. They understood the dangers of soy. Even now most Asians eat very little soy, less than 1-2 percent of total calories. They use it primarily as a condiment to their meals, unlike in the West where it is eaten in relatively large quantities as a replacement for meat and dairy and as a source of protein.[19]

DRUGS

There are literally hundreds of drugs that can interfere with thyroid gland or hormone function. If possible, these drugs should be used sparingly or avoided altogether.

Many drugs contain fluorine or bromine that block iodine absorption and T4 synthesis. Some of these have potentially lethal doses of fluorine or bromine. A few of the most notorious are Redux and Fen-Phen, used to suppress appetite, and Baycol, a cholesterol-lowering statin. Each of these drugs has been pulled from the market after causing a number of deaths and disability.

Beta blockers, corticosteroids, cortisone and other steroids affect the way the body handles thyroid hormones, blocking the conversion of T4 to T3. Large doses of corticosteroids are so effective in reducing T3 levels that they are often used to purposely suppress thyroid function in the treatment of severe hyperthyroidism (overactive thyroid function).

Phenobarbital (anticonvulsant, sedative), phenytoin (antiepileptic), carbamazepine (antiepileptic), and rifampin (antibiotic) induce metabolic degradation of T3 and T4.

Hypothyroidism and subclinical hypothyroidism have been reported in 5 to 20 percent and as much as 50 percent of people taking lithium carbonate, a drug used to treat psychotic disorders. Goiter has been observed in up to 60 percent of those receiving lithium for 5 months to 2 years; hypothyroidism may not be present.

A partial list of other medications that can affect thyroid function: sulfa drugs, antihistamines (Livostin), antidepressants (Prozac, Luvox, Paxil), antacids (Prevacid), antibiotics (Cipro), cholesterol-lowering drugs (Lipitor), antiarrhythmic agents (Cordarone), COPD and asthma inhalers (Atrovent), chemotherapy drugs, ulcer medication (Pro-Banthine), and non-steroidal anti-inflammatory drugs/NSAIDS (Celebrex, Arava, Clinoril, Aspirin). Not all of the drugs in each of these categories have an adverse effect on thyroid function. Ibuprofen (Motrin, Advil), for example, is an NSAID but does not depress thyroid function. Aspirin, another NSAID, is one of the most commonly used drugs in the world and is often prescribed as a blood thinner as well as a pain reliever. Despite it being considered a comparatively benign drug, it has been shown to decrease T4 and T3 levels in the blood. A measurable drop in thyroid hormone levels can be detected after a single dose of aspirin.[20] Chronic aspirin use can lead to reduced thyroid system function.

Several medications, including iron and aluminum-containing products (such as sucralfate, antacids, and didanosine), sodium polystyrene sulfonate, resin binders, and calcium carbonate have been reported to impair the absorption of thyroid hormone medication and decrease its efficacy. If you use thyroid medication it should be taken on an empty stomach for optimal absorption.

Ironically, if you are taking thyroid hormone drugs you may also be iodine deficient. Thyroid hormone therapy exacerbates iodine deficiency. Thyroid drugs increase your metabolism, which increases your cell's requirements for iodine. If you take thyroid hormone drugs without adequate sources of iodine, you could be making a deficiency even worse. Some symptoms of hypothyroidism may improve while others do not—a common occurrence among those on thyroid medication.

IODINE INTAKE
Are You Iodine Deficient?

In the US, health agencies claim most people are iodine "sufficient," meaning they get enough of the nutrient from their diet, primarily from iodized salt. This assumption is based on the RDA of 150 mcg per day. However, this is controversial. According to a number of doctors who have successfully treated thousands of patients with thyroid issues, the RDA is far too low. This level will prevent goiter but not common hypothyroidism or subclinical hypothyroidism, both of which are increasing to epidemic proportions.

The RDA for iodine was established at the lowest level possible to prevent goiter. The need for iodine for optimal thyroid function and the need in other tissues and organs in the body were not even considered. It was just assumed that the RDA provided enough for the entire body. The optimal level of iodine has never been established.

If you have low thyroid function, or symptoms like low metabolism and easy weight gain, the reason may be due to low iodine levels. If you avoid salt like the plague, don't eat much seafood, and live more than 100 miles (160 km) from the nearest coastline, then you might be iodine deficient. Also, if you eat a lot of bread or baked goods, drink a lot of soda or sports drinks, or if you drink fluoridated tap water, you could also be iodine deficient even if you eat seafood and live near the coast.

David Brownstein, MD, who has been researching iodine for the last two decades, states that over 95 percent of the patients in his clinic are iodine deficient. Many other thyroid specialists agree with Dr. Brownstein. The need for iodine is greater now than it has been in the past because we get less in our foods, plus we are exposed to a larger amount and greater variety of iodine blocking substances. The effects of a poor diet, food additives, halogens, goitrogens, drugs, and other conditions that depress thyroid function are amplified in the presence of an iodine deficiency.

Whether you suffer from hypothyroidism or not, chances are, you are iodine deficient. Although iodized table salt is the most common source of iodine, I do not recommend that you get your iodine this way. Table salt has been refined and purified, meaning all of the beneficial trace elements that were originally in the salt have been removed. Sodium aluminosilicate, a source of aluminium, is added to table salt as an anticaking agent. Aluminium is a well-documented neurotoxin and has been linked to increased risk of dementia. You don't want to save your thyroid at the expense of destroying your brain. I recommend using sea salt. Unrefined sea salt contains iodine as well as many other important trace minerals that are naturally found in seawater. Unfortunately, it does not supply enough iodine to satisfy your daily needs, so you still need other sources of iodine in your diet.

You can increase your iodine intake by eating sea vegetables (such as kelp and nori) and ocean fish. Freshwater fish are not a good source. Dietary supplements are also available. Most natural iodine supplements are composed of dried, powdered kelp. Although the exact amount of iodine in kelp supplements varies, since it is a natural product, adults can easily take one to three 600 mg capsules a day. Please note that capsule size is not an indication of iodine content. A 600 mg capsule does not contain 600 mg of iodine. You will need to check the label on each brand to determine the actual amount of iodine in each capsule. Kelp is a traditional food that has been consumed safely for thousands of years. Kelp supplements are very safe, you could easily take several times the dosages recommended without harm.

Kelp is also a rich source of important trace minerals like copper, zinc, manganese, chromium, and dozens of others. Trace minerals are important because they are incorporated into various enzymes used by our bodies. Most people can benefit from these trace minerals because they are generally deficient in the foods that make up our typical diet. Some companies make kelp granules that can be sprinkled on foods like a seasoning.

Lugol's Solution

Most iodine supplements contain iodine in only one form: iodide. However, our bodies actually need iodine in two forms. Iodine (I^2) is one form, while iodide (I^-) is the other. Different tissues of the body require and absorb different forms of iodine. The thyroid gland primarily utilizes iodide. For this reason, potassium iodide was added to table salt. In contrast, breast tissue prefers iodine. Iodine deficiency can alter the structure and function of breast tissue that may lead to breast cancer. Animal studies have shown that iodide (the form in table salt) is ineffective at reversing the precancerous lesions of animal breast tissue, whereas iodine is much more effective. Iodine, but not iodide, also blocks the oxidation of polyunsaturated fats in breast tissue.[21] This is important because oxidation of fats generates free radicals that can damage cells, including delicate DNA, leading to cancer.

The prostate gland concentrates iodine. The skin prefers iodide. Some tissues such as kidneys, spleen, liver, blood, salivary glands, and intestines use both forms. Because different tissues concentrate different forms of iodine, using a supplement that contains both iodide and iodine is preferable to using only one form. This type of iodine supplement is known as Lugol's solution. It is not a brand name, but a term for a mixture of iodine and iodide that has been in use for nearly 200 years.

In 1829 French physician Jean Lugol (1786-1851), was investigating substances that could treat tuberculosis and other illnesses and became interested in iodine. He was experimenting with different forms of iodine. Iodine itself is not very soluble in water. Lugol found that combining potassium iodide with iodine increased its solubility in water. He began using a solution termed Lugol's Iodine that was a mixture of 5 percent iodine, 10 percent potassium iodide, and 85 percent distilled water. Two drops of Lugol's solution (0.1 ml) contained 5 mg of iodine and 7.5 mg of iodide. Lugol recommend two drops per day of his solution to treat infectious illnesses. This provided a 12.5 mg mixture of iodine and iodide. Dr. Lugol's solution was widely available at apothecaries and was routinely prescribed for many different conditions. It was also used as an antiseptic and as a disinfectant in drinking water. In the early 1900s every hospital used it as a disinfectant. For many years it was used extensively and safely in medical practice for treating both hypo- and hyperactive thyroid conditions. The recommended daily intake for Lugol's solutions was 2 to 6 drops, which supplied 12.5 to 37.5 mg total iodine/iodide. Lugol's solution is still available today but at lower iodine concentration (2 percent iodine and 4 percent potassium iodide), so you need 5 drops to get the same 12.5 mg of iodine/iodide that you got from 2 drops of the original solution. The reason for the dilution of the formula was to discourage its use in the illicit production of methamphetamine. Lugol's solution is a dietary supplement that can be purchased at health food stores or online. This solution is not to be confused with iodine tincture, which consists of elemental iodine and iodide salts dissolved in alcohol. Iodine tincture, commonly sold as a first aid antiseptic, is for external use only.

Iodine specialist David Brownstein, MD says he used to treat his thyroid patients using a supplement that contained only iodide and saw only modest success. Some patients improved, but many did not notice any appreciable benefit. When he started using Lugol's solution that contained a combination of iodine and iodide, his results were significantly better. He says this form of iodine is very safe and prescribes doses of 6 mg up to 50 mg a day.

Lugol's solution is taken by putting a few drops in a glass of water. Depending on how much water you use, the solution can give the water a

145

mildly disagreeable metallic taste. Since drop size can vary slightly, dosing using an eyedropper can be inconsistent sometimes. For these reasons, a tablet form of Lugol's solution was developed called Iodoral. Iodoral is preferred by physicians because it is easy to take and provides a consistent amount of iodine. There are two sizes or dosages available, 12.5 mg and 50 mg.

Note that the current RDA of iodine is only 150 mcg (micrograms), which is equivalent to 0.15 mg (milligrams). One drop of Lugol's solution provides 2.5 mg of iodine/iodide or 2,500 mcg, nearly 17 times the RDA. Five drops provides 12.5 mg of iodine/iodide or 12,500 mcg, or 83 times the RDA. In the 1930s during the goiter epidemic in the US, doctors successfully treated patients using up to 36 mg a day of Lugol's solution. Doctors have been using these and even higher doses for nearly 200 years without harm, demonstrating how harmless iodine in this form is, and the inadequacy of the RDA.

Initially, Dr. Brownstein prescribed doses close to the recommended RDA. He was hesitant to use doses higher than 1 mg because some of the research he read speculated that iodine supplementation at this higher level might have adverse effects and even cause hyperthyroid symptoms. However, a further, more exhaustive review of the medical literature failed to prove that iodine in milligram doses was ever shown to be harmful or cause hyperthyroid symptoms.

Our body's requirement for iodine today is higher than it was a few decades ago due the significant increase of halogens and goitrogens in the environment and the decrease in iodine in our foods. Dr. Brownstein and a number of other thyroid experts suggest we get about 12.5 mg daily or 83 times the RDA. He recommends this amount not only from his personal experience in treating thyroid diseases, but from populations around the world that consume large amounts of iodine in their foods and have very little thyroid problems.

Mainland Japanese consume 13.8 mg of iodine per day, which is 92 times the RDA. Japanese living on the coastal areas consume even larger amounts. Most of the iodine comes from the seaweed in their diet. This high amount of iodine doesn't appear to have any harmful effect, in fact, just the opposite. In comparison to people living in the US, they have significantly lower rates of hypothyroidism, goiter, and fibrocystic breast disease, as well as lower levels of breast, endometrial, ovarian, and prostate cancers. They are among the healthiest people in the world, with the longest life expectancy.

Iodine status is known to play an important role in the prevention of breast and other cancers. Japanese women, who have among the highest iodine intake in the world, have the lowest rate of breast cancer. US women, who consume only a fraction of the iodine that the Japanese do, have the highest breast cancer rates. This is not a hereditary trait. When Japanese women move to the US and adopt a diet lower in iodine, they experience a higher incidence of cancer than those living in Japan.[2]

146

In the US, the risk of breast cancer in the 1960s was 1 in 20. Since that time, iodine intake has dropped more than 50 percent and breast cancer rates have increased to 1 in 7.

The thyroid gland itself needs 6 mg of iodine per day.[22-23] This is well above the 150 mcg/day RDA. This is why the RDA is inadequate.

Excess Iodine

Many doctors and health writers warn of the danger of consuming too much iodine believing that any amount over 1.1 mg (1,100 mcg) could be harmful. They cite studies that show reducing iodine intake eases thyroid patient's symptoms or tell stories how thyroid patients' symptoms intensified with iodine supplementation. In some cases, the addition of supplemental iodine caused symptoms of hyperthyroidism in those who had been diagnosed as hypothyroid. Even those who have no thyroid problems are cautioned that taking too much iodine (400 mcg/day or more) may possibly lead to hypothyroidism.[24] It is interesting that the amount cited as being enough to cause hypothyroidism in people with normal thyroid function is only 400 mcg (0.4 mg). This seems strange that in some people adding iodine would cause hypothyroidism and in others it would do just the opposite.

It also seems odd that Lugol's solution has been used by millions of people at doses up to 50 mg/day for the past two centuries without any reported harm. In fact, it has been used successfully to treat both hypothyroidism and hyperthyroidism. The mainland Japanese consume on average 13.8 mg/day without experiencing hyperthyroidism, hypothyroidism, or any ill effect. Coastal Japanese consume as much as 80 mg/day without any apparent harm.[25] Research has shown that the thyroid absorbs up to 6 mg of iodine a day when sufficient quantities are consumed. After observing thousands of patients on iodine supplementation, Dr. Brownstein and others recommend 6 mg to 12.5 mg a day with therapeutic doses up to 50 mg/day. The 1.1 mg limit is based mostly on theory and conjecture, while the 12.5 mg dose is based on real people, in real life, under real conditions.

There are a number of reasons for these discrepancies. Keep in mind that much of the caution about using iodine comes from people who have experienced unpleasant symptoms. One of the most common of these is the claim that it causes hyperthyroidism. It is well established that if there is an iodine deficiency causing low thyroid function, adding iodine into the diet will improve thyroid function. This idea has been taken a step further to suggest that too much iodine will make the thyroid function too efficiently kicking into a state of hyperactivity.

The idea that too much iodine will cause hyperthyroidism is like saying taking too much calcium will make your bones too dense and hard, or eating too much protein will make your muscles too big and strong. You need calcium for building strong bones, but eating excessive amounts of calcium will not overbuild your bones. Likewise, we need protein but eating too much protein will not cause it to magically soak into your muscles and give you a physique like a young Arnold Schwarzenegger. Eating too much iodine will not cause the thyroid to work any faster. The medically recognized symptoms of iodine excess are goiter and depressed thyroid activity—the same as iodine deficiency. In other words, too much iodine doesn't make the thyroid work better or faster but worse, just like an iodine deficiency.

In cases where people report becoming hyperthyroid after taking iodine, they were likely on thyroid medication to treat hypothyroidism. Since they were already hypothyroid, they were probably iodine deficient. Taking supplemental iodine supplied the missing nutrient, allowing their thyroid glands to function more normally and produce more hormones. However, if they were also taking thyroid medication at the same time, the medication now being too strong, would cause them to experience symptoms of hyperthyroidism. The iodine did not cause the hyperthyroidism, the medication did. So when a person on thyroid medication adds iodine, the dosage of their medication needs to be monitored.

Some low-thyroid patients have reported becoming ill or experiencing intensified symptoms when they add supplemental iodine into their diets, fueling the fire that iodine can be dangerous. Some report that doses as low as the RDA were enough to cause them trouble. How is this possible?

Again, iodine is not causing the problem, it is part of the solution. People with low thyroid function are often deficient in iodine as well as being overloaded with goitrogenic substances like halogens and drugs. Adding sufficient amounts of iodine into the diet can initiate a detox or cleansing reaction. Iodine competes with other halogens for binding in the body. If there is a sufficient amount of iodine present, it can have a strong detoxifying effect on the other halogens. Ingesting 12.5 mg to 50 mg of iodine a day crowds out the other halogens, greatly increasing the excretion of fluoride, bromide, and perchlorate.[26-27]

In addition to expelling toxic halogens, iodine supplementation can purge heavy metals as well. In one study to determine the optimal dose of iodine, women supplemented with 12.5 mg elemental iodine daily showed increased urine levels of mercury, lead, and cadmium after just one day.[28] How does iodine increase the removal of toxic metals? Iodine improves thyroid function, boosting metabolism, which improves immune function. As a consequence, iodine can have a pronounced detoxifying effect on the entire body. When these toxins are purged from the body it can bring on a set of symptoms that resemble an illness—diarrhea, nasal discharge, nausea, as well as intensify symptoms associated with hypothyroidism. These symptoms are all temporary, lasting a few days to a couple of weeks. But once the symptoms subside, you will feel better and have fewer harmful substances poisoning your body.

Some of the studies that showed thyroid patients getting worse with iodine supplementation may have been due to a detoxifying effect. Another reason may be caused by a low-fat diet—the type of diet that has become standard in our society for the past 30 plus years. Iodine is lipophilic, meaning it is attracted to fats. This is why butter, egg yolk, and other animal fats can be good sources of iodine. Like with very lean protein, consuming iodine without adequate fat in the diet can be counterproductive (see pages 106-107). Absorption of iodine is improved in the presence of dietary fat and conversely is decreased in the absence of fat. The body needs fat to properly utilize iodine. Adding a source of iodine without added fat in the presence of a low-fat diet could exacerbate low thyroid symptoms, giving the false impression that iodine is harmful even in small amounts. I suspect that many, if not all, of the studies that have shown adverse effects of iodine supplementation are due to combining the extra iodine with a low-fat diet.

Hypothyroidism and hyperthyroidism have been increasing rapidly over the past three decades. At the same time, iodine intake as well as fat intake, have declined. If iodine consumption above 400 mcg really did promote thyroid disorders, we would be experiencing a decrease in these diseases, not an increase.

IODINE LOAD TEST

If you are not deficient in iodine, then you certainly don't need to supplement your diet with more. The only sure way to tell if you have an iodine deficiency is to test your iodine levels. The most common method of doing this is by measuring the amount of iodine in your urine. However, that is not a reliable method because it only measures the amount of iodine that is leaving the body and not what the body is retaining. Exposure to goitrogenic substances, such as bromide and fluoride, will affect how much dietary iodine is actually absorbed, so the urine test is unreliable.

A more accurate method of measuring iodine status is the iodine load test. This test is based on the concept that the greater the iodine deficiency, the more iodine is retained in the body and the less it is excreted in the urine. Iodine binds to receptors throughout the body. If the body's receptors for iodine are sufficient in iodine, a large percentage of the iodine consumed will be excreted in the urine.

The iodine load test involves taking 50 mg of an iodine/iodide supplement (Iodoral). After taking the Iodoral supplement, urine is collected for 24 hours. In an iodine sufficient state, approximately 90 percent of the 50 mg dose of iodine/iodide will be excreted (45 mg) and 10 percent of the iodine would be retained (5 mg). Levels below 90 percent excretion indicate an iodine deficiency.

Jorge Flechas, MD, who has been one of the leading physicians using this method, has found after testing over 4,000 patients that the mean urinary iodine excretion in the US is less than 40 percent. Normal should be 90 percent or above. According to this data, most Americans are not

149

only iodine deficient but seriously deficient. There is a 95 percent chance that you are deficient too. If you are, then your thyroid is underperforming, your metabolism is hampered, and losing weight and keeping it off will be a difficult task regardless of the type of diet used. For this reason, I highly recommend that you get an iodine load test done.

Currently there are three labs in North America doing iodine load testing.

Doctor's Data, Inc.
3755 Illinois Avenue
St. Charles, IL 60174-2420, USA
Phone: 630-377-8139
Toll Free: 800-323-2784
Fax: 630-587-7860
http://www.doctorsdata.com

FFP Laboratories
576 Upward Rd. Suite 8
Flat Rock, NC 28731, USA
Toll Free: 877-900-5556
Fax: 828-697-9020
Email: ffp_lab@yahoo.com

Labrix Clinical Services, Inc.
16255 SE 130th Avenue
Clackamas, OR 97015, USA
Phone: 503-656-9596
Toll Free: 877-656-9596
Fax: 877-656-9756
Email: info@labrix.com

You can contact any of these labs and have them send you instructions and a test kit. You will collect your urine for a total of 24 hours and send a sample of it back to the lab. They will analyze it and discuss the results with you. If you are iodine deficient you will probably be advised to take 50 mg supplemental iodine (Iodoral) daily until your iodine excretion levels are >90 percent, then you will cut back to a daily maintenance level. It usually takes three to six months of iodine supplementation at 50 mg/day before iodine saturation is reached. Most non-obese patients not exposed to excess goitrogens achieve whole body iodine sufficiency within three months. Depending on how deficient you are, you will be asked to do the iodine load test again after a few months to evaluate your progress and determine your iodine status.

If you are on thyroid medications now, you will need to have your doctor monitor the dosage of your medication when you start taking the Iodoral. The added iodine will likely make your thyroid function better. If you experience rapid or irregular heartbeat, nervousness, anxiety, irritability, tremor, sweating, increased sensitivity to heat, difficulty sleeping, fatigue, muscle weakness, changes in menstrual patterns or other symptoms indicative of hyperthyroid activity, you know that you need to reduce your medication.

The added iodine will cause an increased excretion of fluoride, bromide, perchlorate, mercury, lead, and other toxins. During this detoxification process you may experience some unpleasant symptoms of elimination. Not everyone experiences these symptoms. If you do, just let the process run its course. You are not experiencing an illness, just a cleanse. It is not harmful. The symptoms are a natural effect of the cleansing process.

I recommend everyone get an iodine load test done to evaluate their iodine status. This is the only way of knowing if you are iodine deficient or not. If you are, you need to take steps now to correct it. If you don't, it will make losing weight all that more difficult. I recommend you have this done before starting the Coconut Ketogenic Diet.

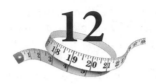

12

Thyroid System Dysfunction

WILSON'S THYROID SYNDROME
A Treatable Thyroid Problem

Linda started gaining weight after she quit smoking. Her weight swelled to the point that she knew she had to do something. She tried losing weight on her own without success. It was frustrating. Realizing she needed help, she went to a weight-loss clinic and started their program. It didn't help. They even accused her of cheating on the diet because she wasn't losing any weight. She tried another weight-loss clinic with a stricter dietary program. After 6 months limited to just 800 calories a day, she lost only 4 pounds (2 kg).

Discouraged and very depressed, she went to an endocrinologist for help. He determined that her thyroid was underactive and prescribed Synthroid, a synthetic thyroid medicine. It wasn't much help. A year later she was even more depressed, constantly tired, had headaches every day, and was still overweight. Her doctor finally told her she would have to live with herself as she was, overweight and tired. She told her doctor that she refused to live the rest of her life this way. He advised her to see a psychiatrist to help her accept the way she was. This caused her to feel even more hopeless, depressed, and discouraged.

Eventually she learned about a condition known as Wilson's temperature syndrome (WTS), also known as Wilson's thyroid syndrome, which could be causing her sluggish metabolism. She began treatment and within a few weeks began to feel more energetic and less depressed. In just a couple of months she lost 40 pounds (18 kg) and her fatigue was completely gone. Depression, fatigue, and headaches were no longer a part of Linda's daily life.

Five years ago Debbie was under an extreme amount of stress. During this time she began experiencing headaches, dry and flaky skin, loss of energy, depression, and weight gain. She had put on weight even though her food intake had decreased. She began to retain fluid and her feet and ankles became so swollen and painful that, at times, it became uncomfortable for her to stand or walk. She knew something was wrong.

At this point she decided to seek medical help. She went to two different doctors and got the same answers. They could find nothing wrong. Her blood tests were normal. They said there was nothing wrong with her thyroid or her metabolism. They couldn't do anything to help her.

She then learned about the Wilson's Thyroid Syndrome Treatment Center and made an appointment. As she filled out the patient information sheet and checked off all the symptoms, she became embarrassed at the large number of symptoms she had that corresponded with those on the list. Her temperature was taken and registered below normal. She told the nurse, "That's okay. It's always low." Her low temperature, however, was a key to her failing health and ballooning weight problem.

Although her blood tests showed her thyroid to be "normal," she did have a thyroid problem. Those with Wilson's thyroid syndrome often display normal blood test readings, yet they don't have normal thyroid system function.

Debbie began treatment, and within a week her symptoms began to disappear. Her family and friends could not believe the immediate changes she was experiencing. She said she had almost forgotten what feeling good was all about.

In Linda's case she was diagnosed with low thyroid, but thyroid medication did little to help alleviate her symptoms. Debbie had no measurable thyroid deficiencies, yet she too suffered from a thyroid system problem. Both were victims of Wilson's thyroid syndrome (WTS). Wilson's thyroid syndrome is a cluster of reversible symptoms caused by dysfunction of the thyroid system. WTS is not easily recognized by doctors because it does not show up on standard blood tests for thyroid gland problems.

Many thousands of overweight people are affected with WTS without realizing it. Aches, pains, and weight gain associated with Wilson's thyroid syndrome are often attributed to aging or some other cause. People can suffer for years with these symptoms without realizing there is a treatment.

Treatment is very simple and in most cases permanent. With hypothyroidism patients must take thyroid medication for life. But Wilson's thyroid syndrome is a reversible condition that can generally be corrected within a few months time. After treatment is over, no further medication is usually necessary. People who have suffered with overweight and other symptoms for 10, 20, 30 years or more have been able to overcome the problem and get on the road to recovery and permanent weight loss.

Thyroid System Disorder

Many overweight people suspect they have a thyroid problem which causes, or at least contributes, to their weight problems. When someone says they have a thyroid problem, what they are generally referring to is the function of the thyroid gland. The thyroid gland, however, is only one part of the thyroid system. A person can have a thyroid gland that is working normally yet still have a thyroid system problem.

The function of the thyroid gland is actually controlled by another gland called the pituitary—a pea-sized organ at the base of your brain. This gland is often referred to as the "master gland" because it produces hormones that regulate the activity of most of your other glands. One of the hormones produced by the pituitary gland is called thyroid-stimulating hormone, or TSH. This hormone stimulates the thyroid to produce and release its own hormones (T4 and T3).

The amount of thyroid hormones circulating in your bloodstream is carefully controlled by a self-regulating process known as negative feedback. When TSH levels increase, it stimulates the production of T4 and T3. As T4 and T3 levels go up, TSH production slows down, which is followed by a drop in thyroid hormones, which in turn triggers an increase in TSH, and the cycle continues. In this manner, the hormones are kept in a delicate a balance. In a sense, the pituitary acts like a thermostat for the body that releases TSH as needed to raise or lower thyroid hormone levels, and consequently control metabolism and body temperature.

When taking a blood test for thyroid hormone levels, it is assumed that these hormones are being properly absorbed and utilized by the cells. If TSH and thyroid hormones levels are within normal parameters, it is interpreted that the thyroid gland (and pituitary) is functioning properly and that there are no thyroid related issues.

Some of the classic signs of hypothyroidism include fatigue, depression, weight gain, cold hands and feet, dry skin and hair, and constipation, among others. Patients suffering with these symptoms may suspect they have low thyroid function and go to the doctor for a diagnosis. The standard method for diagnosing hypothyroidism is a blood test in which TSH and thyroid hormones are measured. A high level of TSH or low thyroid hormone levels indicates low thyroid function. If, however, these hormone levels are within the normal range, the assumption is that the thyroid gland is functioning normally and that there is no thyroid issue. What about the symptoms? Why are they there? Since it is apparent that the patient does indeed have something wrong, the doctor might advise the patient to go home and get more sleep and eat better. If the patient insists that something is wrong, the doctor may conclude that the symptoms are "all in the patient's head" and send her home with a prescription for antidepressants, anti-anxiety drugs, diuretics, antacids, laxatives and other drugs to treat the symptoms. None of these drugs address the real problem—thyroid system dysfunction.

Low metabolism can be the result of either an underactive thyroid gland or a dysfunction of the thyroid system. Blood tests can only determine thyroid gland function. According to Denis Wilson, MD, the first to recognize and successfully treat WTS, most metabolic or thyroid problems are not due to thyroid gland dysfunction, but to thyroid system dysfunction. This is why so many people who suspect metabolic problems have normal thyroid hormone levels. Wilson's thyroid syndrome is a thyroid system problem.

The situation with low thyroid function is similar to that of diabetes. The two most common forms of diabetes are type 1 and type 2. In type 1 diabetes the pancreas gland does not produce an adequate amount of the hormone insulin, which leads to diabetes. In type 2 diabetes the pancreas may produce a normal amount of insulin but the cells have become unresponsive to it. This is called insulin resistance. In both cases, the symptoms are similar.

With low thyroid function you also have two major types of hypothyroidism, you could call them types 1 and 2. As with type 1 and 2 diabetes, one is glandular and the other is cellular. One involves an underactive thyroid gland that is not producing adequate amounts of thyroid hormone. The other, WTS, which could also be called hypothyroidism type 2, the thyroid gland may be producing a normal amount of thyroid hormone but the cells are not able to utilize it properly. In both cases, the symptoms are the same,

The thyroid gland secretes T4 (thyroxin) and T3 (triiodothyronine). Eighty to ninety percent of the hormones released by the thyroid gland are T4. Synthroid, and most other common synthetic thyroid medications, are composed entirely of T4. When someone is hypothyroid (type 1), their thyroid gland is not producing adequate amounts of T4 and T3. They are considered to have a thyroid gland problem.

Many people with low thyroid gland activity are helped by taking medications that supply the body with the thyroid hormone T4. By increasing the blood concentration of T4, the body receives the hormone it needs to keep metabolism up to normal. Taking T4, however, isn't a cure; it's a crutch to assist a thyroid gland that isn't functioning optimally. Thyroid medication must be taken for life.

When T4 is released by the thyroid, it circulates in the blood and is absorbed into cells. Here it is converted into T3. The great majority of the T3 in your body comes from conversion of T4 within the cells. T4 has little biological activity. T3, on the other hand, has four times the activity as T4 and, therefore, has far more impact on metabolism. Thyroid system dysfunction occurs when T4 is not adequately converted into T3. The thyroid may make normal amounts of T4, even overproduce it, but if it is not converted to T3, metabolism will be depressed. This is what happens in Wilson's thyroid syndrome. T4 may be adequate, but T3 is not. Sometimes people with WTS will also have thyroid gland problems as well. Treatment with T4 medications does little good because it isn't converted to the more active T3. This is why

155

a person can be given thyroid medications and experience little or no real improvement.

Multiple Enzyme Dysfunction

The most characteristic feature of WTS is low or unsteady body temperature. In fact, low body temperature is believed to be the primary cause for the symptoms associated with low thyroid function.

Thyroid hormones control the metabolic rate of our cells and our body. Metabolism can be described as the sum total of all the biochemical reactions in the body. Virtually all of these reactions give off heat as a byproduct. This heat, in turn, is what we measure as our body temperature.

Body temperature is one of those things that is tightly controlled. If your temperature goes too high (above 107° F/41.7° C), it can cause brain damage. Likewise, a temperature that is too low (below 90° F/32.2° C) can be just as harmful. The ideal temperature, measured orally, is 98.6° F (37.0° C). This is true for all people regardless of genetic background or individuality. Optimal body temperature is a chemical constant, like water freezing at 32° F (0° C). Whether you are in Alaska or Hawaii, water still freezes at 32° F. Our bodies are structured to function within a very narrow range of temperatures. Any higher or any lower starts to affect body function.

Virtually all of the chemical reactions that take place in our bodies require enzymes for those reactions to occur. These enzymes serve as catalysts to make chemical reactions occur at higher rates than would otherwise be possible, but do not actually become part of the final products produced by those reactions. Enzymes are proteins that depend upon their shape or configuration for their activity. When they are too hot, they become too loose, when they are too cold, they become too tight, and in either extreme the enzymes are not the right shape and cannot function optimally. When body temperature is too low, nearly all of the enzymes function less effectively.

The enzymes in our bodies function optimally at 98.6° F (37.0° C). The farther away from this the temperature gets, the less effective and active enzymes become. Even a variation of a single degree can have a significant effect. If enzyme activity slows down, over time health problems can develop. This is called multiple enzyme dysfunction (MED). Low metabolism can lead to multiple enzyme dysfunction. Dr. Wilson has identified as many as 60 health problems associated with MED. The most common include the following:

Overweight	Fluid retention/swelling
Cold hands and feet	Anxiety and panic attacks
Fatigue	Hair loss
Migraines	Depression
PMS	Decreased memory and
Irritability	concentration

Low sex drive	Hypoglycemia
Dry skin and hair	Frequent or persistent colds
Constipation	Frequent urinary tract infections
Irritable bowel syndrome	Frequent yeast infections
Insomnia	Depressed immunity
Hives	Acne
Itchiness	Arthritis and joint pain
Asthma	Carpal tunnel syndrome
Allergies	Ulcers
Food intolerances/sensitivities	Poor coordination
Slow healing from wounds and injuries	Ringing in the ears
	Acid indigestion
Brittle nails	Infertility
Bruising easily	Irregular periods
Heat and/or cold intolerance	

Chronically low body temperature can be the primary cause or at least a contributing factor for any of these conditions. Those suffering from Wilson's thyroid syndrome won't necessarily have all of these conditions; most will have just a few, while others may have many. I've seen people with at least 16 of the above symptoms (all of which, by the way, were significantly reduced or eliminated by the diet and lifestyle changes discussed in this book).

How can you tell if you have WTS? One way is to check your symptoms with the list above. Are you experiencing any of these symptoms? Many of these symptoms can also be caused by other conditions, such as thyroid gland dysfunction. Some people with mild WTS may have no noticeable symptoms. The best test for WTS is simply taking your temperature. If your body temperature is constantly below normal, enzymes are not working effectively and you probably have a thyroid system problem. If T4 medication is of little or no help, WTS is most likely at fault.

Low body temperature is the most characteristic feature of WTS. Some people may say that their body temperature is "naturally" low, or that it is "normal" for them to have a low temperature. Low body temperature is not normal for anyone. In order for your enzymes to function optimally, your temperature needs to be at or near 98.6° F (37.0° C). This temperature does not vary from person to person. When the temperature does vary, it indicates a metabolic problem.

Feeling hot all the time is not a good indication of body temperature. Many people, particularly if they are overweight, feel hot, yet their temperatures may be below normal. The reason they "feel" hot is that they have become oversensitive or intolerant to fluctuations in temperature. Often, a person who is always unbearably hot in the summer is also frigidly cold in the winter. If you happen to be married to one of these people, you know the conflict that can take place. During the winter one will be constantly turning up the furnace and stacking on blankets at night, while the other turns down the heat and sleeps with little covering. During the summer the roles may reverse. It's a constant battle.

What Causes Chronic Low Body Temperature?

Lisa never had much of a weight problem in her youth, but after the birth of her third child the pounds began to stack up. It was almost like someone turned on a switch for increased fat production. Within just a few years she gained 30 extra pounds. She didn't eat any differently than she used to, but the weight kept piling on. Headaches, irritability, hypoglycemia, and other health problems began to emerge as well. She attributed the excess body fat as simply a consequence of gaining weight during pregnancy and as part of the natural process of getting older. Her real problem, however, was that during her last pregnancy she had developed WTS.

Our body's metabolism has basically three settings—fast, medium, and slow. Metabolism shifts between all three during the day depending on different circumstances. At times our body functions best at high speed, at other times it prefers to go slow. Most of the time it runs at medium, not too fast and not too slow.

Metabolism will shift into high gear in response to certain circumstances. For instance, when we are involved in a physically demanding activity our lungs breathe deeper and faster, our heart rate increases, and a greater amount of oxygen is delivered to our muscles, which is necessary for energy production. If we get an infection and become sick, metabolism increases to accelerate production of antibodies and speed healing and repair.

Metabolism shifts into low gear when we sleep or rest or when food consumption decreases. When we fast or even diet, the body interprets it as a period of starvation. In response, metabolism slows down to conserve energy and ensure survival during the time when food is less plentiful.

A normal, healthy body constantly shifts in and out of all three levels of metabolism. When conditions that cause the body to gear up or gear down are over, metabolism rebounds back to normal. This is the way it's supposed to work. However, in Wilson's thyroid syndrome, when conditions that cause the body to slow down are passed, the body doesn't recover: it becomes stuck in low gear. It can stay stuck for weeks, months, or years. Subsequent events that shift the metabolism into low gear can crank metabolism down even lower. As metabolism slows down, body temperature decreases. This is why some people may have a temperature only slightly below normal while others may be off by two or three degrees.

What causes metabolism to get stuck in low gear? It is a combination of both stress and malnutrition. When we are under stress, the body responds by increasing its metabolism. If you have to take an important test, run a race, or meet a deadline at work, the body responds by pumping up metabolism. As metabolism increases, cellular processes are all shifted into high gear. The demand for energy to fuel these activities increases. The need for vitamins and minerals increases because the enzymes that run all chemical activities in the body depend on these nutrients, so vitamins and minerals are used up at an accelerated rate. If there are enough nutrients in storage, and if the stress is removed after a brief period of time, the body is perfectly able to cope with this shift in metabolism.

A problem arises, however, when stress becomes chronic or severe and the body is undernourished. When stress is frequent or very severe, there is a great demand for vitamins and minerals for the utilization of enzymes. If the needed nutrients are not present, the body senses a situation similar to that of starvation and shifts into low gear. When nutrients become depleted, the body goes into a state of exhaustion and becomes locked in low gear. It does this as a means of self-preservation to conserve energy and nutrients that are vital to maintaining life. Vitamins and minerals are absolutely necessary for the brain, heart, lungs, and other vital organs to function. If these nutrients become too depleted, permanent damage and even death can result. Slowing down the metabolism is a means of self-preservation.

If enough nutrients are not supplied to adequately replenish the body's storehouse, metabolism remains stuck in low gear. Repeated episodes of stress drive metabolism even lower, making it harder to recover. What types of stress can bring about this situation? Any type of chronic or severe acute physical, mental, or emotional stress, such as pregnancy and childbirth, divorce, death of a loved one, job demands, family troubles, surgery, accidents, illness, or lack of sleep can trigger WTS. Eighty percent of those who are affected by WTS are women. This is understandable since the number one cause is pregnancy and childbirth.

During times of stress, the hormone cortisol is released to increase heart rate, fire up metabolism, boost blood sugar levels, and prepare the body for flight or fight. As cortisol levels increase, TSH and thyroid hormones decrease. Even mild stress, which causes slight changes in blood cortisol levels that are within the normal range, can cause significant alterations in thyroid hormone levels.[1]

The lasting effects of stress and undernourishment on thyroid function were demonstrated in a group of young, healthy military cadets. The cadets were subjected to a combination of sleep deprivation, calorie deficiency, and intense physical activity during a 5-day training course. The cadets' thyroid hormone levels declined strongly during the exercise. After the exercise was completed, T4 levels gradually returned to normal within 4 to 5 days, T3 levels, however, remained depressed.[2] Recovery time is dependent on the health and nutritional status of the individual. In older, less healthy individuals, thyroid function would take longer to rebound, especially if there were any nutritional deficiencies.

Malnutrition, or rather subclinical malnutrition, is very common in our society. Eating sweets, refined grains, and other processed foods that have been stripped of much of their natural vitamins and minerals, has created a society of people who are on the edge nutritionally. Pregnant women have an increased demand for good nutrition. The unborn child demands ample nutrients for proper growth and development and will steal them from the mother's body if they are not supplied in her diet. If she doesn't eat properly, her own nutrient reserves can become dangerously depleted. Add on to that the fact that pregnancy can be a very stressful time. Nine months of stress culminate in several hours of arduous labor and childbirth. It is no wonder why pregnancy and childbirth is the number one cause of WTS.

Dieting can worsen WTS. Low-calorie diets, especially those that allow poor quality foods, can be interpreted by the body as starvation. A body already suffering from a lack of good nutrition will shift its metabolism even lower. This makes losing weight harder. When "normal" eating is resumed, weight rebounds, dragging with it a few extra pounds because now metabolism is even lower than it was before.

How Can You Tell If You Have Wilson's Thyroid Syndrome?

Standard blood tests can't detect WTS. Blood tests measure the amount of hormones in the blood, which give an indication of how well the glands are functioning. Blood tests don't measure what's happening in the tissues and cells of the body. In WTS the production of thyroid hormone is often normal, but the processing of that hormone in the tissues can slow down, leading to an imbalance that can leave patients with low body temperature and the classic symptoms of low thyroid function.

Often those who have low thyroid hormone production are also affected by WTS. According to Dr. Wilson there are "far more people with WTS than all other low thyroid problems combined." So WTS is a very common condition. If you suspect a thyroid problem, it is likely WTS.

The way you can tell if you have WTS is to check for the symptoms. Look over the list of symptoms listed on pages 156-157. Do you have any of these? Keep in mind that even one of them is a sign that something is wrong. Illness is not normal and dysfunction is not normal. The body tries to maintain optimal health so long as it is allowed to. When it doesn't have it, something is out of place.

Overweight is one of the most common symptoms associated with WTS. Obviously metabolism is slow and gaining weight is easy. If you are overweight, it may not be simply because you eat too much. Most overweight individuals have thyroid problems that exacerbate their weight problems.

Not everyone who is overweight has thyroid system problems. But a great many do. If you eat little and put on weight, gain weight easily, have been on low-calorie diets in the past, eat junk foods, don't exercise, and experience a lot of stress, then you may have WTS. If you are female and have been pregnant or if you were normal size as a youth and suddenly packed on weight (within a couple of years), you may also suspect WTS.

The strongest indication of WTS is body temperature. If your average daily temperature is consistently below normal, suspect WTS. The late Broda Barns, MD, author of the classic text H*ypothyroidism: The Unsuspecting Illness*, stated, "More information often can be brought to the physician with only the aid of an ordinary thermometer than can be obtained with all other thyroid functions tests combined."

Taking Your Temperature

Simply taking your temperature once during the day isn't a very accurate way to evaluate body temperature. Several factors influence temperature readings such as physical activity, climate, bathing, and eating. Our temperature also fluctuates during the day. Temperature is normally lowest in the morning just as you wake up. As the day progresses, temperature rises, maintains a certain level, and at the end of the day begins to decline. This daily cycle can vary by as much as one degree in a relatively healthy individual. If you take your temperature in the morning you will get a lower than normal value, no matter what your "real" temperature is.

To avoid the lows in the morning and evening you should take your temperature during the day when your metabolism is at its peak. When you measure your temperature at its highest, it should register as normal (98.6° F/37.0° C). For the most accurate evaluation you should take your temperature three times a day and average them together. If your average temperature is normal, it should be at or near 98.6° F.

Dr. Wilson advises taking the first temperature 3 hours after arising in the morning, the second 3 hours later, and the third 3 hours after that. For instance, if you wake up at 6:00 a.m., take your first temperature at 9:00 a.m., the second at 12:00 noon, and the third at 3:00 p.m. For each day, add the readings together and divide by 3 to get the average. Take readings for at least 5 days. For women, body temperature changes during the first few days of the menstrual cycle and the middle day of the cycle, so avoid doing this test at these times.

Temperature should be taken by mouth. Keep the thermometer in your mouth for at least 3 minutes. Foods can affect the temperature of the mouth, so take the reading before or at least 15 minutes after eating or drinking. Also keep in mind that many digital thermometers commonly used have an accuracy of plus or minus 0.2° F (0.1° C).

When you take your temperature during the day, you are recording your body's normal high temperature. It should be 98.6° F (37.0° C) plus or minus about 0.3° F (0.2° C). The farther it is from normal, the greater your chances of WTS. If your average temperature is below 98.3° F (36.8° C), you may have Wilson's thyroid syndrome. Keep in mind, however, that not all low

161

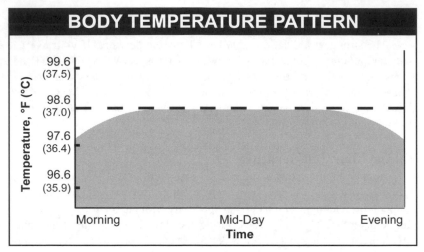

BODY TEMPERATURE PATTERN

Body temperature is normally a little low in the morning and evening. During the day it should be at or near 98.6° F (37.0° C). Those people with WTS usually run about one degree F (2° C) lower throughout the day.

body temperature is caused by WTS. The closer your average temperature is to normal, the less severe your symptoms are likely to be. A person with an average temperature of 98.3° F (36.8° C) may have no noticeable symptoms, while one who has a temperature of 97.5° F (36.3° C) may exhibit many. It is not uncommon for people to have mid-day temperatures as low as 96.0° F (35.5° C) or lower. Dr. Wilson has reported some patients showing signs of WTS with average temperatures as high as 98.4° F (36.8° C), but states that most patients with noticeable symptoms have temperatures of 97.8° F (36.5° C) or less.

If your temperature readings vary significantly, it may also indicate a problem with metabolism. Readings that fluctuate greatly suggest that the body has difficulty maintaining normal temperatures. This can be a sign of possible WTS. It's normal for temperatures to vary 2-3 tenths of a degree under ordinary conditions (not exercising or exposed to extremes in ambient temperatures). If it fluctuates by a degree or more there is clearly a problem. Ideally, your temperature should only fluctuate by 0.6° F (0.3° C) throughout the day under normal circumstances.

If you have a normal temperature reading, yet you experience many of the symptoms associated with WTS, your thermometer may be wrong. Dr. Wilson advises rechecking your temperature using a different thermometer. He claims that if a person has symptoms of WTS, the chances of having a normal temperature are only about 1 in 200. There's a lot better chance that your thermometer is wrong then there is that your temperature is normal.

Treatment

Treatment for WTS is simple. The conversion of T4 to T3 is depressed because enzymes necessary for this process are sluggish due to low body temperature. If the body temperature can be raised to near normal for a period of time, the enzymes will function properly. Simply raising the temperature of the body will improve T4 to T3 conversion. As more T3 is made, metabolism speeds up in response and body temperature increases. At some point, body temperature remains high enough to keep T4 to T3 conversion going at a normal rate. Temperature stays near normal, as it is supposed to, and the body can continue on its own from then on. The entire process can be completed in as little as a few weeks or months. In some cases, where thyroid system dysfunction is more severe, it may take longer. Once the correction is made, body temperature remains normal, metabolism remains normal, and enzymes throughout the body function at a normal rate. The result is recovery from conditions caused by multiple enzyme dysfunction, which includes the loss of excess body weight. When metabolism is where it is supposed to be, excess weight is easier to take off with proper dieting.

How do you raise your temperature? Oral consumption of T3 will raise blood levels of this hormone, which in turn will stimulate metabolism and raise body temperature. T3 must be prescribed by your doctor. Your doctor needs to be familiar with Wilson's thyroid syndrome; not all are and some don't even recognize it as an actual health condition. Before giving you any medication, a blood test will probably be required. If your physician isn't familiar with WTS, the tests may only measure T4 and thyroid gland function.

Most synthetic thyroid medications (e.g., Synthroid, Levoxyl, Levothyroid, etc.) contain only T4, and therefore, are of little value in treating WTS. Synthetic hormone medication, which is by far the most commonly prescribed, is accompanied by some undesirable side effects, one of which is a significant loss of bone calcium. If you take synthetic thyroid hormone medication you should also increase calcium and magnesium supplementation. Natural thyroid medication (e.g., Armour, Nature-Throid, etc.) made from desiccated porcine thyroid, is better because the hormone is essentially identical to that produced by your body and there are few, if any, undesirable side effects. Natural thyroid contains both T4 and the critically important T3. This is the type of thyroid medication you would need to use.

Giving the patient T3 to stimulate metabolism and increase temperature, brings relief to WTS patients. Dr. Wilson has been successful in treating thousands of patients this way. Many other doctors are also treating WTS patients, but not all have the experience, so choose a physician who is familiar with this condition.

The thyroid hormone must be taken each day following a strict time schedule. If the medicine is skipped only once, or even if taken a few hours late, treatment in most cases must start over. When the medicine is not taken on time, the body shifts back into low gear and the process of jump-starting the metabolism must start from the beginning. The reason T3 works is that it keeps the body's temperature elevated at or near normal for a long enough period of time that it allows the body to adapt and continue the process on its own. This means that the temperature during the day must be constantly maintained near normal for several weeks straight for the process to work.

Another drawback to T3 therapy is that if a patient does not address nutritional needs, she can often relapse next time she encounters a stressful situation. In this case, T3 therapy can be repeated. If a stressful situation can be anticipated, low doses of T3 can help prevent relapse. Unfortunately, stress is a normal part of life. We will never be free from it. Our bodies should be healthy enough to handle stress whenever it hits.

T3 therapy is just one way to treat WTS. For severe cases, T3 therapy may be necessary; however, diet and lifestyle changes can also accomplish the same thing without the need of taking prescription medications. Since the WTS responds to a rise in body temperature, any process that can accomplish that goal, when combined with a nutritious diet, has the potential to work. In the following chapter you will learn how to boost your metabolism naturally, without medication, to overcome thyroid system dysfunction, as well as increase your energy level and burn off excess calories.

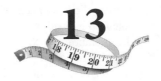

Supercharge Your Metabolism

Don't you hate them—those people who are as skinny as rails and eat like horses? They're full of pep and vitality, gorge themselves on all types of fattening foods and never gain an ounce. You, on the other hand, eat a celery stick and immediately gain five pounds. Why is that? The answer? Metabolism. Your basal metabolic rate (BMR) is slower than theirs. They burn up more calories with the same amount of physical activity as you. They can eat more than you, but weigh less.

Wouldn't it be nice if you could jumpstart your metabolism and kick it into high gear? In this chapter you will learn how to revitalize your metabolism and get it humming along at a more normal, healthy rate.

GOOD NUTRITION

Sandra was overweight, suffered from frequent headaches, irritability, and depression. She always felt cold, lacked energy, and seemed to catch every cold and flu virus that came her way. Her doctor diagnosed her with hypothyroidism and prescribed Synthroid to go along with other medications she was taking to ease many of her symptoms. While the medication helped some, she still didn't feel completely well. Concerned that her diet might be contributing to her health problems, she stopped eating junk foods, sweets, and soy, replaced the packaged, convenience foods she used to eat with fresh vegetables and fruits, and began eating organic meats, eggs, and dairy. In addition to her dietary changes, she added dietary supplements that support good thyroid function. As the changes she made started to take effect and she began to feel better, she gradually weaned herself off the thyroid medication. She is now completely drug-free with normal thyroid function and feeling great. Sandra is one of many people who have been able to reverse a diagnosis of hypothyroidism by simply changing her diet.

Over the past few decades metabolic or thyroid system problems have become commonplace. This rise in incidence suggests that these problems are caused or influenced by dietary or lifestyle choices. The healthier your diet is, the healthier you will be, and the less likely you will have a thyroid system problem. If you have a thyroid system problem, good nutrition is required to correct it.

One of the contributing factors for slow metabolism is malnutrition or, more commonly, subclinical malnutrition. As noted in the previous chapter, poor nutrition combined with repeated episodes of stress can adversely affect thyroid system function, depressing metabolism.

Poor nutrition may also affect thyroid gland health. A lack of vitamins and trace minerals, especially iodine, can adversely affect thyroid gland function. Goitrogens from raw cruciferous vegetables, and soy products especially, depress thyroid gland activity.

The first step in reversing low metabolism is to eat the highest quality foods you can afford. The highest quality foods are not necessarily the most expensive, they are the ones that contain the highest nutritive value and the least harmful additives or byproducts. The lowest quality foods contain the most sugar, the greatest amount of chemical additives, and supply the lowest nutritive value. Generally speaking foods that have had the least amount of processing are of the highest quality. The more processing or refining a food undergoes, the lower in quality it becomes.

The way food is grown also affects its quality. Fruits and vegetables grown in artificially fertilized soils or mineral depleted soils are less nutritious than those grown in rich, organic soils. Organically grown foods are produced in naturally fertilized soils and are not contaminated by pesticides, so they are of a higher quality than non-organic foods.

Meat from grass-fed, organically raised livestock is of higher quality than those from stockyards, fed on corn and soy and pumped up with antibiotics and artificial hormones. Meat from either one of these sources is better than that found in processed meats such as hot dogs and luncheon meats, which are loaded with preservatives, artificial flavor enhancers, and other additives.

The poorest quality foods, those with the least nutrition and often the most chemical additives, also generally happen to be high in carbohydrate like bakery goods, breakfast cereals, desserts, candy, and so forth.

The best foods are fresh vegetables, fruits, meats, eggs, and full-fat dairy that have undergone minimal processing. Always choose fresh foods over packaged. Generally the more processed a food is, the lower its nutritional quality.

A METABOLIC MARVEL
Boost Energy Levels

When someone comes to me and says, "I'm always tired, what can I do to get more energy without taking drugs or using caffeine?" My answer is quick and simple, "Use coconut oil."

When I tell people this, at first they're startled. "Won't that make me fat?" I tell them, "No, coconut oil will give you more energy and help you lose excess weight."

One of the major differences between coconut oil and other fats is the way in which it is digested and metabolized. Coconut oil is different because it is composed predominately of medium-chain triglycerides (MCTs). Most all fats in our diet, whether they are saturated or unsaturated, are in the form of the larger long-chain triglycerides (LCTs). Both vegetable oils and animal fats are composed almost entirely of LCTs. The size makes a big difference.

When we eat foods containing LCTs, the fats are slowly broken down by digestive enzymes into fatty acids (long chain fatty acids or LCFAs), which are small enough to be absorbed through the intestinal wall. As they pass through the intestinal lining they are gathered together and packaged into little bundles of fat (lipid) and protein called lipoproteins. These lipoproteins are sent into the bloodstream, where they circulate throughout the body. As they circulate in the blood, the fats are distributed to all the tissues of the body. With the aid of insulin, some of these long chain fatty acids are shuttled in your fat cells. Excess blood glucose is also converted into long chain fatty acids and stored in fat cells. This is how fat builds up in our fat tissues.

The MCTs in coconut oil, however, are processed differently. Because of their smaller size, MCTs don't require pancreatic enzymes for digestion. By the time these fats reach the intestinal tract they are already broken down into individual fatty acids (medium chain fatty acids or MCFAs) and instead of passing through the intestinal wall like LCFAs, they are immediately absorbed into the portal vein and channeled directly into the liver. Here they are converted into energy to fuel metabolism. MCFAs are not packaged into lipoproteins to the degree that other fats are, so they don't contribute much to your fat cells. Coconut oil goes to the liver to produce energy, not body fat. This difference in the way your body processes MCFAs in coconut oil is very important in respect to metabolism and body weight.

Eating food containing MCTs is like putting high-octane fuel into your car. The car runs more smoothly and gets better gas mileage. Likewise, with MCTs your body performs better. Since MCTs are converted directly into energy, your energy level increases. This energy boost is not like the kick you get from caffeine; it's more subtle but longer lasting. It is most noticeable as an increase in endurance.

The fact that MCTs are digested immediately to produce energy has led athletes to use them as a means to enhance exercise performance. Some studies indicate this to be the case. In one study, for example, investigators tested the physical endurance of mice that were given MCTs in their daily diet against those given LCTs. The study extended over a six-week period. The mice were subjected to a swimming endurance test every other day. They were placed in a pool of water with a constant current. The total swimming time until exhaustion was measured. While at first there was little difference between the groups of mice, those fed MCTs quickly began to out-perform the others and continued to improve throughout the testing period.[1] Tests such as this demonstrated that MCTs had the ability to enhance endurance and exercise performance, at least in mice.

Another study, with human subjects, supports these findings. In this study conditioned cyclists pedaled at 70 percent of maximum for 2 hours, then immediately embarked on a 40K time-trial ride (lasting about an additional hour) while drinking one of three beverages: a MCT solution, a sports drink, or a sports drink/MCT combination. The cyclists who drank the sports drink/MCT mixture performed the best.[2]

Because of these and similar studies, many of the powdered sports drinks and energy bars sold at health food stores contain MCTs or coconut oil to provide a quick source of energy. Athletes and other active people looking for nutritional, non-drug methods to enhance exercise performance have begun using them.

One of the side effects of being overweight is a lack of energy. Part of this may be due to low thyroid function, or simply because carrying about a lot of excess weight is tiring. This encourages inactivity and further encourages weight gain. Coconut oil can give you a boost of energy that will help keep you more active throughout the day and help you burn off a few extra calories.

Many people use coconut oil as a pick-me-up during the day. In the afternoon when energy levels start to drag, taking a spoonful of coconut oil will give you a boost of energy to keep you going for the rest of the day. Some people like to start their day with coconut oil added to their breakfast or to a hot beverage to rev up their engines and get them started. Some add it their coffee or tea, while others take it straight from the spoon.

I can't take much more than a teaspoon or so anytime after about 5:00 pm. It gives me so much energy that if I eat too much in the evening, I'll be wide awake half the night. The effects seem to last a good 6 hours or so. Coconut oil doesn't have this effect on everyone, however. Those people who normally have difficulty sleeping at night, report that consuming the oil in the evening helps them sleep better. Coconut oil promotes better overall health and improves energy balance, so that people who normally have problems sleeping are able to sleep better. Many people report getting a better night's sleep when they add coconut oil into their daily diet regardless of the time of day they eat the oil.

People often express how adding coconut oil into their lives has improved their health. Let me share some comments from a few people who have experienced the energy-boosting effects of coconut oil.

"I started using virgin organic coconut oil three weeks ago and immediately my energy level (which was quite low from my hypothyroidism) increased by approximately 600 percent. Wow! I feel 10 years younger. I have also lost 16 pounds in that time."

Noah Kersey, PhD

"Since I have been using coconut oil in place of other oils I find I have loads more energy compared to before...I used to run out of energy about four hours after waking, I felt terrible. Now, I have energy to last the whole day."

Sue

"I started taking virgin coconut oil faithfully six weeks ago. I am up to 2 ounces a day and I am experiencing fabulous results...I have not had any desire for sweets for over a month. I lost 10 pounds (I was about 30 lbs overweight) and my appetite is back to normal. I feel great and have much more energy."

Bruce W.

"My energy level has increased dramatically to the point where I am willing to exercise to videotapes every day—a new thing for me and desperately needed."

Barbara

"The first week I was very sluggish. I think my body was detoxifying. I have now been on the coconut oil for three weeks and my energy level is incredible."

Donna

"I have noticed an increase in energy. I had low metabolism since I was a teen. I am now 76 years old. I walk for an hour three times a week and the day before yesterday I felt so good that I walked for two hours and felt good. Thank you for opening this wonderful window for me."

Sally

"I didn't even realize how much hypothyroidism was affecting my life till I started on the VCO and suddenly had energy like the Energizer Bunny! I also gave up the white toxins (wheat flour, refined sugar, potatoes, and other high-glycemic index foods) and that, in combination with my VCO consumption has made a tremendous difference in my hormonal balance, mood stability, stamina, and overall energy. And, I'm slowly but steadily losing a little weight without effort. Ya gotta love that!"

Julia

Jumpstart Your Metabolism

Wouldn't it be nice to take a pill that would shift your metabolic rate into a higher gear? In a sense, that is what happens every time we eat. Food affects our basal metabolic rate. When we eat, many of our body's cells increase their activities to facilitate digestion and assimilation. This stimulation of cellular activity, known as diet-induced thermogenesis, equals about 10 percent of the total food energy taken in. Perhaps you have noticed, particularly on cool days, that you feel warmer after eating a meal. Your body's engines are running at a slightly higher rate, so more heat is produced. Different types of foods produce different thermogenic or heat producing effects. Protein-rich foods, such as meat, increase thermogenesis and have a stimulatory or energizing effect on the body. Protein has a much greater thermogenic effect than carbohydrate. This is why when people suddenly cut down on meat consumption or become vegetarians, they often complain of a lack of energy. This is also one of the reasons high-protein diets promote weight loss; the increase in metabolism burns off more calories.

One food that can rev up your metabolism even more than protein is coconut oil.[3] MCTs shift the body's metabolism into a higher gear, so to speak, so that you burn off more calories. This happens every time you eat MCTs. Because of this effect, coconut oil is a dietary fat that can actually promote weight loss!

A dietary fat that burns off weight rather than putting it on is a strange concept for many people to grasp, but that is exactly what happens, so long as calories in excess of the body's needs are not consumed. The reason for this is that MCTs are easily absorbed and are rapidly burned and used as energy. This increase in metabolic activity even fuels the burning of the LCTs.[4] So, not only are medium-chain fatty acids burned for energy production, but they encourage the burning of long-chain fatty acids in the diet as well.[5]

Dr. Julian Whitaker, a best-selling author and well-known authority on nutrition and health, makes an interesting analogy to describe this process. He explains that LCTs are like heavy wet logs that you put on a small campfire. Keep adding the logs, and soon you have more logs than fire. MCTs, on the other hand, are like rolled up newspapers soaked in gasoline. They not only burn brightly, but will burn up the wet logs as well.[6]

Research supports Dr. Whitaker's view. One study compared a high-calorie diet containing 40 percent fat as MCTs to one containing 40 percent fat as LCTs. The thermogenic or fat burning effect of the MCTs was almost twice as high as that of the LCTs—120 calories versus 66 calories. The researchers concluded that the excess energy provided by fats in the form of MCTs would not be efficiently stored as fat, but rather would be burned. A follow-up study demonstrated that MCTs given over a six-day period can increase diet-induced thermogenesis by an amazing 50 percent.[7]

In another study, researchers compared single meals of 400 calories that contained either MCTs or LCTs.[8] The thermogenic effect of MCTs over 6 hours was 3 times greater than that of LCTs. Researchers concluded that substituting MCTs for LCTs would produce weight loss as long as the calorie level remained the same.

Italian researchers showed that after eating a single meal containing 30 grams (2 tablespoons) of MCTs, metabolism in normal weight individuals increased by an impressive 48 percent.[9] In overweight subjects the effects were even more impressive. After a single meal their metabolism increased by an amazing 65 percent! So, the heavier the person, the more effect MCTs have on stimulating metabolism. This is good news for overweight people because it means MCTs can be a useful tool to help boost their metabolism and burn off excess calories.

This metabolic stimulating effect isn't limited to only an hour or two after a meal. Another study by Swiss researchers showed that the effect lasts up to 24 hours![10] That means that after eating a meal containing MCTs, metabolism is elevated and calories are burned off at an accelerated rate for a full 24 hours. That's got to be good news to anyone trying to lose excess weight!

Some people have speculated that the metabolic effects of MCTs may wear down over time with daily use, but this doesn't seem to be the case. The metabolic effect of MCTs doesn't seem to wear off anytime soon, in fact, it seems to get better with continued use. In another study, researchers had subjects consume meals containing MCTs every day for a week. Instead of becoming less effective, metabolism increased by 30 percent by the end of the week.[7] Apparently, MCTs have a cumulative effect. Long-term clinical studies lasting from 4 to 16 weeks show that the metabolic stimulating effects continue to burn off excess calories and promote weight loss for an extended period of time.[11-14]

Fat Deposition

Both animal and human studies have shown that consuming food containing MCTs produces less body fat in comparison to food containing LCTs. In animals, consuming MCTs in place of LCTs results in lower body weight and less fat deposits; even the fat cells themselves are smaller.[15-18] These results have led investigators to propose the use of MCTs as a tool for the prevention and treatment of human obesity.[10, 19-21]

Many studies measure body mass index (BMI) in evaluating weight loss diets and overall health. BMI is a number derived from a person's height-to-weight ratio. It is a much more accurate way of determining a person's body mass because it takes height into account. Obviously a tall person will have more mass than a shorter person and will weigh more even though they may both be considered normal weight. BMI is useful in determining whether a person is overweight, normal, or underweight, and by what degree. In North America and Europe a BMI between 18.5 and 24.9 is considered normal, overweight is 25 and above. (To find your BMI see page 244). These definitions cannot be applied to Asians, who generally have smaller body frames. The Japan Society for the Study of Obesity reports that for Asians, a BMI greater than or equal to 23 indicates being overweight.

In 2001 *The Journal of Nutrition* published a study conducted in Japan which evaluated the use of MCTs in relation to BMI, waist circumference, and percent of body fat. This was a long-term study involving 78 healthy men and women with an average BMI of 24.7.[12] Most of the participants had a BMI over 23—the number at which Asians are considered overweight.

This was a controlled double-blind study—the gold standard for a clinical investigation. A "controlled" diet study is one in which the participants are randomly assigned to receive either the test diet or the control diet. Double-blind means neither the subjects nor the investigators knew which group was which. This way there would be no unintentional prejudice introduced in the investigation. This is why a controlled double-blind trial is regarded as the most reliable type of study.

The subjects were divided into two groups. One group was given a diet containing MCTs and the other group LCTs. The LCTs came from a blend of canola and soybean oils and served as the control. The diet contained 2,200 total calories with 60 grams (540 calories) coming from fat, which included the test oils and the fats naturally in the foods. Total calorie intake and fat intake was stringently controlled under the guidance of dietitians.

Measurements of the subjects' body weight, waist circumference, and body fat were taken before the start of the study and at 4, 8, and 12 weeks. At each of the three stages of evaluation those participants in the MCT group whose initial BMI was 23 or more lost significantly more weight, more body fat, and more inches around their waist then their counterparts in the LCT group. At the end of 12 weeks, those in the LCT group lost on average 10.5 pounds (4.78 kg) and the MCT group lost 13.5 pounds (6.1 kg). Waist circumference in the LCT group decreased by 1.5 inches (3.7 cm) and in the MCT group 2.25 inches (5.7 cm). Body fat, as measured by a CT scan, was also more reduced in the MCT group. Keep in mind that the participants were not on a weight loss diet specifically, they were consuming 2,200 calories, which may have been a little less than some of them normally ate, particularly those who were overweight to begin with. This study demonstrated that MCTs can be used as an effective aid in weight and body fat reduction even when total calorie intake is not drastically reduced, as is common in weight reduction diets.

One interesting observation from this study is the fact that the MCT group lost more body fat around the waist. Measuring waist circumference helps screen for possible health risks that come with overweight and obesity. If most of your fat is around your waist rather than at your hips, you're at a higher risk for heart disease and type 2 diabetes. This risk goes up with a waist size that is greater than 35 inches (88 cm) for women or greater than 40 inches (102 cm) for men. Based on waist circumference, this study suggests that MCTs are superior to LCTs in protecting against heart disease and diabetes.

In addition, total cholesterol and triglyceride levels were reduced in both the MCT and LCT groups, but there was no significant difference between the groups. Even though MCTs are saturated fats, the MCT group recorded improved blood fat levels. This combined with the better results in waist circumference, body fat reduction, and weight loss demonstrate that MCTs are superior to LCTs in terms of reducing excess body fat and lowering the risk of heart disease and diabetes.

Another interesting outcome of this study was that for those participants who were not overweight, there was no significant difference in the measurements between the two groups. This suggests that if a person is already at their ideal body weight and fat percentage, adding MCTs to their diet will not cause them to become too skinny. The more overweight a person is, the more effect MCTs seem to have on fat reduction. In other words, you don't have to worry about becoming too thin by eating coconut oil.

Clinical studies coming out of Japan, China, Philippines, Australia, Canada, Germany, and Brazil comparing MCTs or coconut oil with olive oil, soybean oil, corn oil, canola oil, lard, and other oils composed of LCT have given similar results.[22-29]

MCTs have consistently shown to reduce body fat, waist circumference, and total body weight in comparison to LCTs and have produced better overall blood fat profile—lower triglycerides, lower LDL, higher HDL, and lower cholesterol ratio—all indicating a reduced risk of heart disease.

The source of MCTs used in most of these studies came from fractionated coconut oil, otherwise known as MCT oil. MCT oil is produced by removing all of the long chain fatty acids and unsaturated fatty acids from coconut oil, leaving only medium chain fatty acids, thus the name MCT oil. However, those studies that used unadulterated coconut oil produced the same results as those using MCT oil.[30]

In a few instances, investigators did not achieve the marked results seen in most of the other studies. Some possible reasons for this may be that the investigators used subjects that were normal weight, so the results would not show much change. Another possibility is that the amount of MCTs given to the subjects was not enough to invoke the anticipated response. It appears that a dose of at least 2 or 3 tablespoons a day is required to see the desirable changes in body composition during the study period (usually between a few weeks and a few months in duration). The diet, too, can also have an effect. A low-carb diet is much more effective than a high-carb diet in combination with MCTs or coconut oil.

In addition to stimulating metabolism, MCTs provide another benefit that can aid in reducing fat deposition. Studies show that MCTs and coconut oil improve insulin sensitivity.[31-32] This means that coconut oil can moderate blood sugar and insulin levels, helping to keep them within normal ranges, which is great news for diabetics and others with insulin resistance. Since insulin promotes fat synthesis and storage, moderating blood insulin levels with the use of coconut oil can help reduce fat deposition.

Researchers at the School of Dietetics and Human Nutrition at McGill University in Canada used the data from various studies that measured the metabolic boosting (e.g., calorie burning) and appetite suppressing effects of MCTs on total effective calorie intake. They then calculated what effect replacing all of the LCT based oils in a person's diet with an MCT based oil would have on total calorie consumption. Their most optimistic scenario resulted in a reduction of 346 calories per day. Their least optimistic scenario produced a reduction of 115 calories per day. Theoretically, a decrease of 500 calories a day would result in a weight loss of 1 pound per week. Projecting these calculations over a full year, the researchers estimated that simply switching from using LCT to MCTs would result in a loss of between 12 to 36 pounds (5.4 to 16.2 kg) a year![33] That's a weight loss of up to 36 pounds a year without dieting or changing the types of foods eaten. All that is required to lose the weight is to get an oil change.

Weight loss could be even greater when MCTs are combined with sensible weight-reduction diet; and would be enhanced even further with a low-carb, ketogenic diet.

COCONUT OIL AND LOW THYROID FUNCTION

When I first started writing about the benefits of coconut oil several years ago, people often reported to me how coconut oil had helped them with various health problems. They related how it could increase their metabolism and body temperature, improve digestion, relieve candida overgrowth, improve healing from injury or infection, lose excess weight, and such. I knew that using coconut oil has these effects because they are documented in the medical literature. What surprised me was that people would report improvement from many other conditions not described in the medical journals. I knew the oil was good and had many health benefits, but I was hearing things that I had never seen documented by medical research. I'm naturally skeptical about stories, and I was with these as well. You never know how accurate they are or what other events in a person's life may also have contributed to the results they experience. I made a mental note of them, but paid little attention.

174

I attributed most of these stories to the placebo effect: it was just wishful thinking on their part, or so I thought. What was interesting to me was that many people reported relief from the same conditions—irritability, insomnia, arthritis, PMS, low sex drive, food cravings, and even hypoglycemia, to mention just a few. I still didn't pay much attention and shrugged it off as just a coincidence.

I then learned about the success some doctors were having treating Wilson's thyroid syndrome. Suddenly, all these testimonials now made sense. Standard treatment for WTS involves giving the patient T3 to boost metabolism and raise body temperature. The increase in temperature allows enzymes to function more optimally, thus relieving the symptoms associated with low body temperature and WTS (see list of symptoms on pages 156-157). Coconut oil, used on a regular basis, can also raise metabolism and body temperature and improve enzyme function, thus creating a similar situation. Now I understood why so many people experienced such a wide variety of health benefits by using coconut oil. All of these symptoms are related to low thyroid function. Many people aren't even aware they have thyroid issues and attribute the symptoms to other causes. As thyroid function improves with the use of coconut oil, the symptoms fade or go away.

The advantage to coconut oil is that it's a food, rather than a medicine, and can be used safely without fear of adverse side effects and without a prescription. Coconut oil, combined with a healthy diet, can be a powerful aid to overcoming thyroid problems and associated symptoms. People who experience severe symptoms of hypothyroidism may still need thyroid hormone therapy and should check with their doctors before reducing or discontinuing their medication.

As you recall from Chapter 12, WTS can be caused by excessive stress and poor nutrition. Since coconut oil is a food, it can be eaten every day, which can help prevent relapse if severe stress hits again. Also, eating nutritious foods will supply the body with ample nutrients to protect from nutritional bankruptcy, so the body is better able to cope with stress as it should.

One health professional explained to me that when she first heard about coconut oil she couldn't believe all the claims, but then her own health problems began.

"My thyroid levels were swinging around, but not really high enough to be treated by most allopathic doctors. I felt awful, my hair was falling out, my skin was so dry it itched and cracked, my cholesterol was up, and so was my weight, ever so slowly with every passing month. In addition, my coworkers were amazed at how I can function when I am constantly sick and on antibiotics. I was a mess at a fairly young age. I did some of my own research...and kept coming up with coconut oil. Then I found your website (www.coconutresearchcenter.org) and became more convinced as I accessed the [medical] journals presented. I felt like what was I to lose? Here is what happened after taking coconut oil for several months:

175

Cholesterol dropped, HDL went way up (from 30's to almost 60). My skin is beautiful! I was having rosacea...now it is smooth and clear. My legs feel as if I am a teenager they are so smooth. I even put coconut oil around my eyes as a moisturizer. I love feeling my legs...it is almost as if I have made a discovery...I cannot believe at my age my skin can be so soft and supple. It's almost like having a flashback to my teenage years!...I feel so much more energetic, as if I was 10 years younger. My hair is beautiful and silky and not falling out....My TSH levels are way down into the normal range (not even subclinical hypothyroid anymore). WOW! The first time in over 6 years!"

Experiencing the changes was enough to convince her. The following testimonials provide a few additional examples of what people are experiencing as they have added coconut oil into their lives:

"About two weeks after taking coconut oil I noticed I was toasty warm—the thermogenic property of coconut oil no doubt. Though I've been on thyroid medication for years, it never solved my warmth problem, so the additional warmth on my hands and feet is welcome!"
Sarah

"I had many classic thyroid symptoms prior to using coconut oil, including weight gain, feeling cold, extreme fatigue and brain fog, itchy skin, rashes and acne, brittle nails, hair loss, loss of outer eyebrows (they've grown back), joint pain in my left hand, menstrual problems (periods that were heavy and lasted for two weeks), depression, allergies and asthma, dizziness, swelling in my face (looked very round), and water retention. After starting on coconut oil I'm feeling a remarkable improvement on all fronts. I truly think coconut oil is a miracle substance. I didn't have this improvement on thyroid meds alone."
C.R.H.

"I was stunned when I took my temperature yesterday morning. It was 97 degrees F! For the past two years, it has been 95.5 degrees in the morning. By evening, it was 97.8 degrees! Obviously, the coconut oil is doing something in my body!"
Mary

"I bought some coconut oil for the health benefits, and started it today, as soon as I got it. My temperature (taken as an experiment to see if the oil did raise it) the last few days has been between 97.2° to 97.6° F and after taking the oil it rose to 98.8° F and was still 98.3° F later on in the day. Have to admit this really surprised me, despite having read of it."
Carole H.

"I noticed after one week of taking VCO a substantial improvement in my energy level. My temperature that I tested every morning went from 93-94° F to NORMAL."
Jeri

"For several weeks before starting, I charted my body temps. Rarely did I go over 96°F. I am now never under 97° and more frequently over 98° F. I notice the longer I take it the more my temp is staying higher. My hair was thinning. I see new growth. White hair is darkening and the hair that is coming in is dark. My skin is soft and much less wrinkled. The liver spots on the backs of my hands are fading. My eyebrows are growing in. My nails are long and hard."
Deborah

"My doctor recently called to give me the results of my latest thyroid test, saying it was low again. She said the only time it had been normal in the past year was in July, and asked me what was I doing different then. I couldn't recall. Later it hit me that my in-laws had come to visit around then and my mother-in-law had brought me some coconut oil to try, as she had read about the benefits of it for thyroid problems. I was using it but when I ran out I stopped. I just never bothered to get more…I began religiously taking it again and called my doctor several weeks later to ask to be tested again. Sure enough, a perfect reading of 5! You can imagine my utter joy when hearing this. I continue to take it daily."
Melanie K

"It's only been about three months since I've begun using coconut oil. My skin is like a newborn babe's. My face is lovely and rosy. The bottoms of my feet are like a teenager's (I don't rub it in, I merely ingest it). For the first time in 53 plus years I am WARM as long as I use the coconut oil. And I've lost 11 pounds. My hair is beautiful! As far as I'm concerned virgin coconut oil is my miracle food."
Linda

"Since I started taking the coconut oil my temperature has come up and pretty much stayed in the 98.7° F range! And, it's only been 2 weeks…I have more energy and feel like myself again!"
Rachel

"I eat lots of virgin coconut oil. It has helped my dry skin and boosted my metabolism. It is great to eat a little oil and then get out for my walk where wind chills are within the teens. I am WARM!"
Roxanne

"Thanks to coconut oil my condition is improving. Three months ago my TSH was 20 and the doctor increased by thyroid medication. I got another test done yesterday, after taking coconut oil for three weeks and my TSH has come down significantly to 3.6."

Sam

"I'm a middle-aged woman, 54, hypothyroid, always cold with frosty hands and feet. The thing is, I'm on a natural thyroid, Synthroid didn't work for me. I lead a healthy lifestyle, exercise often, and take plenty of thyroid, so you would think I'd be warm. However, I've always been cold, even the thyroid medication couldn't help that. Nothing helped until I started eating coconut oil. After three days, I noticed a difference, but I was still skeptical. Is it really the coconut oil, I wondered? But after three weeks, there no longer is any doubt."

Sarah L.

"I experienced quite an increase in body temp (taken first thing in the morning). It raised from low 97s to 98.4-98.6° F! I don't feel near as cold as I used too, my energy levels have come back and much more stable. I don't feel the brain fogginess that I was experiencing, my hair is so soft and my nails are growing at a rapid rate! I absolutely love it."

Jen

"My basal and daytime body temperatures have improved steadily over the last 3-4 months and I notice various changes in my symptoms, e.g., my nails are very much stronger, I feel warmer/can cope with change in temperatures better, the pains in my legs have all but disappeared and my missing eyebrow has returned! All good stuff."

Kathy

"I began using virgin coconut oil after reading about it on the Internet. Even though I have hypothyroidism, my weight began to melt off me. This has been such a blessing. My daughter and son-in-law have both experienced weight loss just by adding the coconut oil to their diets. My sister, who also has hypothyroidism, is also experiencing steady weight loss. I've always had such a difficult time with my weight. Now at age 48, and with hypothyroidism, coconut oil has helped me to effortlessly lose 35 pounds! Coconut oil has sparked my fat burning metabolism!

"I've told my doctor's staff all about it and they see the proof every time I come in for my monthly visits. My doctor is amazed; he doesn't know what to think about it. After 37 years of starvation and gaining weight and the heartbreak that comes along with such a futile battle, and all this time the answer for me, my daughter, son-in-law, and sister was coconut oil."

Dana O.

178

Thyroid Medication Reduction

People on thyroid medication can expect to reduce their medication and in some cases get completely off of it. "I no longer take thyroid medication," says Jan H. "I have lost 70 pounds. I have more energy now at age 51 than I did at 20."

Lisa says, "It has only been a couple months now that I have used coconut oil and organic butter exclusively for cooking, baking, anything with heat. Within a few weeks of using the oil, my routine thyroid blood levels were drawn, and for the first time in 12 years, my Synthroid medication needed to be lowered from 150 mcg to 112 mcg. Sorry, but there is absolutely nothing in 12 years that has ever brought my levels down, and now I am hoping to see if they will be lower on the next test, with the hope that I could get off the drug."

If you are taking medication for hypothyroidism, be prepared to lower your dosage. The coconut oil and ketogenic diet will boost thyroid health normalizing thyroid function. As the thyroid starts functioning better, your medication can become too potent, causing the thyroid to become overactive. Hyperthyroid symptoms may develop. If you start feeling nervous, agitated, have difficulty sleeping, or your heart starts racing, you know that you need to reduce your medication.

"I'm 46 years old and have been diagnosed with Hashimoto's thyroiditis," says Carol. "I started using coconut oil a couple of months ago and immediately I began to feel better. It's been miraculous! About a month ago I began feeling dizzy. After some resistance from my doctor (it took 4 weeks), he agreed to retest my TSH, which now is 0.01—putting me in the hyperthyroid range! My doctor reduced my Synthroid dose from 50 mcg to 25 mcg, and said that we'll take it one step at a time, but agreed that I may be able to get off Synthroid and rely exclusively on coconut oil to treat my hypothyroidism."

"My entire family has thyroid disease," says Rischa. "Most of us test within the 'normal' range, while having persistent symptoms." Rischa suffered from years of hypothyroidism despite taking Synthroid plus Cytomel—the most potent form of thyroid medication. When she learned about coconut oil she began taking 2 tablespoons a day, but gradually increased it to 4. Within a couple of weeks she began to experience unusual symptoms. "It hit me like a sledge hammer," she says. "My pulse was racing and a few other fun hyperthyroid symptoms."

She realized that her metabolism was now running too fast. "So I lowered my thyroid meds! I reduced my Synthroid from 225 mcg to about 100 mcg and reduced my Cytomel by half! I felt fine all day and so decided to continue at the reduced dosage. I had read of other people who have regained their health through using coconut oil, and had their thyroids return to normal functioning, even after years of medicating, like me…The results were incredible! I had no idea that this would happen so fast." Under her doctor's watchful eye, she was able to get completely off her medication. "It is like a miracle how different I feel," she says, "I am amazed!"

When Marcy B. sensed her heart racing she headed to the hospital. "I was nervous, aggravated, and my shoulder was hurting. I thought I was having a heart attack." An examination found nothing wrong with her heart but what they did find was totally unexpected—she was suffering from symptoms of hyperthyroidism. "My thyroid had done a flip! I have been hypothyroid for 35 years. Now I am hyperthyroid!" Just a few weeks earlier she had started using coconut oil. She was aware it was supposed to help with low thyroid but was completely shocked at the dramatic results. She asked the doctor about it, but he didn't have a clue. Her prescription for thyroid medication was reduced from 225 mcg to 100 mcg. "I am very pleased that my thyroid is not needing as much medicine," she says.

"Eighteen years ago I was diagnosed with hypothyroidism," says Binky. "I've been on a pretty consistent dosage of 150 mcg of thyroid medication ever since. What happened recently is nothing short of amazing. My thyroid started getting better! As of today, I am at ¼ the dose and I suspect this is still a bit high. It is amazing that this happened."

Coconut oil can work so well in some people at improving thyroid function that some ask: does it ever cause the thyroid to become too active and cause hyperthyroidism? The answer is no. Coconut oil normalizes thyroid function, drugs speed it up. As your thyroid function improves, drugs that you may be taking may no longer be necessary, or they may need to be reduced. Under your doctor's supervision you may gradually reduce your medication as needed.

Some people are able to get off thyroid medications completely, others can get off medication but still need to take coconut oil regularly, others can greatly reduce thyroid medication but still need to take coconut oil. Even those who have had their thyroid glands removed can benefit.

"I have been having a lot of trouble sleeping but I never made the connection," says Nina. "Yesterday I got tested for thyroid levels and my dose is currently too high. Because of VCO, I am able to reduce my thyroid medication. (I have no thyroid gland so I will always need thyroid medication.)"

If you have had your thyroid removed, you cannot make thyroid hormones and must take thyroid medication for life. However, adding coconut into your diet can reduce the amount you need.

METABOLISM BOOSTERS

In addition to coconut oil, there are other ways you can boost your metabolism and jumpstart thyroid activity. This section covers some additional things you can do, along with taking coconut oil, to revitalize your metabolism.

Sunlight

You may wonder why a book on weight loss would include a section on sunlight. Believe it or not, sunlight can help you lose weight! Yes, lying on the beach under the sun is one way your body can shed excess body fat. What a marvelous way to lose weight! Perhaps that's why sunbathers are so thin? It certainly isn't the only reason, but sunbathing can help.

Sunlight has more influence on health than most of us realize. Getting an adequate amount of exposure to full sunlight is critical for the activation of enzymes and the production of certain hormones necessary for many chemical processes that occur in your body. A lack of sun exposure can cause multiple enzyme dysfunction and the undersecretion of hormones that influence metabolism and body temperature. Too little sun can actually contribute to insulin resistance.[34]

Sunlight influences our health by the chemical and electrical activities it ignites in our skin and our brain. For example, when light enters the eye, millions of light-sensitive cells called photoreceptors convert the light into electrical impulses. These impulses travel along the optic nerve to the brain where they trigger the hypothalamus gland to send chemical messages to regulate the autonomic (involuntary) functions of the body. The hypothalamus releases hormones that control the activity of other glands, including the thyroid gland. If the hypothalamus is underactive due to a lack of sunlight, the thyroid gland will also be underactive.

Ultraviolet (UV) radiation from the sun activates enzymes that convert cholesterol into vitamin D. Foods are generally a poor source of vitamin D. The vast majority of the vitamin D in our bodies comes from exposure to sunlight. Low vitamin D levels are common in people with hypothyroidism. Vitamin D is necessary for thyroid hormone production. It must also be present in sufficient quantities inside our cells in order for thyroid hormones to actually affect the cell. This is crucial because without adequate vitamin D there is little thyroid hormone activity. A lack of sunlight and vitamin D can lead to low thyroid function and depressed metabolism.

It's not so hard to recognize the importance sunlight has on health. We see and feel the sun's influence every day. Haven't you ever noticed an increase in energy or a positive mood when you go outside on a bright sunny day? In contrast, you may notice a lack of enthusiasm or feel tired or depressed when it is overcast and dark.

These effects are clearly evident in plants. Shine some light on a dormant plant and it will spring to life. Sunlight activates enzymes in plants, stimulating metabolism, growth, and activity. A lack of sunlight causes plants to go dormant and humans and animals to sleep or hibernate. Without sunlight plants shrivel up and die, and so do we.

During the winter when the sun's rays are less intense and often blocked by clouds, people are known to develop a condition called seasonal affective disorder (SAD), also known as the "winter blues." The symptoms of SAD are depression, irritability, excess sleeping and eating, weight gain, and lowered sex drive. Exposure to sunlight reverses these symptoms.

Your body requires full sunlight. Artificial lighting is not adequate, and research shows it may even be detrimental. Natural sunlight contains a full spectrum of light wavelengths, from infrared to ultraviolet (UV). Each wavelength carries a different level of energy and has a different effect on body tissues. Artificial lighting, both incandescent and fluorescent, lacks the complete balanced spectrum of sunlight.

An analogy can be made between light and nutrients in foods. Natural foods contain a wide variety of vitamins and minerals. When foods are processed, many of these nutrients are removed. Natural sunlight contains a full spectrum of light wavelengths, while artificial light does not. When any wavelength of light is missing, the light becomes imbalanced and can affect health, just as if a food were missing an important nutrient such as vitamin C. That's why artificial lighting is not an adequate replacement for natural sunlight.

Another reason artificial lighting is inferior is because it is far weaker. Most buildings, even with windows, have a light level of 500 lux (lux is the international unit of illumination). Outdoor light has a level of about 50,000 lux, or approximately 100 times more. At night, or in offices where artificial lighting is the only light source, the level drops to 50 lux.

Our body's optimal absorption of vitamins and minerals requires full spectrum sunlight. Windows, windshields, eyeglasses, smog, clouds, and sunscreen all filter out parts of the light spectrum. Research reveals that if some wavelengths aren't present in light, the body can't fully absorb certain nutrients.[35]

Many of us spend 90 percent or more of our time inside buildings or cars, shielded from direct sunlight. Without adequate sunlight, enzyme activity slows down, hormone production tapers off, and nutrients are not properly utilized. The result is a long list of health problems, many of which are the same as for hypothyroidism, including weight gain.

If your metabolism is slow because you don't get enough direct sunlight, taking medications isn't going to help. You need to get out into the sun every day. Sunbathe if you can. Any exposure will be of benefit. I recommend you get at least 15-30 minutes of direct sun every day.

Some people hesitate to go out into the sun for fear of developing skin cancer. Like saturated fat, sunlight has been unjustly criticized in the past as a health hazard. We are warned to avoid overexposure to sunlight because it may cause cancer. Some fanatics even recommend total avoidance of the sun. Research now shows moderate exposure to sunlight is not only harmless, but necessary for good health and can actually protect you from cancer. You don't need to fear sunlight.

A study carried out by the US Navy compared the risk of melanoma— the deadliest form of skin cancer, for different naval occupations. It was

182

discovered that those with indoor jobs had the highest incidence of melanoma, while those who worked at least part of the time outdoors had the lowest rate. In addition, a higher rate of melanoma occurred on the trunk of the body which was covered by clothing, as opposed to the head and arms which are more likely to be exposed to sunlight. The study stated that the location of the melanomas suggest a protective role for regular exposure to sunlight.[36]

Studies also show vitamin D suppresses the growth of malignant melanoma cells. A vitamin D deficiency caused by a lack of adequate exposure to sunlight, therefore, can promote melanoma formation.[37] This is consistent with other studies that have shown that sunlight has a protective effect against many forms of cancer. For example, researchers at Johns Hopkins University Medical School in Baltimore, Maryland, showed that exposure to full-spectrum light, including UV light, is positively related to the prevention of breast, colon, and rectal cancers.[36]

Exercise

One of the best things you can do to boost your metabolism, improve insulin sensitivity, lose weight, and look better is to exercise regularly. Not only will exercise help you burn off fat, it will help you keep it off. Exercise is the strongest predictor of long-term success in weight management. *The Physician and Sportsmedicine* journal reported that 90 percent of women who have lost weight and kept it off exercise on a regular basis. In another study published in the same journal, weight-regain patterns were reported in 40 women who had lost weight in a 16-week treatment program. Over the year that followed treatment, researchers found that the most active third of the participants lost additional weight. The middle third, who exercised about half as much, maintained their full end-of-treatment weight loss. The least active third, in contrast, steadily gained weight throughout the year after treatment.

While engaged in a physical activity, our body's need for energy increases. Consequently, metabolism and the rate at which calories are burned increase. Breathing and heart rate increase, your body becomes warmer, everything is running at an accelerated rate. When sitting down and relaxed, a 150-pound man burns about 82 calories an hour. But when involved in a physical activity, like walking (3 mph/4.8 kph), the rate increases to 225 calories an hour. That's an additional 143 calories that are burned off. Jogging (7.5 mph/12 kph) increases the rate to 510 calories an hour.

Even better: once exercise is ended, metabolism remains elevated and fat continues to be burned at an accelerated rate. Evidence suggests that metabolism is stimulated by about 25 percent for as long as 3 hours after intensive exercise and may still be running 10 percent faster two days later. You will be burning off extra calories even while you're relaxing in front of the television.

Lean, muscular people generally have a higher metabolic rate than out of shape, overweight people. It's not because they were born that way, but because muscle tissue consumes calories at a higher rate than does fatty tissue. The more muscle you have, the more calories your body burns. Each additional pound of muscle uses about 50 extra calories per day. This may not seem like much, but it adds up significantly. In one year that amounts to 18,000 fewer calories worth of fat hanging off your body. This is equivalent to a little more than 5 pounds (2.3 kg) . This is 5 pounds of excess fat that is burned off without any additional effort on your part. One of the best ways to build muscle mass is through weightlifting or resistance training. A typical weightlifting program can add 3 pounds (1.4 kg) of muscle in about 3 months. In 1 year, 3 additional pounds of lean muscle tissue would burn off an extra 55,000 calories or the equivalent of almost 16 pounds (7.2 kg) of fat.

You don't need to join a bodybuilding class, start jogging 10 miles every day or sign up for a high-impact aerobics class to start losing weight. You can do those things if you are physically up to it, but you don't need to. Exercise doesn't need to be a grueling, tedious, or exhausting affair. It can be enjoyable even for those who are unathletic. I recommend starting off with walking, rebounding, or swimming. These are activities most people can participate in, regardless of their fitness level.

Walking outside, especially among trees and foliage, adds a dimension to the activity that increases its enjoyment and allows you to soak up the sunshine and boost your vitamin D levels. On cold or raining days, you can do mall walking. With the abundance of shopping malls, mall walking has become a popular activity, especially with older people. Malls are relatively safe and weatherproof. The shops and people give the walk an added dimension of interest.

Since most people who are concerned about weight loss are physically inactive, I recommend starting out slowly. Walk at a leisurely pace for 15 or 20 minutes the first day you start. Stick to 15 or 20 minutes a day, five to six days a week for the first week. After one week, add 5 minutes to your walk. The following week, add another 5 minutes. Keep adding 5 minutes each week until your walks last a between 30-60 minutes.

Most fitness experts recommend the walking pace to be brisk. This would be 3 miles (4.8 km) per hour or more. Once you're up to 30 minutes a day at a leisurely pace, you can focus on speed. Three miles per hour is not that fast, but it's not leisurely either. Plan your course by driving it in your car and recording the distance. You can judge your speed by how fast you cover the distance you've plotted. At 3 mph you would walk a quarter of a mile every 5 minutes. You cover 1 mile in 20 minutes, a mile and a half in 30 minutes, 2 miles in 40 minutes, and 3 miles in 60 minutes. If you can't go that fast, do whatever you can.

Set goals for yourself and strive for improvement. Your first short-term goal may be to do 20 minutes a day for a week. Another goal would be to reach 30 minutes a day. One of your primary goals should be to strive for 30 minutes a day, 5 days a week, at 3 mph (abbreviated as 30-5-3). The 30-5-3 is a goal everyone should shoot for and maintain as a *minimum* amount of exercise.

Once you've reached the 30-5-3 goal and feel comfortable with it you may consider lengthening out the time, increasing the number of days, or increasing your speed. The Institute for Aerobics Research recommends the following:

Minimum For Moderate Fitness
Women: Walk 2 miles (3.2 km) in 30 minutes or less 3 days a week, or walk 2 miles in 30-40 minutes 5-6 days a week.
Men: Walk 2 miles in 27 minutes or less at least 3 days a week, or walk 2 miles in 30-40 minutes 6-7 days a week.

Minimum For High Fitness
Women: Walk 2 miles (3.2 km) in 30 minutes 5-6 days a week.
Men: Walk 2.5 miles (4 km) in 38 minutes 6-7 days a week.

To add variety to your exercise routine you may want to mix it up a bit by doing different types of exercises on different days—walking, swimming, rebounding, and such. Since muscle mass burns more calories than fat, you might want to add weight training or resistance training into your schedule, as it is the best way to build muscle.

Heat

Saunas or hot baths can elevate your body temperature much like exercise. If the water or steam is hot enough to raise the body's temperature a few degrees, it can remain elevated for a time afterward. The effects of hot baths are short lived, but can be helpful in raising the body's temperature, at least for a couple of hours. During this time, sluggish enzymes will be kicked into high gear and bodily processes will run at a heightened level of activity.

Heat therapy has been in use for thousands of years. The effects of stimulating the metabolism have proven useful in cleansing toxins from the body and speeding recovery from illness. Our bodies' own process of fighting infections involves producing a fever to increase circulation and stimulate cellular and glandular activity.

If you have access to a sauna or steam bath at a spa or health club, take advantage of it. If you don't, a bathtub filled with hot water will also work. Simply sitting in a tub of hot water or taking a hot shower, however, does not work! You need to be completely submerged, except for your head, and the water must be hot enough to raise your body temperature up to about 100° F (37.8° C).

To do this, start filling the bathtub with hot water, but not hot enough to burn yourself. Sit in the tub as it is filling up, keeping the water as hot as you can tolerate. Filling the tub in this way will help your body adjust to the temperature. After the tub is filled to capacity, turn off the water and submerge your entire body, keeping only your head above water. Relax and rest your head on a towel. While you soak and as the water cools, you can drain some out and add fresh hot water to keep the temperature as hot as necessary. Usually as your body adjusts to the heat, you can withstand a little more hot water. Even though you are covered with water, your body will sweat profusely. Remain in the bath for 20-30 minutes.

A major problem with many bathtubs is that they are too small. In order to make this effective, the entire body, except for the head, needs to be submerged. Many bathtubs are not big enough to do this. One solution to this problem is to buy a plastic sheet, available in various lengths at garden supply stores, and drape it over the tub, water, and yourself like a blanket. You do not wrap it around your body or put it in the water with you. It covers the top of the tub to seal in heat. This way if your knees or toes stick out of the water they will still keep warm.

FACTORS THAT AFFECT METABOLISM

Metabolism Depressors
Nutrient deficient diet
Drugs (e.g. sulfa drugs, antihistamines, antidepressants, beta blockers)
Consuming excessive amounts of raw cruciferous vegetables
Consuming soy products, with the exception of fermented soy
Low-calorie diets
Low-fat diets
Consuming excessive amounts of sugar and other simple carbohydrates
Fluorine (e.g. toothpaste, mouthwash, tea, non-stick cookware, tap water)
Bromine (e.g. baked goods, soda, insecticides)
Iodine deficiency

Metabolism Stimulators
Eating a wholesome diet containing a wide variety of nutrients, including
   fat and protein
Drinking adequate water to prevent dehydration
Coconut oil
Consume sources of iodine regularly (e.g. sea salt, sea food, supplements)
Regular exercise
Regular exposure to sunshine
Occasional sauna/hot baths
Adding hot peppers and cayenne pepper into the diet

Keep the plastic off your face. The head should be left exposed to cool air. This will allow you to remain in the water longer, gaining the full benefits. If you get a headache, the water is too hot. Cool it down with some cold water and apply a cold wet washcloth to your forehead as you soak. You want to heat your body up to about 100° F (37.8° C). This is only 1.4° F (0.8° C) above normal. A healthy person can easily handle temperatures up to 104° F (40° C), so there is no need to worry about overheating yourself at 100° F. Use a thermometer to regulate your temperature. If you get too hot, cool down the tub. If you're not hot enough, add more hot water.

Even though you are submerged in water you will do a lot of sweating. The sweat glands can secrete nearly a full pint of water in 15 minutes, so you need to drink plenty of water. Drink a full glass of water before bathing and another glass afterwards. Do not drink cold water because it will cool your body down. Sweating removes salt and minerals from the body, so you should make sure to replenish them by eating an adequate amount of sea salt and taking a mineral supplement afterwards.

To take full advantage of your elevated temperature created by the bath, avoid activities immediately afterwards that will cool you down, such as going out in cold air or consuming cold foods or beverages. Hot baths are relaxing. It is best to do this in the evening so you can relax or go to bed afterwards.

Heat therapy can have a dramatic effect on the body. Those who have multiple sclerosis, hyperthyroidism, hypertension, or serious heart conditions should consult a health professional before trying it.

Chili Peppers

Have you ever broken out in a sweat after indulging in some fiery hot chili or a taco that had a little too much hot sauce? The heat your mouth feels when you indulge in spicy Mexican, Thai, and Indian cuisines comes from chili peppers. There are hundreds of varieties of pepper ranging from the mild bell pepper and the moderately hot poblano, to the hotter jalapeno and the super hot habanero. What makes chilies so hot is a heat-generating compound called capsaicin. The more capsaicin the pepper has, the hotter it is. Bell peppers have none, habaneros have a lot.

If scientists wanted to create a pill that could instantly boost metabolism and encourage the burning of excess calories, they would have to look no further than the chili pepper. Rather than eating them in pill form, chilies are combined with other foods as a flavoring. They can be consumed fresh, dried and powdered, or minced or juiced to form a sauce. Adding a little powdered cayenne pepper to your foods is a convenient way to spice up your meals and reap the benefits these little chilies have to offer.

Chili peppers are thermogenic foods, meaning they are foods that create heat. Calories are simply a measure of heat. When you eat chili, you turn up the body's metabolic furnace and burn more calories. Spicy foods can speed

187

up your metabolism for up to five hours after eating, enough to keep your internal engines running in a higher gear until your next meal.

In addition to burning off more calories, spicy foods moderate the effects that carbohydrates have on blood sugar levels. After eating a spicy meal, blood glucose levels are significantly lower than they are after the same meal without the chilies.[38] This effect has led some researchers to propose the use of chilies as an aid in moderating insulin resistance and in treating type 2 diabetes.[39]

That's not all. Eating spicy foods can also help you eat less by curbing your appetite. When chili pepper is added to meals, hunger is satisfied sooner and a desire to eat is delayed for a longer time afterwards. In one study, for example, subjects who were fed a breakfast with red chilies ate less during the meal and less at lunchtime in comparison to subjects who ate the same food without the peppers. Even when the breakfast was loaded with carbohydrate, which normally digests so quickly that hunger quickly returns, the chili prolonged the feeling of satiety.[40]

Studies have shown that chili peppers provide many health benefits; in addition to boosting metabolism, moderating blood sugar and insulin levels, and curbing appetite, which can all aid in weight loss, they have shown to have strong antioxidant properties, fight inflammation, improve digestion and nutrient absorption, reduce risk of heart attack, and protect against stomach cancer.

Can't tolerate spicy hot food? Don't worry. You don't need to use so much that it sets your tongue on fire and brings tears to your eyes. Smaller, more manageable portions can still work wonders, and over time, you will develop a greater tolerance and appreciation for the heat. If you are unaccustomed to eating spicy foods, you can start off slowly. Sprinkle a little cayenne pepper on your eggs, meat, or vegetables and add more as your tolerance grows. Eating spicy foods is certainly not a requirement for losing weight on a ketogenic diet, but for some people it can be helpful, especially for those who are suffering with low thyroid function and need that metabolic boost.

WHAT ARE PEOPLE SAYING?

"I've gone from tears and a life of despair over my weight, to a young, healthy, vibrant 34-year-old," says Danielle Johnson of Sault Sainte Marie, Canada. At 360 pounds, doctors told Danielle that she was at risk for heart disease and a host of other life-threatening problems. She tried all the weight loss diets—Slim Fast, Nutrisystem, Weight Watchers, South Beach, Relacore, and others without success. "I was desperate to find the answer to my lifelong weight problem," she said. "Then I discovered the coconut cure." A healthy low-carb diet, coconut oil, spicy foods, and apple cider vinegar kicked her metabolism "through the roof," she says. In just the first week she lost 13 pounds. "I'm running around here doing housework like a maniac and I can't sit still. My metabolism is so revved up and my cravings have totally vanished."

Super metabolism and easy weight loss were not the only benefits she was experiencing, many chronic health problems were also beginning to disappear. "I no longer feel the aches and pains from fibromyalgia associated with my weight. I am a type 2 diabetic and my blood glucose levels have dropped significantly. I also notice that the white powder on my feet that diabetics often get, has also disappeared. I can't say enough about this cure. It's not hocus pocus, like some may believe. I was a skeptic at first, like most, but I opened up my mind to it because I'd tried so many other treatments for my obesity. I figured it was worth a shot. I was currently on a waiting list for gastric bypass surgery, which I will no longer be needing."

Danielle takes 3 tablespoons of organic raw apple cider vinegar along with her coconut oil every day, before each meal. "I have abolished sweeteners and have turned to stevia to sweeten my tea just a little. Last but not least, I incorporate hot peppers and cayenne pepper into my diet. This tactic raises my body's basal temperature and kick starts my metabolism. I've noticed that I no longer have a problem with acid-reflux or constipation. I have lost that bloated, distended feeling—it's truly wonderful."

Here are a few more comments from people who have added coconut oil into their daily lives.

"I have been sticking with your plan for thyroid health. About three days ago (three weeks into the plan and 6 weeks into using coconut oil) I just started feeling so much better. My energy level is so high now; much, much higher than it has been in my whole life (54 years). I have really come out of my slump. I thank you from the depths of my heart. This is such a miracle for me. I will continue with your plan using it as a lifelong guide."
Stephanie G.

"My temperature was very low (95 degrees F). I just told everyone I am a 'cool' person. When I found that a sluggish thyroid can lower the body temperature I wanted to do something about it. I found out about coconut oil and started consuming it (3-4 tbsp with my meals). And in one week (I am not exaggerating), my always low temperature began to rise. It is normal now. Sometimes it ranges from 98.2 -98.6 degrees F now. I must say I could not believe the thermometer. So I am really sold by this coconut oil thing."
Jessie

"I was diagnosed with Hashimoto's and was put on Synthroid. Once I started the drug I still felt hypothyroid and I was still pretty tired. I started taking the VCO about 2 months ago and I became hyperthyroid. So my doctor took me off the Synthroid and the hyperthyroid went away in about

2 days and now all I do is the VCO…I have energy like you cannot believe. And before even on the Synthroid I was still sleeping way too much and felt tired most of the time…It seems to have jumpstarted my thyroid into working on its own again. My doctor was quite impressed and is now recommending it to all his patients."

Danne H.

"I have been carrying around quite a few extra pounds for years and was caught up in the yo-yo dieting cycle. I made lifestyle changes which mean eating healthy and exercising regularly, but never really saw a consistent weight loss. I had thyroid tests run and they were always "normal." Well, a few weeks ago I started adding coconut oil to my diet and a miracle has happened. I've been losing two pounds a week without really trying , which tells me that my thyroid function wasn't as "normal" as they told me it was. I have more energy and just feel better."

Irene

"Virgin coconut oil is working for me. My second (six-month delayed) thyroid test results came back with levels improved and in the safe zone. Coconut oil, apart from making me feel so much better, has saved me from thyroid medication. My doctor was extremely skeptical about using coconut oil (it's in his never to be used basket) and was surprised at not only the thyroid results but also my improvement in cholesterol levels and blood sugar levels. Still skeptical about coconut oil, he could only say, 'Whatever you are doing, keep doing it.'"

Cleve

"My temp has continued to rise and this morning was up to 97.5° F (from a pre-VCO low of 96.2 only 10 days ago)…I've been eating a low-carb, high-fat diet for three years, so am no stranger to satiety from plenty of good fats in my meals, but I'm struggling to include 3.5 tbs VCO because it makes me over-full for hours and hours! I've tried cutting back with other foods, which helps a bit, but I can still barely face dinner five hours after lunch!"

Katy

"I feel fantastic! This is the first time in years that I have felt well and healthy. I have been troubled with hypothyroidism for 5-6 years now, and NOTHING has worked until now. As you can imagine, I am ecstatic! I keep thinking that the next day I will again feel badly, and have no energy, so far that has not happened. I have lost 4½ pounds last week. That in itself is a wonderful sign that this plan is working."

Pat

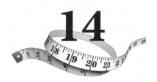

14

Drink More, Weigh Less

"Drink plenty of water." You've probably heard that advice a hundred times, but do you follow it? How much water do you drink each day? I mean real water—pure water without flavorings, sweeteners, and other chemicals added. Three glasses? One glass perhaps? Maybe none at all? That's fairly typical. As incredible as it may sound, one of the reasons you may be overweight is because you don't drink enough water.

Of all the food and beverages we consume, water is by far the most important. Although it contains no calories and provides no energy, it is considered our most vital nutrient. Our bodies require a constant source of water throughout the day in order to maintain bodily functions and to sustain life. We can live for several weeks and even months without other nutrients, but if completely deprived of water we would die of dehydration in a matter of days. A lack of adequate water is, in essence, a death sentence.

Approximately 60 percent of our body weight is from water. Every function inside the body is regulated by and depends upon water. Water must be available in sufficient quantities to adequately transport nutrients, oxygen, hormones, and other chemicals to all parts of the body. Water lubricates our joints, protects our brain, facilitates digestion and elimination, and provides the medium in which all chemical reactions in the body occur. Water is so important to the proper function of the body that even a small reduction from normal can have a dramatic effect on your health.

Water has another very important purpose. It is necessary in the right amount in order to regulate and manage weight. Many people are overweight because they don't drink enough water. Yes, part of the reason you may be overweight is because you don't drink enough pure, clean water. Diets that ignore fluid intake or that cause the loss of water are dangerously unhealthy!

Dieting should improve health, not destroy it. A proper diet that recognizes the importance of water can help you lose weight and improve your health.

THE ELIXIR OF LIFE
The Discovery Made in Prison

Surprisingly, the importance of water in weight management and health in general was discovered by Dr. Fereydoon Batmanghelidj while he was serving time at Evin Prison in Iran. After graduating from medical school in London and working for a time in England, Dr. Batmanghelidj returned to Iran, where he was born, to help the people of his country. In 1979 a violent revolution swept a new government into power. Almost all professional and creative people who had stayed in the country were rounded up and jailed as political prisoners. Dr. Batmanghelidj was among them.

The prison in which he was placed was built to hold only 600, but quickly overflowed with 9,000 inmates. Trained medical personnel were scarce, so Dr. Batmanghelidj was given the responsibility of caring for the sick. The prisoners' health was not a high priority with the new government, and consequently, medical supplies were woefully inadequate.

Dr. Batmanghelidj wasn't there long when an inmate racked with excruciating stomach pain was brought to him. The man was suffering from peptic ulcer disease and pleaded for something to stop the pain. Dr. Batmanghelidj had nothing at his disposal that would help. The cries of agony from the man were so disturbing that in desperation Batmanghelidj gave him two glasses of water. He simply didn't know what else to do. To his surprise, within minutes the man's pain disappeared. He told the patient to drink two glasses of water every few hours. The man did so and remained free from pain and disease for the rest of his time in prison.

This was Dr. Batmanghelidj's introduction to the role water can play in health and healing. Had medications been available they would have been used and Dr. Batmanghelidj would probably have never discovered the dangers of chronic dehydration and the importance of water.

Sometime later, after a few medications became available, a similar experience occurred with another inmate. Walking past a jail cell Batmanghelidj spotted a man curled up on the floor of his cell semi-conscious crying in pain. He had an ulcer that was nearly killing him. Batmanghelidj asked the inmate if he had done anything to relieve the pain. He said he had taken three Tagamets and a full bottle of antacid, but the pain only got worse. Remembering his previous experience, Dr. Batmanghelidj gave the man two glasses of water. Within 10 minutes the pain subsided. He had him drink another glass and within four minutes the pain stopped completely. This patient had taken a huge amount of ulcer medication without results, but after drinking only three glasses of water the pain was gone and he was up socializing with his friends.

192

These instances prompted Dr. Batmanghelidj to start researching the effects of water on health. For nearly 3 years he treated countless numbers of patients for a variety of illnesses using ordinary tap water and nothing else. The government, impressed with his work, released him from prison. He immediately immigrated to the United States where he continued his research and wrote a book titled Your Body's Many Cries for Water. Dr. Batmanghelidj claims that many of the degenerative illnesses we suffer from today are to a large extent caused by chronic dehydration. He has treated many thousands of patients with water and has witnessed complete recovery of those suffering from an assortment of conditions such as high blood pressure, migraine headaches, arthritis, asthma, back pain, chronic constipation, colitis, heartburn, chronic fatigue syndrome, and even obesity. Yes, overweight problems can be treated with water.

Dr. Batmanghelidj claims that every single one of these conditions can be caused by dehydration. Severe dehydration is so destructive it causes quick death. But chronic low-grade dehydration causes disease which can lead to a slow death. Health deteriorates so slowly we don't realize what's happening. We attribute it to age. He maintains that most of us are chronically dehydrated because we don't drink enough water. Dehydration causes damage to cells which leads to inflammation, swelling, and pain. Each individual's response to dehydration differs depending on his or her own chemical and physical makeup. For some it manifests itself first as arthritis, and in others migraine headaches. Arthritis occurs when joints become dehydrated and tissue damage occurs. Back pain occurs when discs between vertebrae become dehydrated: as a result, bones and muscles twist out of alignment, causing stress.

A study published in the British Medical Association journal *Annals of the Rheumatic Diseases* (July, 2000) found that people who drank more than 3 cups of coffee a day were twice as likely of getting arthritis as those who drank less. This study confirms Dr. Batmanghelidj's observations. Rheumatoid arthritis is more prevalent in coffee drinkers because coffee has a dehydrating effect. Arthritis is considered incurable by conventional medical standards, yet Dr. Batmanghelidj has done what seems to be the impossible. He's cured many people of arthritis by simply having them drink more water and less coffee, tea, and other beverages.

Other researchers have noted that drinking too little water increases the risk of kidney stones, breast cancer, colon cancer, bladder cancer, obesity, mitral valve prolapse (a heart condition), and physical and mental health.[1]

Chronic Dehydration

The US Institutes of Medicine recommends that we should drink at least eight glasses of water a day. This is the amount the body loses from perspiration, respiration, and elimination every day. This is the minimum amount you should consume each day.

We often hear the recommendation of drinking eight glasses of water a day, but how big is a glass? Is it 4 ounces, 8 ounces, or 12 ounces? The amount of water you need depends on your size. A large person needs more water than a smaller person. A general rule of thumb is to drink 1 quart (1,000 ml) of water for every 60 pounds (30 kg) of bodyweight. A 120-pound (55 kg) person, therefore, needs to drink at least 2 quarts (2,000 ml) of water a day. A 210-pound person needs 3½ quarts (3,300 ml). Also, if you are physically active, if you live in a dry or hot climate, if it is summer, or if you eat foods or beverages that have a diuretic effect, then you need to drink more than this. Most people don't drink enough and suffer from mild chronic dehydration.

Chances are, you are chronically dehydrated right now. But you may say, "I'm not dehydrated, I drink lots of fluids during the day and don't feel particularly thirsty." That's just the problem! You don't have to feel thirsty in order to be dehydrated. As a consequence, most of us don't drink enough, and what we do drink is usually coffee, soda, or some other beverage rather than water.

The sensation of thirst, like many other physiological processes, becomes less active as we age.[2] This doesn't mean we don't need as much water when we're older; it means we don't have the urge to drink as much as we should. As a result, many older people are dehydrated without even knowing it. Dehydration is so common among the elderly that it has been identified as one of the most frequent causes for hospitalization for people over 65. In one study, half of those hospitalized for dehydration died within a year of admission. Even though these patients knew dehydration was a problem for them, they still weren't drinking enough. Without the sensation of thirst, we tend not to drink.

While the elderly are most at risk, they aren't the only ones who suffer from chronic dehydration. Often, we become so busy at work and in our everyday lives that we don't take the time to satisfy thirst. We put it off until it's more convenient. Ignoring the thirst reflex dulls this sensation. We become so accustomed to ignoring the body's subtle signals of thirst that we don't realize we are becoming dehydrated. So even relatively young people can and do become chronically dehydrated.

Another problem is that we often satisfy thirst with beverages rather than water. Many people mistakenly believe that coffee, tea, soda, and juice are just as good as water. They're not. Keep in mind that it's water that the cells of your body need and want, not soda pop. If you drink caffeinated beverages to quench your thirst you are not satisfying the body's need for water. Caffeine and sugar will cause the body to become more dehydrated. If the beverage is again consumed to quench thirst, the problem can escalate. For every beverage you drink, you need to add at least half as much extra water to your 8 glass requirement just to stay equal; if you don't, you will become dehydrated. Only water hydrates the body and cures dehydration.

A study by the National Research Council revealed that on average, women (ages 15-49) drink a mere 2.6 cups (615 ml) of water a day.[3] Most of their fluids come from beverages. This finding suggests that a large portion of women may be chronically dehydrated. Another study performed by researchers at Johns Hopkins Hospital in Baltimore discovered that as much as 41 percent of men and women ages 23-44 are chronically dehydrated to one degree or another.[4] Some food consumption surveys indicate that as much as 75 percent of the population (all ages) is chronically mildly dehydrated.

Dehydration of as little as a one percent decrease in body weight, results in impaired physiological function, including cardiovascular performance and temperature regulation.[5-7] Normally, a sensation of thirst manifests after the body has reached a level of dehydration of 0.8-2 percent loss of body weight.[8-9] At this point the body is in a mild state of dehydration. If this situation persists, it can become chronic. Even mild chronic dehydration is dangerous and has many adverse effects on body function and performance. Studies have shown that a two percent loss of water results in significant reductions of arithmetic ability and short-term memory.[10] If a 150 pound (68 kg) person loses two percent of his or her body weight (3 lbs/1.3 kg), mental as well as physical performance will decrease by 20 percent.[11-12]

Usually drinking a glass or two of water can relieve mild dehydration. If the level of dehydration is greater than three percent of body weight, complete rehydration requires more than just drinking a glass of water. Complete rehydration in this case would require many glasses of water over an 18-24 hour period.[13]

The role of water in maintaining good health has been recognized since ancient times. Hippocrates, the father of medicine, recommended increasing the consumption of water to treat and prevent kidney stones. Doctors today also recommend drinking more water for the same purpose. Approximately 12-15 percent of the population will develop kidney stones at some time in their lives.[14-15] The prevalence of kidney stones is higher in those who are chronically dehydrated. While several factors, such as age and climate, may influence stone formation, adjusting water consumption is a simple preventative measure that has proven successful since the days of Hippocrates.

It appears that if you want to avoid cancer, or at least some forms of cancer, you should be drinking plenty of water every day. As simple as it sounds, just drinking five glasses of water can reduce the risk of colon cancer by 45 percent, urinary tract cancer (bladder, prostate, kidney, testicle) by 50 percent, and breast cancer by 79 percent.

One of the most common problems associated with chronic dehydration is constipation. A healthy, well-hydrated individual should have a full bowel movement at least once, if not twice, a day. If you eat three meals a day, then you need to eliminate a minimum of once a day. The process should be quick and easy. If it is a strain to eliminate or takes more than a few minutes, then you are constipated.

In the colon (the endmost segment of the intestinal tract) a certain amount of water is normally extracted from the feces to facilitate excretion. When the body becomes dehydrated the amount of moisture removed is increased, in order to slow down water loss. A greater amount of water than normal is removed from the feces traveling through the colon. As a consequence, fecal matter becomes excessively dry and hard, slowing down elimination. The result is constipation. The solution is simple: drink more water.

Another common symptom of chronic dehydration is pain and cramping. Muscle fatigue, spasms, and cramping occur more frequently when the body is dehydrated.[16] Most of us have had the painful experience of a leg cramp during heavy physical activity. Exercise causes a high rate of perspiration, which can easily lead to dehydration which, in turn, promotes muscle cramps.

Many people experience chronic neck and back pain. They go to the doctor to get pain killers or to the chiropractor to fix subluxations (misalignments in the spine caused by muscle spasms and cramps). The chiropractor will relax the muscles and realign the bones, but if the cause was due to chronic dehydration, the muscles will eventually cramp up again and the person is soon back in the chiropractor's office getting another adjustment. Drugs and spinal adjustments cannot cure dehydration.

Fatigue, headaches, fuzzy thinking, and loss of strength or coordination are all consequences of dehydration. It's interesting how often when we get a headache, it is simply due to a lack of water. Most people, instead of drinking water to relieve their headaches, will take pain pills like aspirin or Tylenol. These pain killers haven't solved the problem; the body is still dehydrated. All they did was deaden the nerves carrying the pain sensation, masking the symptom of dehydration which was brought about by your body to get your attention and tell you it needs more water. It is amazing how many people can relieve their headaches within 15 minutes or so by simply drinking a large glass of water, rather than relying on pain pills. The water solves the problem rather than covering it up by deadening the nerves.

Dehydration and Insulin Resistance

One of the consequences of dehydration is insulin resistance. Insulin resistance promotes excess insulin secretion. Insulin is a fat storage hormone, and will cause you to convert more of your food into fat. Dehydration causes transitory or temporary insulin resistance. If dehydration becomes chronic, it can lead to chronic insulin resistance, and thus promote weight gain.

When your blood vessels lose water, the sugar in your blood becomes more concentrated, the higher your blood sugar concentration, the more insulin resistant you become. The more insulin resistant you are, the higher your blood sugar becomes. It's a vicious cycle. When you have high blood sugar, your body tries to remove the excess glucose from your bloodstream by filtering it through the kidneys and washing it out of the body, which causes frequent urination. Whenever you eat sugar or any carbohydrate, it will raise your blood sugar and increase urine volume. Thus, you will become even more dehydrated.

In addition to drinking water throughout the day, you should also drink water with your meals to avoid carbohydrate induced dehydration. Water adds volume to meals and helps satisfy hunger. It also provides the medium in which foods are properly digested and absorbed. Some people claim that drinking water with meals will dilute the digestive enzymes, thus reducing their effectiveness. This is not so. Drinking water with meals actually increases enzyme efficiency, so long as you don't drink excessive amounts. Water is almost immediately absorbed through the stomach wall, which will promote the secretion of digestive enzymes and acids that will improve digestion. You can see how quickly water travels from your stomach to your bloodstream on a hot day. When you are very hot and dehydrated and drink a glass of water, within about 5 minutes you will begin sweating profusely. In just a few minutes the water can travel from your stomach, into your bloodstream, and produces sweat. Water does not stay in the stomach long.

Water is essential for proper digestion and enzyme activity. For example, take a bowl of water, stir it, and add a few drops of food dye. The dye immediately begins to dissimulate throughout the entire bowl. Within seconds the entire bowl of water is colored by the dye. Fill a second bowl with cooked oatmeal add enough water to make it mushy. Stir it and add in a few drops of food dye. What happens? The dye stays in little puddles. It does not spread throughout the bowl. This is analogous to food in the stomach. The dye represents the digestive enzymes. These enzymes must come into contact with each particle of chewed food in order for the enzymes to do their job and break it down. If the chewed food does not have enough water mixed into it, the enzymes cannot migrate and reach all the food particles and do their job. Consuming adequate amounts of water will dilute the food enough to allow proper mixture of enzymes with the food.

If you just don't like drinking water with your meals, you can drink a full glass of water 5 or 10 minutes before eating. This will give your body the fluids it needs to properly digest the food and will help fill the stomach, taking the edge off your hunger and start the process that signals satiety.

DRINK MORE WATER, LOSE MORE WEIGHT

Water is the ultimate diet drink because it contains zero calories, suppresses appetite, boosts metabolism, and helps remove fat. Yes, drinking water can help you take off fat! Studies have shown that decreasing water consumption causes an increase in fat deposition, and an increase in water intake has the opposite effect.

197

The kidney's job is to filter waste from the blood and maintain electrolyte and pH balance. The kidneys need plenty of water to perform their function properly. If water isn't available, the blood becomes too congested and the kidneys can't do their job effectively. Since maintaining a chemical balance is vital to health, the liver jumps in and takes on the task performed by the overworked kidneys. This, in turn, puts undue stress on the liver, which must continue to perform all of its regular duties as well. One of the jobs of the liver is to convert fat into energy for the body. But if the liver is struggling under excessive stress from helping the kidneys, it can't function at optimal levels either. Less fat is converted into energy and more fat remains stored as fat. So when you drink more water, the kidneys and liver are able to function more efficiently, and more fat is metabolized and removed.

If you don't normally drink water, you must be getting your fluids from some other source. No other fluid can adequately replace water and most of the beverages we drink actively contribute to weight problems.

A major key to losing weight is to replace all the beverages you ordinarily drink with plain water. Most beverages contain empty calories. That is, they provide little nutritive value but lots of calories. The more beverages you drink, the more calories you consume. A 16-ounce glass of orange juice contains 220 calories. A 12-ounce can of soda has about 150 calories. Water, on the other hand, has zero calories. By drinking water in place of these other beverages, you consume fewer calories.

We tend to eat about the same amount of food and get the same amount of calories each day. The calories in drinks, however, are all added calories. Regardless of how much or how little you drink between meals, you will eat about the same amount of food. Studies have shown that drinking sugar-laden drinks has little effect on how much people eat at a meal. No matter how many beverages we drink, we still eat the same amount. Drinking water instead of beverages can significantly reduce the number of calories you consume each day.

You may think to yourself, "I drink low-calorie beverages so it's okay." It's not. Eating and drinking foods containing artificial sweeteners is not a good idea. They stimulate the sweet tooth, keeping addictions alive and thriving. A person who becomes accustomed to eating and drinking artificially sweetened foods and beverages establishes a bad habit that leads to overeating, particularly of nutritionally poor foods and drinks.

Another problem with sweet or appetizing beverages is that they stimulate the salivary glands and trick the body into thinking it's going to receive food. The body gears up to handle a hearty meal, but all it gets is a liquid, which is digested almost immediately. The body now is primed to receive solid food and you begin to feel "hungry." Consequently, you end up snacking and consuming needless calories.

Beverages, whether they are low-calorie or not, can also make you thirsty and cause you to want to drink more. For example, caffeinated drinks like coffee and soda have a diuretic effect. You may drink a soda to quench your thirst and gain immediate temporary satisfaction, but the caffeine will draw water out of the body, causing you to urinate more frequently and become thirsty again. If you satisfy this thirst with another soda, the cycle repeats itself. You gradually become more and more dehydrated while consuming more and more soda and more calories. If you satisfied your initial thirst with water instead of soda, you would not become thirsty again as quickly and you would not consume any calories or artificial flavors, caffeine, and other chemicals that stimulate the taste buds and encourage addiction.

An interesting study on coffee was carried out using 12 healthy men and women. They were all coffee drinkers, but abstained from drinking or eating anything containing caffeine for five days before the study. They were then allowed to drink six cups of coffee per day. The researchers found that when the subjects drank coffee, they excreted more water in their urine than they consumed in their foods, so that they had a net loss in water. Total body water decreased by 2.7 percent. Despite this level of dehydration, only two of the subjects experienced thirst.

Water should replace all alcohol, coffee, black and green tea, soda, juice (which is often packed with additional sugar), and flavored drinks. The ones you should avoid the most are those that contain sugar, caffeine, or alcohol. These are the ones highest in calories and producing the strongest diuretic or dehydrating effects.

This doesn't mean you can never drink these beverages. If you must drink a beverage now and then, make sure you follow it with an equal amount of water. As a general rule of thumb, for every cup of coffee, tea, or soda you drink, you need to drink at least half that much again in water. But don't count this water as part of your daily water requirement. You still need to drink another eight glasses of water a day. Alcohol poses the biggest problem because it requires eight times its volume in water for metabolization. So if you drink 1 ounce of alcohol, you need to follow it with 8 ounces of water.

Just drinking water can boost your metabolism and cause you to burn off additional calories. Researchers from Germany and Canada found that when you drink 17 ounces (500 ml) of water, your metabolic rate shoots up by about 30 percent. This increase in metabolism was observed within 10 minutes after drinking the water, reached a maximum after 30-40 minutes, and lasted for more than an hour. Based on these measurements, the researchers estimated that increasing your current water ingestion by 1.5 liters (1.5 quarts) a day would burn off an additional 17,400 calories a year, or the equivalent of a weight loss of 5 pounds (2.4 kg).[17] While 5 pounds is not a lot, it is 5 pounds less of excess fat that is not hanging on your body.

The weight loss effects of drinking water can be enhanced even more if the water is chilled. The definition of a calorie is the amount of energy it takes to raise the temperature of 1 gram of water 1 degree Celsius. Considering that the definition of a calorie is based on raising the temperature of water, it is logical to say that your body burns calories when it has to raise the temperature of ice water to your body temperature. When you drink a glass of ice water and it goes through your body and comes out as urine, the temperature of the urine is same as your body. Therefore, your body must be raising the temperature of the water and calories must be burned.

Ice water is 0° C (32° F), body temperature is 37° C (98.6° F), there are 473.18 grams in 16 fluid ounces (473 ml), and it takes 1 calorie to raise 1 gram of water 1° C. So in order for your body to raise the temperature of 16 ounces of ice water to 98.6° F (37° C), it needs to expend 17.5 calories of energy. If you drink 2½ quarts (2,395 ml) of ice water a day, you will burn off an extra 87.5 calories a day or 31,937.5 calories per year, which is the equivalent to a weight loss of over 9 pounds (4 kg). If you are already drinking 1 quart of water a day and add 1½ quarts and drink it chilled, you can experience a total weight loss of 14 pounds (6.4 kg) a year just from drinking water! Talk about easy weight loss. This is just another reason why you should replace the beverages you normally drink with cold water.

If your goal is to lose weight and keep it off, you should try to get into the habit of drinking only water (except perhaps for special occasions). Once you develop this habit you will begin to prefer water over other drinks because it satisfies thirst better. Often people will say they don't like to drink water. What they are really saying is that they are addicted to the chemicals in drinks and they need to satisfy those cravings. Even one soft drink a day can have a significant impact on weight.

Simply substituting water for other drinks can have a remarkable impact on your health and weight. For example, Donna Gutkowski replaced the six to eight cans of Mountain Dew she was drinking each day with water. As a result, she lost 35 pounds of excess weight. "I'm able to wear clothes that I thought would never touch my body again." Speaking of her upcoming wedding she says, "I can walk down the aisle looking better than I have looked in 15 years."

Bob Butts says, "I easily took off 15 pounds without trying. I eat whatever I want...I can honestly say that you have made losing weight an easy thing to do. I know of two brothers, one lost over 100 pounds and the other lost 30."

YOU'RE NOT HUNGRY, YOU'RE THIRSTY

Most of us don't always recognize the body's signals for thirst. It is often misinterpreted as hunger and we end up eating when our body is actually crying for water. Oh sure, when you get cotton mouth you know you are thirsty, but by the time the body starts exhibiting this symptom you have become seriously dehydrated. Dry mouth is a sign of severe thirst. This stage of dehydration ordinarily could have been prevented if you paid attention to your body's earlier cries for water.

The first sign of thirst is a subtle desire to drink. If we ignore this sensation we become more dehydrated. The body is forced to resort to other means to motivate us to drink. The next sign to appear is an empty feeling in the stomach. When the body becomes desperate for water, prompting feelings of hunger may motivate eating foods that would supply enough liquids to prevent dehydration. The body isn't really hungry, it's thirsty. If you continue to ignore the body's signal or if you eat foods that don't supply the needed water, you will develop a dry mouth. A dry mouth is an unmistakable signal that the body needs water. It can be accompanied by fatigue, light-headedness, or headache. By this time, you are very dehydrated and symptoms are severe.

A very important concept you need to understand is that if you become hungry between meals, it most likely is a sign you are thirsty, not hungry. You have ignored earlier signals of thirst and now the body is crying out for water. The only way to satisfy thirst is with water. Often we make do with something else such as coffee, soda, or a snack of some sort, which may bring immediate satisfaction but in the long run will make matters worse.

Part of the diet described in this book is to recognize the fact that feelings of hunger between meals are almost always signals that our bodies need water, not food and not beverages. Limit your eating to your regular mealtime. Between meals when you feel "hungry," drink a glass of water. The water will surprisingly satisfy your hunger. The liquid in the stomach will fill it up, producing a feeling of satiety. The feeling may only last an hour or two, but that's okay because by then your body needs another drink of water anyway. So give it another drink. Do this throughout the day. When you feel hungry, drink water.

This way you will get your required amount of water each day without trying or forcing yourself to drink. As you begin drinking more water, your sensation of thirst will become stronger or actually become reactivated and you will be more aware of your need for water. This will help you satisfy thirst before the body has to resort to a sensation of hunger or dry mouth.

Simply drinking water between meals can be very effective in cutting unwanted pounds without discomfort often associated with dieting. Dr. Batmanghelidj says, "I know a man who weighed 480 pounds. He lost 290 pounds in one year by drinking water whenever he felt hungry. He had to have two operations to remove the loose skin. Another man lost 156 pounds in a year and a half. He reduced 14 pants sizes. A 15- to 45-pound weight loss with water is possible with minimal effort." Wow! What phenomenal results from simply drinking water.

SALT AND MINERALS

When your body loses water through perspiration, urination, and such, you also lose electrolytes (minerals) important to your health. Two of the most important minerals are sodium and chloride.

201

Sodium and chloride are the fifth and sixth most abundant minerals in the human body. A 130 pound (60 kg) human body contains 90 grams each of sodium and chloride, or about 36 teaspoons total. Only calcium, phosphorous, potassium, and sulfur are found in larger quantities.

Sodium is essential in maintaining normal fluid balance and acid-base balance, and assists in nerve impulse transmission. Chloride is also essential in maintaining normal fluid balance and acid-base balance, and is necessary for proper digestive function. A chronic deficiency in these minerals can cause growth failure in children, muscle cramps, mental apathy, loss of appetite, and poor digestion. An acute deficiency caused by excessive perspiration, vomiting, or diarrhea can lead to a severe electrolyte depletion, resulting in coma and death. Athletes competing or working out in hot temperatures often fall victim to electrolyte depletion due to heavy sweating. Many have ended up in the hospital and a number have died. For this reason, sports drinks or rehydration beverages have become popular. Next to water and sugar, the most abundant ingredient in these beverages is sodium chloride (salt).

For many years medical "experts" have told us to limit our salt (sodium) intake. Although they acknowledge the need for salt in the diet, they assume that we eat too much, and have convinced the world that everyone needs to lower their salt intake. Lowered salt intake, they theorize, would lower blood pressure, which should automatically lower the risk of heart attack. Over the past 30 some years we have cut back on salt consumption by 65 percent, yet it has made no impact on the rates of high blood pressure or heart attacks.[18] In fact, the rate of people with high blood pressure is increasing. Something apparently is wrong with the theory.

According to Jan Staessen, MD, PhD and colleagues at Department of Cardiovascular Diseases, at the University of Leuven, Belgium, the theory is wrong. His team of investigators found that only the systolic blood pressure (the top number) slowly rises over time with increased salt intake. But this rise does not translate into an increased risk for high blood pressure or for heart attacks. They found just the opposite, lower salt intake is associated with higher heart and blood vessel disease and increased incidence of death. In fact, in their studies the death rates got progressively worse as the salt intake got progressively lower.[19] Staessen says, "Our current findings refute the estimates of computer models [based on theories] of lives saved and health care costs reduced with lower salt intake. They also do not support the current recommendations of a generalized and indiscriminate reduction of salt intake at the population level [for everyone]."

The available evidence shows that significant cuts in salt consumption can result in small reductions in blood pressure for some people, while increasing the risk of number of other health problems for the vast majority of the population. In addition to Staessen's studies, researchers from other institutions have shown that salt intake below our current level of consumption may increase the risk of insulin resistance, metabolic syndrome, congestive heart failure, diabetes, dehydration, and mortality.[20-22]

Don't be afraid of eating salt because it might raise your blood pressure. A summary of all studies on high blood pressure and salt has shown that in people with normal blood pressure, adding salt has no harmful effect. In people who have high blood pressure, only about three percent are affected by salt. Of these three percent, it is believed that they have high blood pressure because they are chronically dehydrated. Dr. Batmanghelidj's research has shown that drinking more water can lower high blood pressure, and he has been very successful in this area. Also, the ketogenic diet will help lower blood pressure as well, so using salt into your diet will not have an adverse effect on your blood pressure.

The US National Research Council advises limiting daily salt intake to less than 6 grams (1 teaspoon of salt = 5.69 grams). An international salt study, which included over 10,000 subjects from 32 countries, showed an average consumption of 9.9 grams of salt a day. Some populations, however, consume much more than this. For example, in some parts of Japan where salty foods are popular, salt consumption can average an incredible 26 grams or more a day.[23] The national average in Japan is 11.4 grams a day. Despite the high salt diet, the Japanese have one of the highest life expectancies in the world and a relatively low rate of high blood pressure and heart disease.

Salt can also help detox the body by aiding in the removal of toxic halides. The chloride in salt is part of the halide family. Chloride can competitively inhibit bromide and help the kidneys excrete bromide and fluoride.[24-25] In fact, years ago doctors would treat bromine toxicity by administering therapeutic doses of salt in order to wash bromine out of the body. A low salt diet will exacerbate bromine and fluoride toxicity. When lab rats are subjected to a low salt diet, the half-life of bromine is prolonged by 833 percent as compared to rats given a normal salt diet.[24]

Daily Loss of Water (ml)

Mode of Loss	Normal Temperature (68°F/20°C)	Hot Weather	Prolonged Heavy Exercise
Skin	350	350	350
Respiration	350	250	650
Urine	1400	1200	500
Sweat	100	1400	5000
Feces	100	100	100
Total	2300	3300	6600

Source: *Textbook of Medical Physiology*, 8th Ed, Arthur C. Guyton. 1991, W.B. Saunders Company.

Unless your doctor has given you a sound reason why you shouldn't eat salt, there is no reason to restrict your salt intake. Ten grams a day (a little over 2 teaspoons) appears to be quite safe for the vast majority of the population, even for those who are sensitive to salt or sodium, as long as they drink enough water to stay hydrated. I recommend that you use sea salt because it contains many trace minerals, ordinary processed salt does not. Like sodium and chloride, trace minerals are washed out of the body so they, too, must be replenished. Dietary trace mineral supplements made from sea water or other sources could also be of value in replenishing trace minerals. These supplements are usually sold in liquid form and are available in most health food stores.

Because of the presences of fluoride and other contaminants in the water, home purification systems have become popular. While this may solve one problem, it may cause another. Purified water has been stripped of much of its mineral content and will absorb minerals in the body and pull them out. Drinking this type of water could even create a mineral deficiency. So if you drink distilled or filtered water, you need to make a special effort to consume more sea salt and take trace mineral supplements.

If you experience muscle cramps while on the Coconut Ketogenic program, it may mean that you need more water or more minerals. To avoid muscle cramps, make sure you are using an adequate amount of sea salt in your foods and that you are taking a magnesium supplement (400-1,200 mg/day). One of the best sources of magnesium is a product called magnesium oil. It really is not an oil, but a water-based solution of magnesium chloride. You rub the solution on any area of your skin. When you rub it onto the skin it feels very slippery like it is made of oil—thus the reason for the name. Magnesium is absorbed more easily into the body when it is applied on the skin this way. Magnesium taken orally can have a strong laxative effect on some people. Sometimes when they start the Coconut Ketogenic Diet they experience diarrhea. This effect is often caused by the supplemental magnesium. Using magnesium oil and rubbing on the skin will generally prevent this problem. The drawback to the magnesium oil is that you don't know exactly how much magnesium you absorb. However, this really isn't a problem because you absorb more magnesium this way than you get from a dietary supplement. Most people are magnesium deficient.

YOU NEED A SYSTEM

Most adults need to drink about 2½ quarts (2,400 ml) of water a day, but few people actually do. You can't rely on guesswork. Just knowing that you need to drink plenty of water a day doesn't accomplish it. We tend to forget or overestimate the amount we do drink, especially when we consume beverages. People go all day without a single drink of pure water, yet feel they've gotten all the liquids their bodies need. They could not be further from the truth.

If you kept a record of how much water you drink, you would find that more than likely you do not get enough. You may think you are drinking plenty of water, and may drink more than you ordinarily would, but for most people it would still be short of the recommended one quart (1,000 ml) for every 60 pounds (30 kg) of body weight.

To help you get your minimum daily recommended amount you should use a system where you can keep an accurate record of how much you consume. One idea is to keep a small notebook and record every glass of water you drink during the day and make sure before the day is over that you get your full amount. Don't wait until just before bedtime and try to down two quarts of water or you will be up all night. Make sure you drink throughout the day.

I think the best method is to fill one or more containers in the morning with the amount of water you're going to drink during the day. Drink the water throughout the day with the goal of emptying the container before retiring at night. You may have to use two or more containers so you can carry one with you when you go to work.

I don't recommend that you drink other beverages, especially coffee, tea, or soda, but if you do, then add half as much water to your daily ration. If you keep strictly to this regime you won't drink many additional beverages because you will be downing so much water you won't want anything else to drink.

Keep in mind that the recommended daily amount is a minimum. This is equivalent to the amount of water we lose in urine, feces, perspiration, and respiration each day. You're just replacing what's lost. You can drink more than this if you need to, and in certain circumstances you will want to. If you exercise or if your climate is dry or hot, you may need more water. How much should you add? It all depends on the amount of water you lose. A way in which you can determine that is to observe the color of your urine. If it is a dark yellow or amber color, you're dehydrated and need to drink more. You want your urine to be a very pale yellow, almost clear in color. Other signs or symptoms of dehydration include dry mouth, weakness, lightheadedness, headache, muscle cramps, constipation, and not sweating during warm weather.

In summary, the important concepts you need to remember from this chapter are:

- Drink water instead of beverages.
- Drink whenever you feel thirsty.
- Drink when you feel "hungry" between meals rather than eating snacks.
- Drink a minimum of 1 quart (1,000 ml) of water per day for every 60 pounds (27 kg) of body weight.

- If you drink anything other than water, add half as much water to your daily water requirement.
- Set up a system to assure that you get your full recommended daily water requirement.
- If the climate is hot or dry or if you exercise heavily, increase your water intake.
- Check the color of your urine to determine if you need more water.

I often ask people if they are drinking enough water and they say, "Sure, I drink three quarts of water a day." But they are still dehydrated. Why? Because it's 98° F (36.7° C) outside and they're losing more water than usual. People often neglect to account for the environment, and although they drink three quarts of water a day, they may still not be getting enough.

In the summer, especially if you live in a hot, dry climate, you need to increase your total daily water intake by about a quart (1,000 ml). If you exercise heavily or drink other beverages, add more. This may sound like a lot of water, but your body needs it. Keep in mind, especially if you drink distilled or filtered water, to add a little more salt into your diet.

At a temperature of 68° F (20° C), a sedentary adult loses about 2,300 ml (2.4 quarts) of water a day. In hot weather, the loss is about 3,300 ml (3.5 quarts), and with prolonged heavy exercise, the loss can be as much as 6,600 ml (7 quarts) of water. You can see that in warm weather or if you are physically active, you have to significantly increase your water intake to compensate for water loss. If you exercise and perspire heavily, you may need to almost triple the recommended daily allowance of water.

Other factors that increase water loss are a diet high in protein, alcohol, caffeine, sugar, and diuretic drugs and herbs; or eating a lot of dry, dense foods such as crackers, pretzels, chips, dried fruit, jerky, granola, etc. Dry, dense foods demand additional water. Living in a high-altitude environment also increases water loss, because it is drier at higher elevations.

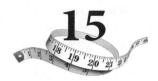

15

Low-Carb, High-Fat Eating Plan

CONTROLLING CARBOHYDRATE INTAKE

"I lost 17 pounds taking coconut oil. I did nothing else but add it to my skillet for dinner some (not all) nights and maybe in a few other experimental recipes. As a matter of fact, I had stopped exercising during this weight loss."
Malikah

"After taking a small amount of the VCO every day for the last 3-4 months, I am now delighted to say that I have lost over 31 pounds in weight. I can hardly believe it, but I am now back to size 12 from being size 18 and feel so much better for it!"
Rose

Many people like Malikah and Rose report that simply adding coconut oil into their diets brings about effortless weight loss. The reasons for this is because coconut oil boosts metabolism, increases energy levels and promotes greater physical activity, curbs appetite, diffuses sugar cravings, and improves thyroid function. However, just as many people say that they don't notice any appreciable weight loss when they add coconut oil into their normal daily diet. Why the discrepancy? There are a number of reasons for this apparent inconsistency.

For one, you can't expect to lose weight if you add coconut oil into your diet and continue to eat hydrogenated and other bad oils. You need to replace these oils in your diet with coconut oil; that's when you start seeing a difference. You should also add enough coconut oil into your diet to make a metabolic impact. Adding 1 or 2 teaspoons isn't going to have much effect.

You need to add 3 or more tablespoons to see an effect. Also, if you eat a high-carbohydrate diet filled with sweets and refined grains, and continue to do so even after adding coconut oil, you are not likely to see much or any weight loss.

To see significant weight loss, the carbohydrates have got to go, or at least be reduced. Coconut oil works best with low-carb diets, especially when it is the primary source of fat in the diet. The most effective way to lose weight is with a very-low-carb, high-fat, coconut oil-based, ketogenic diet or a Coco Keto Diet as I sometimes refer to it.

The classic ketogenic diet limits carbohydrate intake to about 2 percent of total calories consumed. This equates to approximately 10 grams of carbohydrate a day. Fat comprises up to 90 percent of calories and protein makes up about 8 percent. This is a very difficult diet to follow and many people can't endure it for long.

In contrast, the Coconut Ketogenic Diet is much more palatable and easier to follow. Most people can show measurable ketones in their urine by restricting carbohydrate intake to 40-50 grams. This would produce a mild ketogenic effect. Some people who are more carbohydrate sensitive need to cut this down even further. In the Coconut Ketogenic Diet, carbohydrate consumption is limited to 30 grams per day (6 to 8 percent of calories). At this level the vast majority of people show ketones in their urine, indicating they are in ketosis. Fat takes up about 70 to 80 percent of the daily calories and protein about 15 to 20 percent. As a general rule of thumb, protein intake should be limited to about 1.2 grams for every 1 kg (2.2 lb) of normal or desirable body weight (see height and weight table on page 245 to find your desirable body weight).

You do not need to worry about counting total calories consumed. Your primary goal is to keep track of the carbohydrate you eat, limiting it to no more than 30 grams. This makes the diet simple and easy to follow. Since as much as 58 percent of the protein you eat can be converted into glucose, you do not want to over-consume high-protein foods either. This is not a high-meat or high-protein diet, it is a high-fat diet. Your protein intake should be adequate, but modest. Fat calories take the place of the missing carbohydrate calories.

A person can live on this diet indefinitely. It is not lacking in nutrients. It provides all the nutrients needed for good health. Consider the fact that the Eskimo traditionally lived, and even thrived, on a diet consisting totally of meat and fat. Their diet was as much as 80 percent fat. Carbohydrate from plant foods constituted less than 1 percent of their total calories. They were healthy without diabetes, Alzheimer's, Parkinson's, cancer, heart disease, or any other degenerative disease common in our high-carb society today. This new diet allows many more plant foods, greater variety, and more nutrients then the traditional Eskimo diet. It is probably a far healthier diet than you have ever eaten before.

208

You do need to calculate every gram of carbohydrate you eat. This is very important. You do not want to estimate or guess, as this will decrease the effectiveness of the program. As you gain experience, you will be able to prepare meals without actually calculating each gram of carbohydrate; a diet diary will be helpful in keeping track of carbohydrates in frequently eaten foods. But for the first few months you need to pay particular attention to stay strictly within your carbohydrate limit.

All fats are free foods; meaning there is no limit on the amount you are allowed to eat. You are encouraged to use as much fat as possible in meal preparation. Forget the lean cuts of meat, eat fatty meats and eat all the fat, including the skin on chicken and other fowl. Eat all the meat drippings after cooking. Add more fat when possible. The added fat makes foods taste better. You will be expected to add more fat, primarily coconut oil, to your foods. You will be surprised how good vegetables taste when they are smothered in meat drippings, butter, or coconut oil. If you weren't a fan of vegetables before, you will become a veggie lover now that you can spruce them up with fat. Most fresh meats, fish, fowl, are essentially carbohydrate-free. Eggs and cheese contain very small amounts. Processed meats, however, often contain sugar or other fillers as well as preservatives and other food additives.

Use the Nutrient Counter in the appendix to calculate the amount of net carbohydrate in your meals. The term "net carbohydrate" refers to carbohydrate that is digestible, provides calories, and raises blood sugar. Dietary fiber is also a carbohydrate, but it does not raise blood sugar or supply calories, so it is not included. Most plant foods will contain both digestible carbohydrate and fiber. To calculate the net carbohydrate content, you subtract the fiber from the total carbohydrate. The Nutrient Counter in the appendix lists net carbohydrate of various whole foods. You can figure out the net carbohydrate content of mixed packaged foods yourself. The Nutrition Facts label on packages show the amount of calories, fat, carbohydrate, protein, and other nutrients per serving. On this label under the "Total Carbohydrate" heading, you will see "Dietary Fiber." To calculate the net carbohydrate content, subtract the grams of fiber listed, from the grams of total carbohydrate.

The Nutrient Counter lists the most common vegetables, fruits, dairy, grains, nuts, and seeds. To find foods not on the list, including many popular packaged and restaurant foods, go online to www.calorieking.com. On this website, type in the food you are looking for and you will get a listing of everything included on a Nutrition Facts label. To find the net carbohydrate content, you must go through the same steps you do with any Nutrition Facts label and subtract the fiber from total carbohydrate listed. There are several websites that provide the carbohydrate count on various foods. Another good one is www.carb-counter.org.

In order to stay under your carbohydrate limit for the day, you will want to eliminate or dramatically reduce all high-carb foods in your diet. For instance, a slice of white bread contains 12 grams of carbohydrate. Just two slices will bring you close to your 30 gram limit. Since all vegetables and fruits contain carbohydrate, you would be restricted to eating only meat and fat for the rest of the day in order to stay under your limit—which is not a good idea. A single medium-size baked potato contains 32 grams of carbohydrate—more than a day's allotment. An apple has 18 grams, an orange 12 grams, and a medium-size banana 25 grams. Breads and grains contain the highest amount of carbohydrate. A single 4-inch (10 cm) pancake without any syrup or sweeteners has 13 grams, a 10-inch (27 cm) tortilla has 34 grams, and a plain bagel has 57 grams. Candy and desserts are just as high in carbohydrate and provide almost no nutritional value, so they should be completely eliminated from the diet. All breads and most fruits are very limited if not totally eliminated.

Vegetables, however, are much lower in carbohydrate. One cup of asparagus has 2 grams, a cup of raw cabbage 2 grams, and a cup of cauliflower 2.5 grams. All types of lettuce are very low in carbohydrate: a cup of shredded lettuce has only about 0.5 gram. You can easily fill up on green salad and other low-carb vegetables without worrying too much about going over your carbohydrate limit.

Although fruit normally is fairly high in carbohydrate, a limited amount can be consumed. Fruits with the lowest carbohydrate content are berries such as blackberries (½ cup contains 3.5 grams of carbonydrate), boysenberries (½ cup contains 4.5 grams), raspberries (½ cup contains 3 grams), and strawberries (½ cup, sliced, contains 4.5 grams). Any fruit, vegetable, or even grain product can be eaten, as long as the portion size is not so big that it puts you over your carbohydrate limit. Since most fruits, starchy vegetables, and breads are high in carbohydrate, it is best to simply avoid them altogether.

Let's look at a typical low-carb meal plan. Net carbs for each item are listed in parentheses.

Breakfast

Omelet made with 2 eggs (1 g), 1 ounce of cheddar cheese (0.5 g), ½ cup sliced mushrooms (1 g), 2 ounces of diced sugar-free ham (0 g), and 1 teaspoon of chopped chives (0 g), cooked in 1 tablespoon of coconut oil (0 g). Net carbohydrate count: 2.5 grams.

Lunch

Tossed green salad with 2 cups shredded lettuce (1 g), ½ cup shredded carrot (4 g), ¼ cup diced sweet bell pepper (1 g), ½ medium tomato (2 g), ¼ avocado (0 g), ½ cup shredded cabbage (1 g), 3 ounces chopped roasted chicken (0 g), 1 tablespoon roasted sunflower seeds (1 g), topped with 2 tablespoons of olive oil-based Italian dressing, without sugar (1 g). Net carbohydrate count: 12 grams.

Dinner

One pork chop (0 g) cooked in 1 tablespoon of coconut oil (0 g), 4 spears cooked asparagus (2 g) with 1 teaspoon of butter (0 g), 2 cups cooked cauliflower (3 g) topped with 1 ounce of Colby cheese (0.5 g) with various herbs and spices (0 g) to enhance flavor, ½ cup strawberries topped with ¼ cup whipped cream (6.3 g). Net carbohydrate count: 11 grams.

Total net carbohydrate consumed in the above three meals is 25.5 grams, which is 4.5 grams under the 30 gram daily limit. As you see from this example, the diet provides a variety of nutritious foods.

In comparison, let's look at the carbohydrate content of some typical unrestricted meals. A typical breakfast might include a 1 cup serving of Frosted Flakes cereal (35 g) with ½ cup serving of 2% milk (11.5 g). Total carbohydrate count comes to 46.5 grams. A single serving of this cold cereal, which is very typical in carb content, exceeds the 30 gram limit by 16.5 grams. Obviously, cold cereals are not a good option for those following a low-carb, ketogenic eating plan.

Most people realize that cold breakfast cereals are not the healthiest of foods. People eat them because they are convenient, quick, and generally tasty. People certainly shouldn't eat them for their nutritional content. Hot whole grain cereal is considered a better choice. While a bowl of hot oatmeal is more nutritious than an equal portion of cold cereal, the carbohydrate content is about the same. A one cup serving of cooked oatmeal (21 g), with 1 tablespoon of sugar (12 g) and ½ cup of 2% milk (11.5 g) provides a total carbohydrate count of 44.5 grams.

A typical lunch might include a MacDonald's Big Mac hamburger (42 g), one medium fries (43 g), and a 12-ounce soda (40 g) providing a whopping 125 grams of carbohydrate, more than 4 day's worth of carbohydrate on our ketogenic diet.

A typical dinner might include three medium-size slices of pepperoni pizza (97 g) and a 12-ounce soda (40 g), providing 137 grams of carbohydrate, again more than 4 full day's worth.

Most typical meals are carbohydrate-rich. Consequently, the average American (or European or Australian) consumes in excess of 300 grams of carbohydrate a day. The best way to avoid excess carbohydrate is to make your meals at home using fresh, low-carb ingredients.

Does this mean you can't have pizza anymore? You will have to make some difficult decisions. Do you want pizza or do you want to lose that spare tire around your middle? It's your choice. If you are thinking that eating pizza, or ice cream, or soda, or whatever is not going to hurt, then you are addicted to these foods. The sure sign of addiction is to ignore sound reason in favor of satisfying cravings. You need this diet to break those addictions.

This ketogenic eating plan really doesn't forbid any type of food, it only sets limits on how much you eat. So, you can eat pizza occasionally, especially on the maintenance part of the program, but restrict the portion size and make adjustments in the other foods you eat so that your daily carbohydrate consumption remains within the limits of the program.

It is not a good idea to be too indulgent by eating one high-carb meal in anticipation of eliminating all carbs from the other two meals to make up for it. Let's assume you splurge by eating a piece of pie with 28 grams of carbohydrate. That leaves you with just 2 grams of carbs for the rest of the day. You would have to eat almost nothing but meat for two meals to make up for it. Even if you managed to do this, it is not a good idea. The 28 grams of carbohydrate consumed all at once is going to affect your blood sugar and ketone levels. The reason for limiting carbohydrate consumption in the first place is to avoid large influxes of sugar into your bloodstream, as this is what throws the body out of whack. It is best to divide your carbohydrate consumption over all three meals so that no single meal contains more than half of a day's total allotment.

Obviously you cannot gorge yourself on pizza or ice cream as you may have as a teenager. The body is very sensitive to carbohydrates. A single candy bar can be very destructive. The sugar it contains is enough to block the formation of ketone bodies and significantly lower ketone levels, not to mention what it does to blood sugar levels.

Food preferences can and do change. As you begin to eat more vegetables, especially when combined with butter, cheese, and rich sauces, they will become more satisfying than the junk foods you used to eat.

You are encouraged to eat fresh, raw salads several times a week. A variety of tossed green salads can be made by simply changing the type of vegetables, toppings, and dressings you use.

Homemade salad dressings are generally the best. If you use a store bought dressing, avoid those with added sugar. Check the Nutrition Facts label for carbohydrate content. See Chapter 17 for dressing recipes.

Very simple dinners may consist of a serving of your favorite meat— roast beef, roasted chicken, lamb chop, baked salmon, lobster, etc.—served with a side dish or two of raw or cooked vegetables, such as steamed broccoli topped with butter and melted cheddar cheese.

You are encouraged to eat full-fat foods, butter, cream, coconut oil, the fat on meat, and chicken skin. Fat is good for you. Fat satisfies hunger and prevents food cravings. Desires for sweets will greatly diminish. Because fat is filling, hunger can be satisfied with less food, so total calorie consumption should decline.

BASIC FOOD CHOICES
Meats

You can eat all fresh red meats—beef, pork, lamb, buffalo, venison, and game meats. All cuts of meat such as steaks, ribs, roasts, chops, and ground beef, pork, and lamb can be consumed. Red meat from organically raised, grass-fed animals without hormones and antibiotics is preferred. Leave the fat on the meat and eat it.

Processed meats that contain nitrates, nitrites, MSG, or sugar should be avoided. This includes most lunch and processed meats like hot dogs, bratwurst, sausage, bacon, and ham. However, processed meats with only herbs and spices added are allowed. Read the ingredient labels. If they don't contain chemical additives or sugar, they are likely okay to use. If they contain only a small amount of sugar and no other chemicals, you may still use them if you take into account the sugar and add it to your total carbohydrate allotment for the day. If you eat breaded meats or meatloaf you must account for the carbohydrate content.

All forms of fowl are allowed—chicken, turkey, duck, goose, Cornish hen, quail, pheasant, emu, ostrich, and all others. Do not remove the skin; eat it along with the meat. It is often the tastiest part. All eggs are allowed.

All forms of fish and shellfish are allowed—salmon, sole, trout, catfish, flounder, sardines, herring, crab, lobster, oysters, mussels, clams, and all others. Wild-caught fish is recommended over farm raised. Fish roe or caviar is also allowed.

Most fresh meats do not have carbohydrate, so you can eat them without doing any calculations on carbohydrate content. The only exceptions are some shellfish and eggs, which do contain a small amount of carbohydrate. A large chicken egg, for instance, contains about 0.5 grams of carbohydrate. Processed meats often have added carbohydrate, so you will need to calculate the carb content using the Nutrition Facts label on the package.

One of the things many people miss when they go on a ketogenic diet is the crispy snacks they used to eat—the pretzels, chips, and crackers. These, of course, are too high in carbohydrate and often contain unwanted additives. A zero-carb alternative is fried pork rinds, sometimes also called pork skins. Pork rinds are made from the layer of fat under the animal's skin. As the fat is rendered off, only the protein matrix is left. These crispy treats can be eaten as snacks, used in place of croutons in salads, crushed and used as breading in frying fish or chicken, or as a topping on casseroles or other dishes.

Dairy

Some dairy products are relatively high in carbohydrate, while others are low. A cup (236 ml) of whole milk contains 11 grams of carbohydrate; 2% has 11.5 grams and 1% has 12 grams. As you can see, as the fat content decreases, carbohydrate content increases.

A cup of full-fat plain yogurt contains 12 grams of carbohydrate and a cup of fat-free yogurt 19 grams. Sweetened vanilla low-fat yogurt has 31 grams and fruited low-fat yogurt has 43 grams.

Most hard cheeses are very low in carbohydrate. Soft cheeses have a little higher carb count but are still not bad. Good cheese choices include cheddar, Colby, Monterey, mozzarella, gruyere, Edam, Swiss, feta, cream cheese (plain), cottage cheese, and goat cheese. An ounce of cheddar cheese has only 0.5 grams. A full cup of cheddar cheese contains a mere 1.5 grams. A cup of cottage cheese has 8 grams; a tablespoon of plain cream cheese contains 0.5 grams. Whey cheese and imitation cheese products have a much higher carb content and should be avoided.

Heavy cream has a little over 6 grams per cup. Half and half contains 10 grams per cup, so you would want to stick with full-fat cream. A tablespoon (14 g) of sour cream has 0.5 grams.

You can eat most cheeses and creams without overloading on carbs, but be careful with milk and yogurt. Sweetened dairy products like eggnog, ice cream, and chocolate milk should be avoided.

Fats and Oils

Fats and oils contain no carbohydrate, so you can eat as much as you like. Some fats are healthier than others. Choose fats from the "Preferred Fats" category below. All of these oils are safe for food preparation. Steer away from the "Non-Preferred Fats" and never use them in cooking. Completely avoid the "Bad Fats," all foods that contain them, and foods cooked in them such as fries and battered fish.

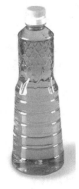

Preferred Fats	**Non-Preferred Fats**
Coconut Oil	Corn Oil
Palm Oil/Palm Fruit Oil	Safflower Oil
Palm Shortening	Sunflower Oil
Red Palm Oil	Soybean Oil
Palm Kernel Oil	Cottonseed Oil
Extra Light Olive Oil	Canola Oil
Extra Virgin Olive Oil	Peanut Oil
Macadamia Nut Oil	Walnut Oil
Avocado Oil	Pumpkin Seed Oil
Animal Fat (lard, tallow, meat drippings)	Grapeseed Oil
Butter	**Bad Fats**
Ghee	Margarine
MCT Oil	Shortening
	Hydrogenated Vegetable Oils

Vegetables

You are encouraged to eat plenty of vegetables. Most vegetables are relatively low in carbohydrate. A half cup each of cooked cabbage, asparagus, broccoli, mushrooms, and green beans provides a total of less than 9 grams

214

of carbs. You could eat nearly three times this amount every day along with other appropriate low-carb foods and stay within the 30 gram limit.

Salad greens provide the greatest bulk with the least amount of carbs. Lettuce has 0.5 gram of carbohydrate per cup. A tossed salad consisting of two cups of lettuce, 1 cup of mixed low-carb vegetables, and 1 cup of medium-carb vegetables plus a tablespoon or two of Italian dressing could easily come to under 8 or 9 grams of carbs. You can add on cheese and meat without seriously affecting the total carb count.

Vegetables are listed below according to their relative carbohydrate content. Vegetables with 6 grams of carbohydrate or less per cup are listed in the low-carb group. Some of these vegetables, particularly the leafy greens, have much less than 6 grams. The average carbohydrate content for the vegetables in the low-carb list is about 3 grams per cup. Most of the vegetables you eat should come from this group.

The medium-carb vegetable group has between 7 and 14 grams of carbohydrate per cup. These vegetables should be eaten in moderation. Eating too many can easily go over the 30 gram limit. A cup of chopped onions contains 14 grams of carbohydrate. However, it isn't often you would want to eat this much onion. A couple of tablespoons or less is more likely. A tablespoon of chopped onion has less than 1 gram of carbs.

Starchy vegetables are packed with carbohydrate. One medium-sized baked potato delivers a whopping 32 grams of carbohydrate. While no vegetable is strictly off-limits, it makes sense that you would want to avoid eating these types of vegetables as a general rule. One serving can eat up an entire day's worth of your carbohydrate allowance.

Most types of winter squash are high in carbohydrate. Two exceptions are pumpkin and spaghetti squash, which have about half the amount of carbohydrate as other squashes. Spaghetti squash gets its name from the fact that after it is cooked, it separates into strings resembling spaghetti noodles. These "noodles" can be used as a replacement for noodles in some pasta dishes. For example, a low-carb spaghetti dish can be made by topping the spaghetti squash "noodles" with meat and sauce.

Fresh corn is listed in the high-carb category. Technically, corn is not a vegetable, it is a grain, but it is typically eaten like a vegetable. Corn contains about 38 grams of carbohydrate per cup.

Soybeans and soybean products, like tofu and soy milk, contain substances that slow down metabolism so they are not desirable foods for those who are interested in weight loss. The antithyroid chemicals in soy are neutralized during fermentation. So fermented soy products are okay. These include tempeh, soy sauce, and miso. All other soy products should be avoided.

Low-Carb Vegetables (less than 7 g/cup)

Artichoke
Avocado
Asparagus
Bamboo Shoots
Bean Sprouts (mung bean)
Beet Greens
Bok Choy
Broccoli
Brussels Sprouts
Cabbage
Cauliflower
Celery
Celery Root/Celeriac
Chard
Chives
Collard Greens
Cucumber
Daikon Radish
Eggplant
Endive
Fennel
Green Beans
Herbs and Spices
Jicama
Kale

Lettuce (all types)
Mushrooms
Mustard Greens
Napa Cabbage
Okra
Peppers (hot and sweet)
Radish
Rhubarb
Sauerkraut
Scallions
Seaweed (nori, kombu, and wakame)
Sprouts (alfalfa, clover, broccoli, radish)
Sorrel
Spinach
Snow Peas
Summer Squash
Taro Leaves
Tomatillos
Tomato
Turnips
Water Chestnuts
Watercress
Wax Beans
Zucchini

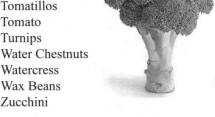

Medium-Carb Vegetables (between 7-14 g/cup)

Beets
Carrot
Kohlrabi
Leeks
Onion
Parsnip
Peas
Rutabaga
Soybean (edamame)
Spaghetti Squash

High-Carb Starchy Vegetables (over 15 g/cup)

Chickpeas (garbanzo)
Corn (fresh)
Dry Beans (pinto, black, kidney, etc.)
Jerusalem Artichoke
Lima Beans
Lentils
Potato
Pumpkin
Sweet Potato
Taro Root
Winter Squash (acorn, butternut, etc.)
Yams

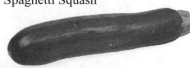

Fruits

A few fruits can be incorporated into the diet if eaten sparingly. Berries have the lowest carbohydrate content of all the fruits. Blackberries and raspberries contain about 7 grams per cup. Strawberries, boysenberries, and gooseberries have a little more, about 9 grams per cup. Blueberries, however, have a much higher carb content, 17 grams per cup. Lemons and limes are also low in carbs, containing less than 4 grams per fruit. Most other fruits typically deliver about 15 to 30 grams of carbohydrate per cup.

With careful planning you can incorporate some low-carb fruits into your diet. Because of their high sugar content, fruits should always be eaten in moderation. Choose fresh fruits over canned or frozen. With fresh fruit you know exactly what you are getting. Canned and frozen fruits often have added sugar or syrup.

Dried fruit is extraordinarily sweet because the sugar is concentrated. For example, a cup of fresh grapes contains about 26 grams of carbohydrate while a cup of dried grapes (raisins) contains 109 grams. Dates, figs, currants, raisins, and fruit leathers are so sweet that they are little more than candy.

Low-Carb Fruits
Boysenberries
Blackberries
Gooseberries
Lemon
Lime
Cranberries (unsweetened)
Raspberries
Strawberries

High-Carb Fruits

Apple	Melons
Apricot	Mulberries
Banana	Nectarine
Blueberries	Orange
Cherries	Papaya
Currants	Passion fruit
Dates	Peach
Elderberries	Pear
Figs	Persimmon
Grapefruit	Pineapple
Grapes	Plum
Guava	Prunes
Kiwi	Raisins
Kumquat	Tangerine
Mango	

Nuts and Seeds

At first, you might think of nuts and seeds as being high in carbohydrate, but surprisingly they are only a modest source. For example, one cup of sliced almonds contains about 9 grams of carbohydrate. A single whole almond supplies about 0.10 gram of carbohydrate.

Most tree nuts deliver about 6-10 grams of carbs per cup. Cashews and pistachios pack a higher carbohydrate punch of 37 and 21 grams per cup respectively.

Seeds are generally more carbohydrate rich than nuts. Both sesame seeds and sunflower seeds contain about 16 grams per cup.

Black walnut, pecan, almond, and coconut contain the lowest carbohydrate content of all the common nuts and seeds. One cup of shredded raw coconut has only 3 grams of carbohydrate. One cup of dried, desiccated, unsweetened coconut has 7 grams. Canned coconut milk has about 7 grams per cup. In comparison, whole dairy milk delivers 11 grams per cup. Coconut milk can make a suitable lower carb substitute for dairy milk in most recipes.

All nuts and seeds can be used as toppings on vegetables and salads if the serving size is limited to a tablespoon or two. When eaten as a snack it is best to stick with the low-carb nuts. The nuts in the low-carb category below contain less than 10 grams of carbohydrate per cup. Those in the high-carb list have 11 grams or more per cup.

Low-Carb Nuts and Seeds	High-Carb Nuts and Seeds
Almond	Cashew
Black Walnut	Peanut
Brazil Nuts	Pine Nuts
Coconut	Pistachio
English Walnut	Pumpkin Seed
Hazelnut (Filbert)	Sesame Seed
Macadamia	Soy Nuts
Pecan	Sunflower Seed

Breads and Grains

Breads and grains are among the highest sources of carbohydrate. You generally need to eliminate all breads, grains, and cereals. This includes wheat, barley, cornmeal, oats, rice, amaranth, arrowroot, millet, quinoa, pasta, couscous, cornstarch, and bran. A single serving can eat up all or most of the day's carbohydrate allotment. A large soft pretzel contains 97 grams of carbohydrate, a cup of Froot Loops breakfast cereal supplies 25 grams, and a cup of Raisin Bran cereal contains 39 grams. A cup of Cream of Wheat with a half cup of milk and a spoonful of honey comes to 48 grams of carbohydrate.

Whole grain breads and cereals are more nutritious and have a much higher fiber content than refined breads; however, the carbohydrate content is almost the same. A slice of whole wheat bread delivers about 11 grams of carbohydrate, while a slice of white bread has 12 grams. Not a big difference. A small amount of flour or cornstarch can be used to thicken gravies and sauces. One tablespoon of whole wheat flour contains 6 grams of carbohydrate. A tablespoon of cornstarch contains 7 grams. This must be calculated into your daily total carbohydrate allotment, so you don't want to use too much. Cornstarch has greater thickening power than wheat or other flours so a smaller amount can be used to accomplish the same effect.

A non-carb thickening option is to use cream cheese, which will impart a cheesy flavor to the gravy or sauce. Another non-carb and tasteless thickener is xanthan gum, a soluble vegetable fiber commonly used as a thickening agent in processed foods. A similar product is ThickenThin not/Starch thickener. This product can be used to thicken sauces the way cornstarch or flour do, and since it is made from fiber, it has no net carbs. Both ThickenThin not/Starch and xanthan gum powder are available at health food stores and online.

A limited amount of coconut flour can be included in the diet. Coconut flour is not a grain but is derived from coconut meat. It can be used to make wheat-free breads and baked goods. It contains no gluten, it has a higher fiber content than wheat bran, and is very low in digestible carbohydrate, making it an excellent low-carb replacement for wheat flour.

Beverages

Beverages are among the biggest contributors to diabetes and obesity. Most beverages are loaded with sugar and provide little or no nutrition. Sodas and powdered drinks are no more than liquid candy. Even fruit juices and sports drinks are primarily sugar water. One cup of orange juice contains 25 grams of carbs. Vegetable juices are not much better. Many beverages contain caffeine, which is addicting and encourages the overconsumption of sugary beverages. Many people habitually down five, six, or 10 cups of coffee or cans of cola a day. Some people don't even drink water, relying solely on beverages of one type or another for their daily fluid needs. It would be best to avoid caffeinated beverages. Caffeine mimics the effect of sugar on blood glucose levels by stimulating insulin release.[1]

The absolute best beverage for the body is water. When the body is dehydrated and needs fluids, it requires water, not a Coke or a cappuccino. Water satisfies thirst better than any beverage without the added baggage of sugar, caffeine, or chemicals.

Water is by far the best option and I encourage you to make it your first choice. You can spike the water—or club soda, which is basically carbonated water without sweetening or flavoring—with a little fresh lemon or lime juice to give it flavor. Another option is unsweetened essence-flavored seltzer water. Unsweetened herbal teas and decaffeinated coffee are essentially carb-free. Stay away from all artificially sweetened low-caloric soft drinks. Artificial sweeteners carry health risks and keep sugar cravings alive and active.

Dehydration increases blood sugar concentration and exacerbates insulin resistance. Most people are slightly dehydrated most of the time. People often ignore their body's internal signals of thirst until dehydration is well under way. This situation is compounded the older you get because the sense of thirst declines with age.

Condiments

Condiments include herbs, spices, garlic, salt, seasonings, salt substitutes, vinegar, mustard, horseradish, pickle relish, soy sauce, hot sauce, fish sauce, and the like. Soy sauce is permitted because it has been fermented. Most condiments are allowed because they are used in such small quantities that the amount of carbohydrate consumed is insignificant. There are a couple of exceptions, however. Ketchup, sweet pickle relish, barbecue sauce, and some salad dressings are loaded with sugar. In many cases you can find low-carb versions. You need to read the ingredient and Nutrition Facts labels on all prepared foods.

Most salad dressings are made with polyunsaturated vegetable oil. A better choice is an olive oil-based dressing or a homemade dressing. See Chapter 17 for dressing recipes and ideas. Vinegar and olive oil or vinegar and water make excellent dressings. Vinegar is especially good because it has shown to improve insulin sensitivity and to lower blood sugar levels by as much as 30 percent after a high-carb meal.[2] The effects of vinegar have been compared favorably to metformin, a popular medication used for blood sugar control.[3] Incorporating a little vinegar into your diet would be beneficial.

Mayonnaise is an excellent high-fat condiment made from a blend of oil and eggs. Unfortunately, all the commercial brands of mayonnaise are made primarily of polyunsaturated vegetable oil. Even the so-called olive oil based mayonnaise are composed primarily of soybean or canola oils. However, you can make your own healthy mayonnaise from coconut oil. See Chapter 17 for recipes.

Sugar and Sweets

It is best to avoid all sweeteners and foods that contain them. One of the signs of carbohydrate addiction is a craving for sweets. The so-called "natural" sweeteners such as honey, molasses, sucanat (dehydrated sugarcane juice), fructose, agave syrup, and such are not much better than white sugar. All foods containing artificial sweeteners and sugar substitutes such as aspartame, Splenda, xylitol, and sorbitol should also be avoided. Although stevia is considered to be a healthier alternative to most other sweeteners, it can keep sugar cravings alive if used too often. If you need to add just a little sweetening to something, stevia is prefered. One good thing about stevia is that if you use too much, it produces a bitter aftertaste. For this reason, you can use a little to slightly sweeten fruit or beverages. Use it sparingly and definitely not every day.

All sweeteners, even the natural ones, feed sugar addiction. When the tongue senses sweetness, it doesn't make a difference if it is from granulated sugar, or Splenda; cravings for sweets are maintained. When you are tempted, your willpower will be tested. Once you break down and eat a forbidden sweet, it will be easier to repeat the action the next time temptation arises and, before you know it, you are hopelessly trapped in the clutches of carbohydrate addiction.

Once you break your addiction to sugar, sweets lose their control over you. They become less appealing. You can take them or leave them. They no longer control you; you control them. If you do indulge, you decide when and where. You are in charge.

In packaged foods, sugar can appear under a variety of names. Listed below are some of the different names for various types of sugar.

Agave	Glucose	Molasses
Barley malt	High fructose corn syrup	Saccharose
Brown rice syrup	Honey	Sorbitol
Corn syrup	Lactose	Sorghum
Date sugar	Levulose	Sucanat
Dextrin	Maltodextrin	Sucrose
Dextrose	Maltose	Treacle
Dulcitol	Mannitol	Turbinado
Fructose	Maple sugar	Xylitol
Fruit juice	Maple syrup	Xylose

SMALL FATTY SNACKS

If you start to feel hungry in the middle of the day, the reason may not be because of hunger but of thirst. When you get hungry, think first of drinking a glass of water; this is often enough to satisfy these feelings. If water isn't satisfying enough, you can eat some low-carb, high-fat options that I call "fatty snacks."

While you are in ketosis, your appetite will be suppressed enough that you may feel like skipping a meal or two each day or simply replace a meal with a small snack. Since fat is the major source of energy in this diet, you need to make sure your snack is loaded with fat. Adding fat to your snacks will make them more filling and more sustaining, allowing you to skip meals without feeling hungry.

Snacks should be high in fat to ensure that you get all the fat you need every day to maintain your metabolic advantage, even when you skip full meals. Each low-carb snack should include at least 2 to 3 tablespoons (28 to 42 grams) of added fat. For example, combining otherwise low-fat vegetables like carrots and celery with a high-fat dip will create a satisfying fatty snack.

The base for dip can be made from peanut butter, cream cheese, or sour cream. One tablespoon of peanut butter has 8 grams of fat and a tablespoon of plain cream cheese 5 grams of fat. This is not nearly enough fat, but you can boost the fat content by combining them with coconut oil. A tablespoon of coconut oil contains 14 grams of fat. Two tablespoons of peanut butter mixed with 1 tablespoon of coconut oil supplies a combined 30 grams of fat with only 4 grams of carbohydrate. Adding celery, cauliflower, or cumber for dipping will contribute only 1 to 2 more grams of carbohydrate. Pork rinds are great with dips and have zero carbs.

Another crispy low-carb snack is nori—a seaweed. Nori is popular in Japanese cooking and is used as the wrapper for sushi. It is commonly sold dried and roasted in paper thin 8 x 8-inch (20 x 20-cm) sheets. Nori has a mild salty seafood flavor. It can be cut into bite-size squares and eaten like chips. It is usually purchased in a package containing several sheets. One sheet has essentially zero carbs. Nori is low-fat, so you must add a source of fat.

Low-carb nuts such as almonds, pecans, macadamia, and coconut make good snack foods. A quarter of a cup of these nuts supplies about 2 grams of carbohydrate and 14 to 25 grams of fat. You can increase their fat content by toasting them in butter or coconut oil.

Meat, cheese, and eggs are other good snack foods. A 1-ounce slice of cheese has about 9 grams of fat and 0.5 grams of carbs. Eggs have about 8 grams of fat and half a gram of carbs. Meat has no carbs, unless it is processed, and about 6 grams of fat per ounce. Some simple snacks are deviled eggs, string cheese, cucumber "boats" filled with tuna salad, and sliced cheese and ham together with a little mustard or sour cream or rolled around some fresh sprouts and mayonnaise.

One of my favorite fatty snacks is coconut oil mixed with an equal amount of cottage cheese. It can be eaten plain or you can add a few berries to sweeten it up a bit. For more ideas and recipes for fatty snacks see Chapter 17.

Store-bought protein bars are popular with low-carbers. I don't recommend them. They are nothing more than glorified candy bars and sweetened with artificial sweeteners or sugar substitutes. They are just a form of processed junk food.

DIET DIARY

Get a notebook and keep a diet diary. In your diary you will record everything you eat—all meals and snacks. Faithfully record what you eat at each meal and snack, the time of day you eat, and the number of grams of carbohydrate, fat, and protein, and total calories. You do not need to record salt or spices since their nutrient content is minimal. Although water does not contain any nutrients or calories, you may want to record the amount you drink so that you can make sure you are getting enough each day.

222

Date: June 5, 20___

8:00 am
8 ounces (235 ml) water

9:30 am/Breakfast
2 scrambled eggs
3 strips nitrite-free bacon
3 tablespoons coconut oil
12 ounces (355 ml) water
Carbohydrate 1 g, Fat 65 g, Protein 22 g, Calories 677

12:00 noon
12 ounces (355 ml) water

2:00 pm/Snack
3 tablespoons cottage cheese
3 tablespoons coconut oil
2 ounces (56 g) raspberries
12 ounces (355 ml) water
Carbohydrate 4.5 g, Fat 42.5 g, Protein 6.5 g, Calories 426

4:00 pm
12 ounces (355 ml) water

5:30 pm/Dinner
1 pork chop (3 oz/85 g)
2 cups asparagus
1 cup salad (tomato, cucumber, vinegar, herbs)
1 tablespoon olive oil
2 tablespoons butter
12 ounces (355 ml) water
Carbohydrate 13 g, Fat 61.5 g, Protein 32.5 g, Calories 735

7:30 pm
12 ounces (355 ml) water

Daily Total
Carbohydrate 18.5 g, Fat 169 g, Protein 61 g, Calories 1,838
Water 80 oz (2,365 ml)

Above is an example of what you might enter in your diet diary on any given day. You may also want to enter you weight and body measurements.

You can also record favorite low-carb recipes, changes in your body measurements, BMI, and weight as well as thoughts about how you are feeling and any improvements you experience in your health.

Keeping an accurate diet diary is far more important and useful than most people tend to think. While it may seem like it will take a lot time, it will actually save you time in the long run by giving you the total nutrient values of meals you frequently eat (so you don't have to recalculate them each time). It will also provide you with an invaluable record of everything you've eaten, keeping you aware of what you are eating, helping to keep you in bounds, give you clues where you can improve or refine the diet, and how to spot trouble. Do not try to rely on memory! Unless you have a photographic memory, you will not remember all the data. During the course of the program you will be changing the amount of carbohydrate you consume, you need to know what you have been eating and how to adjust it properly. Keeping a diet diary is a requirement!

Keeping a record makes you aware and accountable for what you eat. This is a great motivating tool. Studies show whether you are on a ketogenic diet or some other type of diet, keeping a diet diary is a powerful tool in your weight loss efforts. A study involving 1,685 middle-aged men and women over a six-month period found those who kept diet diaries lost nearly twice as much weight (18 pounds/8 kg) as those who did not keep a diary (9 pounds/4 kg).[4]

If the diary helps you to lose twice as much weight, isn't it worth it? You don't have to keep the diary forever, only until you reach your goal weight and during the transition period from the weight loss phase of the program to the maintenance phase. The diary will become even more important to you during your transition to the maintenance phase as you customize the diet to your own personal needs.

DIETARY SUPPLEMENTS

At first glance, because many foods are restricted, including some healthy foods, it may seem that the diet could be lacking in nutrients. That is not the case. This diet supplies all the nutrition a person needs to be healthy.

For some reason, people tend to assume that meat and fat are nutritionally poor foods. That is far from the truth. Meat provides plenty of nutrition. In fact, it is an excellent source of many vitamins and minerals, supplying some essential nutrients not easily obtainable from plant sources, such as vitamins A, B_6, and B_{12} as well as CoQ10, zinc, and other nutrients. Fat, as discussed earlier, enhances the absorption of vitamins and minerals. In fact, this diet will supply you with far more nutrients than you had when the bulk of your diet consisted of low-fat, empty calorie foods.

This is not a meat heavy diet. It includes plenty of natural, whole plant foods, both raw and cooked. The amount of meat you eat will probably remain about the same as you are eating now, unless you are a heavy meat eater, in which case, your meat consumption will probably decrease. Most of the added nutrition you will get will come from a better quality, nutritionally dense source of carbohydrate—fresh vegetables. You will be eating more vegetables than you probably have in your entire life. You could call this a vegetable-based diet supplemented with ample fat and adequate protein.

You do not need to take dietary supplements to make up for any missing nutrients because there aren't any that are missing. If you are already taking supplements and would like to continue them, you can.

Despite everything that has just been said, I do recommend certain supplements. This isn't a requirement, but it is strongly suggested. The reason for this is that most people are deficient in many essential and supportive nutrients. Adding certain vitamins and minerals will help to make up for nutritional deficiencies and speed your progress. The supplements should be taken for at least the first few months of the program. By then, nutrient reserves should be restored and the foods in the diet should provide adequate nutrition so that supplementation is no longer necessary. Some nutrients, such as vitamin D, magnesium, and possibly iodine should be continued indefinitely. The vitamin D requirement is best satisfied by getting at least 30 minutes of full body mid-day sun exposure three times a week or 20 minutes a day with head, arms, and legs exposed daily. During the winter when this is not feasible, a dietary supplement may be necessary.

The nutritional supplements can support fat metabolism, enhance insulin sensitivity, support thyroid function, and aid in weight loss. For example, the mineral chromium is essential for the proper action of insulin, which affects blood sugar levels and the rate of fat storage. There is no RDA established for chromium. However, the Food and Drug Administration (FDA) has indicated that 50-200 mcg to be a safe and probably adequate daily dose and this amount is generally what is included in multivitamin and mineral supplements. Actually, you can safely take two or three times this amount.

Getting an adequate amount of vitamin C into your diet can help in your weight loss efforts. In a placebo controlled double blind study, obese subjects were divided into two groups. One group was given 3,000 mg of vitamin C daily and the other a placebo. After 6 weeks, the group that received the vitamin C lost, on average, nearly three times as much weight as the placebo group—5.7 pounds (2.6 kg) versus 2.1 pounds (1 kg).[5] The RDA for vitamin C is a meager 60 mg/day; this is enough to prevent scurvy, but is not optimal. A better daily dose for overall health is 1,000 to 3,000 mg.

Your new diet should include an iron-free all-purpose multiple vitamin and mineral supplement containing vitamins A, B_1 (thiamin), B_2 (Riboflavin) B_6, and B_{12}, folic acid (folate), niacin, manganese, zinc, and other basic nutrients. It should supply the Recommended Dietary Allowance (RDA) of each nutrient. Make sure it contains no iron. Contrary to popular belief, most people are not iron deficient but get too much iron. It is added to many

VITAMINS AND MINERALS

Vitamin/Mineral	US RDA	Recommended
Vitamin A	3,000 IU	
Vitamin B_1 (Thiamin)	1.5 mg	
Vitamin B_2 (Riboflavin)	1.7 mg	
Vitamin B_3 (Niacin)	20 mg	
Vitamin B_6	2.0 mg	
Vitamin B_{12}	6 mcg	
Vitamin C	60 mg	1,000 mg
Vitamin D	600 IU	2,000 IU
Vitamin E	30 IU	400 IU
Folate	0.4 mg	
Calcium	1,200 mg	
Magnesium	400 mg	800-1,200 mg
Selenium	70 mcg**	
Pantothenic acid	10 mg*	
Biotin	30 mcg*	
Chromium	50-200 mcg*	200-500 mcg
Copper	2.0 mg*	
Manganese	5.0 mg*	
Molybdenum	250 mcg*	
Zinc	15 mg	
Iodine	150 mcg***	500-1000 mcg

*FDA estimated safe and adequate intake.

**If you suspect you have low-thyroid function you might consider increasing your selenium intake to 200 mcg per day.

*** If you have had an iodine deficiency, as determined by an iodine load test, you may take up to 12 mg per day as a maintenance dose.

processed foods and most refined grain and cereal products. Excess iron has been linked to increased risk of heart disease. Unless you have been diagnosed with an iron deficiency, you should avoid adding it with a supplement. If you cannot find an iron-free multiple vitamin and mineral supplement at your local store, you can get it over the Internet. Take at least the RDA of the major vitamins and minerals each day. In addition, I recommend higher amounts of certain vitamins and minerals because of their antioxidant and metabolic benefits.

ADDING MCTS INTO YOUR DIET
Types of Coconut Oil

As you have learned about the many benefits of coconut oil, it should be obvious that this extraordinary food can play a central role in your fight against flab. Therefore, understanding how to incorporate it into your daily life is important. The simplest way to do this is to prepare your foods with it. Coconut oil is very heat stable, so it is excellent for use in the kitchen. You can use it for any baking or frying purpose. In recipes that call for margarine, butter, shortening, or vegetable oil, use coconut oil instead. Use the same amount or more to make sure you get the recommended amount in your diet.

Not all foods are prepared using oil, but you can still add oil into the diet. For example, add a spoonful of coconut oil to hot beverages, soups, sauces, and casseroles, or use it as a topping on cooked vegetables and even meats.

Although I recommend that you consume coconut oil with foods, you don't have to prepare your food with it or add it to the food. You can take it by the spoonful like a dietary supplement. Many people prefer to get their daily dose of coconut oil this way. If you use a good quality coconut oil, it tastes good. Many people don't like the thought of putting a spoonful of oil, any oil, into their mouths. It may take some people a little time to get used to it.

When you go to purchase coconut oil at the store there are two primary types to choose from. One is virgin coconut oil and the other is refined, bleached, and deodorized (RBD) coconut oil. Virgin coconut oil is made from fresh coconuts with very minimal processing. The oil basically comes straight from the coconut. Since it has gone through little processing, it retains a delicate coconut taste and aroma. It is delicious.

RBD coconut oil is made from copra (air dried coconut) and has gone through more extensive processing. During the processing all the flavor and aroma have been removed. For people who don't like the taste of coconut in their foods, this is a good option. RBD oil is processed using mechanical means and high temperatures. Chemicals are not generally used. When you go to the store, you can tell the difference between virgin and RBD coconut oils by the label. All virgin coconut oils will state that they are "virgin." RBD oils will not have this statement. They also do not say "RBD." Sometimes they will be advertised as "Expeller Pressed," which means that the initial pressing of the oil from the coconut meat was done mechanically, without the use of heat. However, heat is usually used at some later stage in the refining process.

Many people prefer the virgin coconut oil because it has undergone less processing and retains more of the nutrients and the flavor that nature put into it. This is why it maintains its coconut flavor. Because more care is taken to produce virgin coconut oil, it is more expensive than RBD oil.

Most brands of RBD oil are generally tasteless and odorless and differ little from each other. The quality of the different brands of virgin coconut oil, however, can vary greatly. There are many different processing methods used to produce virgin coconut oil. Some are better than others. Plus, the care taken also affects the quality. Some companies produce excellent quality coconut oil that tastes so good you can easily eat it off the spoon. Other brands have a strong flavor and may be nearly unpalatable. You generally cannot tell the difference just by looking at the jar. You have to taste it. If the oil has a mild coconut flavor with a mild coconut smell and tastes good to you, then that is a brand you should use. If the flavor is overpowering or smells smoky, you might want to try another brand.

Coconut oil is available at all health food stores, many grocery stores, as well as on the Internet. There are many different brands to choose from. Generally, the more expensive brands are the best quality, but not always. The cheaper brands of virgin coconut oil are almost always of inferior quality. All brands, however, have basically the same culinary and therapeutic effects and are useful.

If you purchase coconut oil from the store, it may have the appearance of shortening, being firm and snow white in color. When you take it home and put it on your kitchen shelf, after a few days it may transform into a colorless liquid. Don't be alarmed. This is natural. One of the distinctive characteristics of coconut oil is its high melting point. At temperatures of 76° F (24° C) and above, the oil is liquid like any other vegetable oil. At temperatures below this, it solidifies. It is much like butter. If stored in the refrigerator, a stick of butter is solid, but let it sit on the countertop on a hot day and it melts into a puddle. A jar of coconut oil may be liquid or solid depending on the temperature where it is stored. You can use it in either form.

Coconut oil is very stable, so it does not need to be refrigerated. You can store it on a cupboard shelf. Shelf life for a good quality coconut oil is 1 to 3 years. Hopefully, you will use it long before then.

MCT Oil

Most of the health benefits associated with coconut oil come from its medium chain triglycerides. If MCTs are so good, then it might be reasoned that a source that contains more than coconut oil may be even better. Coconut oil is the richest "natural" source of MCTs, but there is another source that contains even more: MCT oil. Coconut oil consists of 63 percent MCTs, while MCT oil is 100 percent. MCT oil, which is sometimes referred to as fractionated coconut oil, is produced from coconut oil. The 10 fatty acids that make up coconut oil are separated out and two of the medium chain fatty acids (caprylic and capric acids) are recombined to form MCT oil.

One of the advantages of MCT oil is that it provides more MCTs per unit volume than coconut oil. It is tasteless and, being liquid at room temperature, can be used in cooking or as a salad dressing. The disadvantage of MCT oil is that it is more likely to cause nausea and diarrhea than coconut oil. So there is a limited amount that can be used without experiencing this side effect.

The medium chain fatty acids in MCT oil are quickly converted into ketones. Blood ketone levels peak 1½ hours after consumption and are gone after 3 hours. The conversion of the mixed MCTs in coconut oil into ketones is slower. Ketone levels peak at 3 hours after consumption of coconut oil, but remain in the blood for about 8 hours. MCT oil may give a quicker and higher peak in ketosis, but fizzles out much sooner.

The biggest difference between coconut and MCT oils is the melting point. MCT oil has a much lower melting point, around 38° F (3° C), so it stays liquid even when refrigerated. The benefit with this is that it can be used in making salad dressings or be stirred into chilled beverages. When coconut oil is poured on a cold salad it "freezes" and hardens almost immediately. When stirred into a cold beverage the same thing happens. MCT oil, on the other hand, remains liquid. This characteristic makes MCT oil a good choice for salad dressings and for making mayonnaise.

Another type of oil you may find at the market is a type of coconut oil called "liquid" or "winterized" coconut oil. This is coconut oil that has the longer chain fatty acids removed. It is very similar to MCT oil in its fatty acid profile, but with a slightly greater mix of different fatty acids. It, too, has a lower melting point than ordinary coconut oil and can be used on cold foods without hardening.

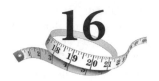

The Coco Keto Weight Loss Program

THE COCONUT KETOGENIC PROGRAM

There are three phases in the Coconut Ketogenic Diet. The first phase is a 2 to 8 week low-carb induction period that allows you to prepare for the second, or ketogenic, phase of the program. Depending on the foods you choose to eat, you may or may not get into ketosis during this initial phase. During the second phase, you actually go into full ketosis where you will lose the majority of your unwanted weight, reach your goal weight, and experience dramatic beneficial changes to your metabolism, blood chemistry, and overall health. In the third and final phase you can relax some of the restrictions, decrease total fat consumption, and increase carbohydrate and calorie intake. You continue to eat sensibly but can include more fruit and higher carb foods, if desired. This is the phase of the diet where you maintain the progress you have made and continue to improve your overall level of health. Your diet at this stage will include a wide selection of meats, cheeses, diary, nuts, and vegetables, tasty fats and sauces as well as some fruits and reasonable amounts of higher carbohydrate vegetables and possibly even some grains. You should remain at this stage indefinitely. With the variety of delicious foods you get to eat, this won't be difficult, it is a diet that can be maintained and enjoyed for a lifetime.

While you may be anxious to start losing weight on this program, make sure you read this entire chapter first, there are some things you need to do before you actually begin the program.

Phase 1: Low-Carb Induction

The purpose of the Induction Diet is to prepare you both physically and mentally for the ketogenic portion of the plan. Because the dietary changes you are about to make may be significant, jumping straight into the program can be difficult. The Induction Phase allows you time to ease into the program, become accustomed to eating more fat, adapt to burning fat rather than sugar, and learn how to prepare and enjoy eating the low-carb way.

One of the major characteristics of the Coconut Ketogenic Diet is the consumption of coconut oil. You are encouraged to eat at least 3 tablespoons (45 ml) of added oil at each meal. Read that last sentence again carefully; this is not 3 tablespoons a day, but for each meal. This is a lot of oil, but that is what this diet is all about. The 3 tablespoons do not have to be coconut oil, they can be any oil, but coconut oil is preferred and it should be the dominant oil in this diet.

After visiting your doctor and getting your blood work done (see page 240 for details), you should start immediately adding coconut oil into your diet. Go to your local health food store or online and purchase several jars of coconut oil. It doesn't matter what brand or type of coconut oil you use. Most of the brands will be labeled "Virgin," "Extra Virgin," or "Expeller Pressed." Any of them will do. Start using the oil in your everyday cooking now. In recipes that call for butter, margarine, vegetable oil, or shortening, use coconut oil instead. At first, try to consume at least ½ tablespoon (8 ml) of coconut oil at each meal. If you eat three meals a day, you should be getting at least 1½ tablespoons (22 ml) of coconut oil a day. Use the oil in your food preparation and add more if you need to after the food is prepared.

Some people are more sensitive to adding fat into their diet than others. The reason for this is that many people have cut back on fat consumption due to the hysteria in our society against eating fat. Because people have limited their fat intake, their digestive systems are not conditioned to processing the amount of fat that is required on this program. Adding fat into the diet may cause some people to experience nausea or diarrhea.

To avoid this as much as possible, it is advised that you start now to prepare your digestive system for the increased fat by adding the coconut oil to your meals. When fat consumption increases, your body naturally steps up production of fat-digesting enzymes. As your body adjusts to the added fat, you can increase your fat consumption without experiencing any side effects. These side effects are less likely to occur when you eat a very low-carbohydrate diet. Keep in mind that emptying the bowels once or twice a day does not indicate diarrhea; this is how a healthy colon should work. Your bowels will be working better and possibly more often on this diet.

Most people are able to add 2 tablespoons (30 ml) of coconut oil immediately into their daily diet without experiencing any problems whatsoever. However, every person is different; some will experience a little diarrhea with 1 tablespoon a day, while others can take 5 or 6 tablespoons (75-90 ml) right from the start without problem. Everyone can build up their tolerance for oil by gradually working it into their diet. You should start doing this now. Getting the body accustomed to processing a higher intake of fat is the primary purpose for the Induction Phase.

If you can handle ½ tablespoon (8 ml) of coconut oil per meal (1½ tablespoons per day) without problem, after a few days increase your dosage to 1 tablespoon (15 ml) and then to 2 tablespoons per meal. If this is too much for your digestive tract at this time, go back to 1 tablespoon for another few days or weeks, if necessary, and then try again. Gradually work toward consuming 3 tablespoons of coconut oil with each meal.

As you are adjusting to the increased fat intake from the coconut oil, you should be eating low-carb meals. Calculate how much carbohydrate is in each meal. Build up a file of tested low-carb recipes and meal plans that you enjoy. Limit your total carbohydrate intake to no more than 30 grams a day. Start keeping a diet diary and record what you eat and even your favorite low-carb recipes. Keep an accurate record of the carbohydrate content in everything you eat. You may also want to keep track of the amount of fat, protein, and calories you eat as well. Use the recipes in Chapter 17 to help you with meal planning.

At this stage, you don't need to worry about the number of calories you are consuming. Eat until you are satisfied, but not stuffed. At first, you may increase your protein intake a little to make up for the reduction in carbohydrates. Add as much protein-rich foods you need to satisfy your hunger. When you get into Phase 2: Ketogenic Weight Reduction, you will work on cutting down on your calories and possibly protein consumption.

After two weeks of using coconut oil and eating low-carb meals, if you are able to handle at least 2½ tablespoons of coconut oil added to each meal without any digestive distress, you can increase your added fat per meal to 3 tablespoons and jump into Phase 2 full speed. If you still feel a little queasy with the added fat, stay at this low-carb phase until 2½ tablespoons of added fat per meal feels comfortable. Unless you have already had experience with low-carb eating, it may take you 1 or 2 months before you feel comfortable enough to move to the next phase. You don't need to be in a hurry, even in the induction phase you should see your weight melting away. For some people, it may take 3 to 4 months before they are comfortable enough to move on to the Ketogenic Weight Reduction phase, and that's okay. Progress at you own pace.

If after 4 months you still cannot handle 3 added tablespoons of oil per meal, your problem is most likely due to poor digestion, your digestive system is underactive and you are not producing enough digestive enzymes to properly digest your food. In this case, it will be helpful for you to take a digestive enzyme supplement with each meal. Make sure the supplement contains lipase, this is the enzyme that breaks down fat. It should also include proteases, which are protein digesting enzymes. Take the supplement immediately after eating. Although, it can be taken as much as an hour or two after a meal and still be useful.

232

Some people add coconut oil into their diets by taking it by the spoonful, like a dietary supplement. You don't need to do this. The body is better able to digest fat if it is eaten along with other foods. When you start the diet, consume the coconut oil as part of your meals. Over time as your body adapts to the increased fat intake, you can, if you desire, take the oil by the spoonful.

You should drink 1 quart (1,000 ml) of water for every 60 pounds (30 kg) of body weight each day and more during hot weather. This amounts to about 2½ quarts (2,400 ml) for most people or roughly 8 glasses of water a day. You should add at least 1 teaspoon of sea salt to your diet for every 2½ quarts (2,400 ml) of water consumed.

Start taking a multiple vitamin and mineral supplement, with an additional 400-800 mg of magnesium, 500 to 1,000 mg vitamin C, and possibly some additional vitamin E and chromium. Get regular mid-day sun exposure or take a vitamin D supplement that supplies the equivalent of 2,000 IU/day. If you believe you have low-thyroid function you should consider increasing your iodine intake to 1,000 mcg or more and selenium to 200 mcg per day.

Start a regular exercise program. You should do some type of physical activity three to six times a week. Going for a 30 minute walk is fine. Do more if you are physically able.

In summary, the Low-Carb Induction phase includes the following:

- Eat no more than 30 grams of carbohydrate per day.
- Gradually work up to eating 3 tablespoons of added oil at each meal.
- Coconut oil should be the primary fat in your diet.
- Take a daily multiple vitamin and mineral supplement, including additional magnesium.
- Get exposure to the sun every day or take a vitamin D supplement that provides 2,000 IU.
- Drink about 8 glasses of filtered water per day. Avoid drinking tap water.
- Add at least 1 teaspoon of sea salt to your foods daily.
- Become involved in a regular exercise program.
- Keep a diet diary.

In this phase, there is no restriction on the amount of meat you can eat or the total number of calories consumed. As you increase the fat content of your diet (working toward 3 tablespoons per meal), your appetite should diminish and you will naturally want to decrease the amount of food (especially meat) you eat, which will also reduce your calorie intake.

Although no foods are actually forbidden, it is wise to avoid all grains, cereals, pasta, breads, sweets, desserts, potatoes, dry beans, and other high-carbohydrate vegetables, as well as most fruits. You can eat a limited amount of fruit, just make sure to keep track of the total amount of carbohydrate you eat. A little stevia can be added from time to time, but keep it on an occasional basis, not every day.

In addition to doing all of the above, you should also avoid all artificial sweeteners, caffeine and caffeinated beverages, hydrogenated vegetable oils (including shortening and margarine), all soy products (with the exception of limited amounts of fermented tamari sauce, soy sauce, miso, and tempeh), fluoride and fluoride containing products (including fluoridated water), and, if you can, all drugs that interfere with weight loss or thyroid function. If you have thyroid problems you should also limit your consumption of raw cruciferous vegetables. Whenever possible, eat organic meat, dairy, eggs, and produce. Reduce the stress in your life. Exercise is a great stress reducer.

Phase 2: Ketogenic Weight Reduction

This is the part of the program where you will lose most of your excess weight. Your primary goal is to limit your total daily carbohydrate intake to 30 grams or less. You need to calculate every gram of carbohydrate you eat—do not guess! You need to calculate the carbohydrate grams in foods so that you know exactly how much you are eating. The Nutrient Counter in the appendix will guide you. Add up all the grams of carbohydrate in all the foods you eat including eggs, cheese, and meats. Although these foods usually have only a small amount, if you eat a lot of them, that amount can become significant. Lunch meats and cured meats often have sugar added so you need to read the ingredient labels even for packaged meats.

Ideally, fat should comprise at least 60 percent of your daily calories and preferably 70 to 80 percent. The Nutrient Counter also contains calorie data on various foods so you can determine precisely how much fat you are eating. To calculate the percentage of fat calories you eat each day, use the following formula:

Total fat calories consumed ÷ total calories consumed = percent of fat calories

For example: if you consume a total of 1,800 calories for the day and 1,200 of those calories came from fat, the formula would read: 1,200 ÷ 1,800 = 0.67 or 67 percent. Your fat intake comprised 67 percent of your total calories for the day. By making this calculation you can adjust the fat content of your meals to achieve the desired percentage.

This procedure is great if you like doing the math and want to figure your exact fat intake each day. However, most people don't want to bother with all the math. To simplify the process, I recommend that you just add 3 tablespoons (45 ml) of oil to each of your meals. This way, you will generally get about 60 to 80 percent of your calories from fat each day.

If you skip a full meal and eat a light snack instead, include 2 to 3 tablespoons of oil with that snack. The 3 tablespoons you eat per meal can

234

be coconut oil or another fat, but coconut oil should make up the bulk of the added fat in your diet.

In addition to the 3 added tablespoons of fat, you are encouraged to eat additional fat. Eat the natural fats in your foods. Choose fatty cuts of meat. Don't be afraid of the fat. Enjoy the flavor. Use fat and oil liberally in cooking, frying, baking, and all your food preparation needs. Eating fat is going to help you feel full, prevent hunger, condition your body to burn off stored fat, and promote weight loss.

For example, if you cook a pork chop, use 3 tablespoons of oil to fry the chop, the same if you fry a hamburger patty or a fish fillet. If you use coconut oil, the meats and seasonings you use give the oil a wonderful savory flavor and acts like a rich sauce that you would eat with your meat and the accompanying vegetables. If you don't use the oil in cooking, you can add it to your food afterwards. For instance, if you eat baked chicken with steamed vegetables, add the oil to the cooked chicken and vegetables. You add the coconut oil like you would butter to hot foods. You can even mix oils. Combine coconut oil with butter or olive oil. With a garden salad add enough oil-based salad dressing to equal 3 tablespoons of oil to get your full meal's worth of fat.

You don't always have to combine the full 3 tablespoons of oil with the meat and vegetables. Instead you can use a smaller portion of oil in the preparation of the food and add a fatty snack to make up for the rest. For instance, if you use only 1 tablespoon of oil for cooking, you can get the remaining 2 tablespoons of oil by adding the Cinnamon Cream Drink to your meal. In this case, the fat in the snack comes from cream. Or in place of the drink, have a dessert snack made of cottage cheese, coconut oil, and berries; I call this Coconut Cottage Cheese with Berries. Another option is a mini soup which you can consume like an appetizer immediately before the main meal. These are the same types of snacks you would eat in place of a meal. The amount of fat in the snacks can vary from 1 to 3 or more tablespoons of oil each. You can decide how much fat to use. This way you can make sure you get your minimum dose of oil for every meal. You will find these and other fatty snack recipes in Chapter 17.

One of the major benefits of the ketogenic diet is that it depresses hunger and allows you to cut back on calories without feeling deprived or miserable. You reduce your calories by choice not by force. You should consciously reduce the amount of food you eat on this diet. Do not eat simply because it is your regular time to eat. Eat only when you are truly hungry. Since your appetite will decrease, you will likely end up skipping meals. If you are not hungry for breakfast, skip it. Don't force yourself to eat simply because it is your usual time to eat. If you eat breakfast but are not hungry when lunchtime comes, skip it. If you do get hungry later in the day have a small snack instead of a full meal, just enough to tide you over until dinner.

Rollups or cottage cheese and coconut oil blend make excellent snacks (see Fatty Snack recipes in the following chapter). Although you do not need to count calories, you may want to calculate this to see how many calories you are eating just for comparison purposes (see table on the following page). The Appendix provides the calorie count for most foods you will be consuming. Try to limit yourself to no more than two full meals a day, and if you are still hungry add a small fatty snack. You may even get by with one meal and one or two fatty snacks.

Regardless of how many meals and snacks you eat per day, you should consume around 6 to 9 tablespoons (98-126 g) of added fat daily to keep your metabolism up and prevent your body from going into starvation mode. This is added fat, not total fat. Total fat intake will be higher. Remember, fat is the fuel that drives your metabolism. You need to eat an adequate amount, even on a calorie restricted diet to keep your internal engines running at peak performance. This means you should eat some fat at different times of the day and not all at one meal.

Your diet will consist primarily of meat, fish, fowl, eggs, butter, cream, vegetables, and select fruits, nuts, and oils. You are encouraged to eat a healthy amount of vegetables, both raw and cooked. Eat plenty of raw green salads. Limit your protein consumption to approximately 70 to 90 grams per day. This is not a strict rule, but a guideline to avoid eating too much protein.

Protein intake varies depending on your height and ideal body weight. You can use this formula: 1.2 grams of protein for every 1 kg (2.2 lb) of body weight. Use the weight chart on page 245 to find the proper weight for your height. To make the calculation, multiply your ideal weight (in kilograms) by 1.2. If your normal or ideal weight for your height is 125 pounds (57 kg), you should limit your protein intake to 68 grams (57 × 1.2 = 68) a day. This is the maximum amount that should be eaten, not the minimum. You can eat less if you like. If your normal healthy weight is 150 pounds (68 kg), you should limit your protein intake to 82 grams. If your normal weight is 180 pounds (82 kg), you should limit your protein intake to 98 grams. Keep in mind, this is protein intake, not meat intake. Contrary to popular word usage, protein and meat are not synonymous terms.

Every ounce (28 g) of lean beef or chicken delivers about 9 grams of protein; an ounce of fish provides about 7 grams of protein. Fatty meats have less protein. Prime rib, which is marbled in fat, has a little more than half as much protein as lean sirloin steak, and I might add, tastes a lot better. A typical serving size of cooked meat weighs 3 ounces (85 grams) and contains 27 grams of protein; this is about the same size as a deck of playing cards. Based on ideal body size, most people following this diet should limit their meat consumption to about 6 to 9 ounces (170 to 255 grams) or the size

CALORIES NEEDED PER DAY TO MAINTAIN DESIRABLE WEIGHT

Gender	Age	Sedentary*	Moderate Activity*	Active*
Female	19-30	1800-2000	2100-2300	2400-2600
	31-50	1800-1900	2000-2100	2200-2400
	51+	1600-1700	1800-1900	2000-2200
Male	19-30	2400-2600	2700-2900	3000-3200
	31-50	2200-2400	2500-2700	2800-3000
	51+	2000-2200	2300-2400	2500-2800

*Activity level: Sedentary includes light physical activity associated with typical daily living with little or no regular exercise routine. Moderate activity equates to exercising (walking, swimming, aerobics, etc.) 4-5 hours per week. An active person exercises the equivalent of 6-8 hours a week.

This table is based on a typical mixed diet of fat, carbohydrate, and protein. The number of calories you need per day depends on your age, height, and activity level. For simplicity, average height (men 69.5 in/177 cm, women 64 in/163 cm) is assumed. If you are taller than average you would need a few more calories, if you are shorter you would need a little less. Generally, consuming more calories than that listed above would cause weight gain, consuming less would lead to weight loss.

of two to three decks of playing cards per day. If the meat is fatty, the size can increase to about 8 to 12 ounces (227 to 340 grams). This is cooked weight, not raw. Again, this is not a strict rule, but a helpful guideline. Let your hunger be your guide.

If you are following the program and eating the recommended amount of fat yet still feel the need to eat three meals a day, that is a sign that you are probably eating too much protein. You are eating more protein than your body needs and the excess protein is being converted into glucose and affecting your blood glucose and insulin levels, stimulating hunger. Cut back on your protein consumption. This will put you deeper into ketosis and further curb your appetite.

In addition to all the bulleted items indicated in Phase 1: Low-Carb Induction outlined above, Phase 2 includes the following:

- Consume at least 3 tablespoons of added oil at each meal, and 2 to 3 tablespoons with each snack (essentially get at least 60 percent of your daily calories from fat).
- Consume at least 7 tablespoons (98 g) of added fat per day, most of which should be coconut oil.
- Eat only when hungry and reduce normal calorie consumption.
- Limit your daily meat intake to about 6 to 9 ounces/170 to 255 grams if lean, and 8 to 12 ounces/227 to 340 grams if fatty, cooked weight.

Some people have what Robert Atkins, MD, the author of *Atkins New Diet Revolution*, calls metabolic resistance to weight loss. Those with metabolic resistance have a very difficult time losing weight and easily gain weight. They are the ones who can reduce their total calorie intake to 1,000 calories or less per day and not lose any weight or may even gain weight. Metabolic resistant people are highly sensitive to carbohydrate. A portion of any carbohydrate they eat is converted into fat and stored, even if their total calorie intake is so low that they are literally starving. They often are diabetic or prediabetic but not always. They may have normal fasting blood glucose levels, yet produce a high amount of insulin immediately after eating, leading to fat storage. Low-fat, high-carb diets are a nightmare for these people. A very low-carb, ketogenic diet is their only hope for successful weight loss. A high-fat, ketogenic diet is essential in order to condition their bodies to burn fat rather than store it.

If on this diet you don't see the improvements you were expecting, you may be one of those who are metabolically resistant to weight loss. This doesn't mean you can't lose weight on this diet, it means that you will need to fine tune it. If you aren't losing weight by limiting your carbohydrate intake to 30 grams per day, you may need to lower it to 25 or even 20 grams a day. A very few number of people who are extremely metabolic resistant may need to reduce it a little more than this to experience consistent weight loss.

Phase 3: Low-Carb Maintenance

Once your weight has dropped to within your target range you are ready to move on to the Low-Carb Maintenance Phase. Unlike most diets that people go on for a brief period of time to lose weight and then abandon as soon as they have reached their goal or tire of it, this diet is a lifestyle change. People usually go on diets as a temporary fix and once they have reached their goal, they abandon the diet and go back to eating the way that caused them to gain weight in the first place. Weight loss is viewed like a bus ride; you get on it to reach a destination and once you are there, you get off. This is why diets don't work. You will never lose weight permanently by getting on and off diets. To keep the weight off permanently, you cannot go back to eating sugar, grains, and other carbohydrates like you did before.

In order to keep the weight off, you need to make a permanent change to your diet. This really isn't as hard as you might think because you get to eat all the delicious foods that are taboo on low-fat diets. In Phase 3: Low-Carb Maintenance, you will relax the restrictions somewhat and allow more healthy carbohydrates into your diet. You will be able to eat more fruits, higher carbohydrate vegetables, perhaps some whole grains or breads and even a treat now and then. But you should never go back to eating sweets, sugar, and refined carbohydrates like you did before. Unfortunately, once you start eating white bread, sugar, and sweets, they can quickly reactivate addictions and enslave you and before long, your weight will be right back where it was before. While the Coconut Ketogenic Diet can help you lose excess weight and greatly improve your overall health, it cannot erase the tendency for carb addiction. This can only be controlled by abstinence. Like an alcoholic, a sugarholic is always at risk and must be careful.

One of the unique characteristics about the Low-Carb Maintenance diet is that it is customized for each individual. It is not one set of rules for all, but provides general guidance to suit the needs and unique metabolic state of each person.

Once you meet your weight loss goal, you will transition from a ketogenic diet to a more moderate low-carb diet. First, reduce the total amount of fat you eat, instead of adding 3 tablespoons of fat for each meal, cut it down to about 1 tablespoon per meal. Second, you can start eating a little more carbohydrate. I recommend more vegetables or a limited amount of higher carb vegetables. You don't want to add too much too soon or you will start to gain weight. Almost everyone who has, or has had, a weight problem is sensitive to carbohydrate. However, the degree of sensitivity varies from person to person. Some people can eat a moderate amount of carbohydrate without much effect on their weight, while another person can eat just a few grams and gain weight. You need to find precisely how much carbohydrate you can tolerate before you start to gain weight.

Start by adding 5 grams of carbohydrate to your daily diet. If you had been eating no more than 30 grams of carbs per day, increase this to 35 grams per day. Monitor your weight every day. After a week, if you are still losing weight or at least not gaining any weight, increase your carbohydrate intake to 40 grams. Increase the total amount of carbohydrate you eat by 5 grams per week until you start to gain weight. At this point, cut back by 5 grams. This will be your carbohydrate limit. For example, if you start gaining weight when you hit 55 grams of carbohydrate per week, then your carbohydrate limit is 50 grams. You can eat less than 50 grams, of course, but that is as much carbohydrate as your body can tolerate before it starts converting the carbs into body fat. This point will be different for each person. Some people will be able to increase their carbohydrate limit to 80 or 100 grams per day, while others, particularly those with extreme metabolic resistance, may have to limit themselves to 30 or 35 grams and, in some cases, 25 grams or less. Most people will fall somewhere between 40 and 80 grams a day. At this point, the diet is no longer ketogenic, but it is low-carb. If you continue to use coconut oil as your primary source of fat, you will still benefit to some degree from the ketones produced from the medium chain fatty acids in the coconut oil. Your hunger will be lessened, you will have better energy, maintain higher metabolism, and all the other benefits associated with coconut oil.

As you become familiar with calculating the carbohydrate content of foods, you will likely stop counting the number of carbs in every meal and depend more on your diet diary and a visual estimation based on your experience. This is fine. However, portion sizes often tend to get larger over time or the amount of higher carbohydrate foods increases. You may notice that you are gaining weight. Don't let it get out of hand. Start calculating the exact number of grams of carbohydrate you are eating. You will probably find that you have gone over your limit, so you will need to cut back. To lose the few extra pounds you may have gained, simply go back to 30 grams of carbohydrate again. After you lose the weight, go back to your previous carbohydrate limit and be a little more careful about the added carbs. In this manner, you can maintain your proper weight indefinitely.

BEFORE STARTING THE PROGRAM
Get A Medical Checkup

Regardless of your age or level of health, I recommend that you get a medical checkup before starting the program. The reason for this is partly to make sure you are physically capable of making a dramatic change to your diet, but more importantly, to get a record of your current level of health.

You should already have had your iodine levels tested, preferably with the iodine load test (as recommended in Chapter 11) and be taking iodine supplements, if necessary. When you have your medical checkup, record your blood pressure. Get your blood chemistries done so that you have a record of your fasting blood glucose level, high sensitivity C-reactive protein (hs-CRP), triglycerides, HDL, Total Cholesterol/HDL ratio, and Triglyceride/HDL ratio.

All of these measurements are needed in order to establish a baseline for comparison. After several weeks on the program you will have your blood work done again so you can compare your results and evaluate your progress. This step is very important! It will provide you with the proof that the program is improving your overall health and that the increased fat you will be consuming is not causing you any harm. It also provides documented proof you can show to your doctor or to anyone who is skeptical about this program. These records will also help to encourage you to keep with the program and continue progressing and improving.

A common concern about replacing carbohydrates with fat is how it is going to affect cholesterol levels. If you have read the earlier chapters, then you know this is not a problem. Cholesterol numbers will improve. All blood markers will improve.

Don't worry about total cholesterol or even the so-called "bad" LDL cholesterol. There are two types of LDL cholesterol: a "good" LDL and a "bad" LDL. Most tests don't differentiate between the two and lump them together under LDL, so this reading is meaningless.

Be aware that total cholesterol may rise a bit or fall—it doesn't matter either way since total cholesterol is not a good predictor of heart disease or ill health. The cholesterol ratio—total cholesterol divided by HDL cholesterol—is universally accepted as a far more accurate indicator of heart disease risk. Likewise, your triglyceride/HDL ratio is also a more accurate indicator. Your HDL, cholesterol ratio, and triglyceride ratio are the numbers that have any real meaning as far has risk of heart disease is concerned.

Do not wait until a week or two after you start the program to have your blood work done. It must be done before you start. If you wait until after you start the program, you may see some values that are not to your liking and complain that the program is not working. For example, your HDL may be low, around 35 mg/dl, and you may blame the new diet for the low reading. Yet when you started the program your HDL may have been only 25 mg/dl. So although it is low, it has improved. But you would never know this unless you have a record of this marker before going on the program.

Stay on the program for at least 2 to 3 months and then go back and get your blood work done again. The longer you are on the program the better will be your results. It is important that you get your blood work done by the same doctor and that he or she use the same laboratory, as results may vary somewhat from lab to lab.

Use the chart on the following page to see where you stand and evaluate your progress. Here is what you can expect to happen. Your blood pressure, if too high at the start of the program, will be lower. If your blood pressure was normal, it will remain normal. Your fasting blood sugar level will be lower. Triglycerides will be lower, HDL cholesterol will be higher, both your total cholesterol/HDL and triglyceride/HDL ratios will be lower, your level of inflammation (C-reactive protein) will be lower. All of these changes are positive and indicate better blood sugar control, improved insulin sensitivity, reduced risk of heart disease, better circulation, less oxidative stress, reduced inflammation, and better overall health. All these changes show that the program is working! Keep going. The numbers will continue to improve.

Get your blood work done as soon as possible, even before you finish reading this book. You want to have this data available so that you can begin the program as soon as possible. But do not start until your blood work is completed.

Atherosclerosis (hardening of the arteries) is an inflammatory process. Diabetes is also associated with chronic inflammation. C-reactive protein (CRP) is a protein found in the blood that indicates the presence of inflammation. Normally there is no CRP in blood. A measure of 1.0 mg/l or less is desirable. When CRP is above 10 mg/l, it suggests an active infection or chronic inflammation.

There are two types of blood tests for CRP. Both tests measure the same molecule, but one test is more sensitive than the other. The high sensitivity CRP or hs-CRP is the test you want. It measures very small amounts of C-reactive protein in the blood and is used most frequently as a means to assess potential risks for heart problems or diabetes, which are commonly associated with low-grade chronic inflammation. High sensitivity CRP is generally measured in the range of 0.5 to 10 mg/l. The regular CRP test is ordered for patients at risk for acute infections or chronic inflammatory diseases and measures a range from 10 to 1000 mg/l. The scale below is based on recommendations by the American Heart Association to assess risks for heart disease.

Blood Test Reference Values

Blood Pressure (mm Hg)

Systolic (top number)	Diastolic (bottom number)	Status
<90	<60	Low
90-99	60-65	Low Normal
100-130	66-85	Normal
131-140	86-90	High Normal
141-159	91-99	High
>159	>99	Very High

Fasting Glucose

mg/dl	mmol/l	Status
75-90	4.2-5.0	Normal
91-100	5.0-5.5	Borderline High
101-125	5.6-6.9	High (early diabetes)
>125	>6.9	Very High (established diabetes)

High Sensitivity C-Reactive Protein (hs-CRP)

mg/l	Status
< 1.0	Optimal
1.0-3.0	Average
3.1-10	High
>10	Very High

Blood Lipids
HDL Men

mg/dl	mmol/l	Status
<40	<1.0	Low
40-60	1.0-1.6	Average
>60	>1.6	Optimal

HDL Women

mg/dl	mmol/l	Status
<50	<1.3	Low
50-60	1.3-1.6	Average
>60	>1.6	Optimal

Triglycerides

mg/dl	mmol/l	Status
<130	<1.5	Desirable
130-150	1.5-1.7	Normal
150-199	1.7-2.2	Borderline High
200-499	2.3-5.6	High
>499	>5.6	Very High

Total Cholesterol/HDL Ratio
Men

Ratio	Status
< 3.4	Optimal
4.0	Below Average
5.0	Average
6.0	Above Average
>9.5	High

Women

Ratio	Status
< 3.3	Optimal
3.8	Below Average
4.5	Average
5.5	Above Average
>7.0	High

Triglyceride/HDL Ratio

Ratio	Status
<2 .1	Optimal
2.1-3.9	Average
4.0-5.9	High
>6.0	very high

In the United States, blood sugar and cholesterol readings are usually given in milligrams per deciliter (mg/dl). In Europe they are commonly given as millimoles per liter (mmol/l).

Body Measurements

The primary goal of dieting is to lose excess body fat. This is generally determined and monitored by measuring one's weight. Body weight, however, isn't the only form of measurement and is not necessarily the most accurate. Your body weight changes constantly even during a single day depending on how much and what you eat and drink, your level of physical activity, the temperature and humidity, and the presence of health issues that may cause you to retain water or be constipated. Your weight may fluctuate by a few pounds every day and from day to day. Even though you follow a diet to the letter, you may weigh more one day than the previous day. This can be discouraging but it is normal. For this reason, I don't recommend that you weight yourself every day. Limit it to just two or three times per week. This way you will get a better overall picture of your progress, without getting discouraged when some days the scale doesn't change or even goes up. For the best accuracy, weigh yourself at the same time of day. I suggest in the morning before eating breakfast, every few days. To give you an idea what you should weigh according to your height, refer to the table on the following page.

A tool often used to measure a person's body fat is the body mass index (BMI). This number is determined by taking the ratio of a person's height-to-weight. A BMI number between 18.5 and 24.9 is considered normal or desirable. People with BMI numbers lower than this are considered underweight and those with higher numbers are considered overweight. You can calculate your BMI using the following formula:

$$BMI = weight\ (kg)/height^2\ (m) = weight\ (lb)/height^2\ (in) \times 703$$

BMI	Status
<18.5	Underweight
18.5-24.9	Normal
25.0-29.9	Overweight
>30	Obese

While BMI can be a useful tool, it isn't completely accurate. It does not take into account muscle mass, body frame, or age.

Another tool that more accurately gauges changes in body fat is a simple measuring tape. Body measurements can a very useful way to track your progress. Many times you will see a loss in inches even if the bathroom scale isn't moving. The Coconut Ketogenic Diet can bring about remarkable improvement in your body measurements. The most important measurement is the circumference of your waist because it most closely reflects your risk of diabetes and heart disease. If you only monitor one measurement, this is the one you should focus on. To correctly measure your waist, stand erect and

Desirable Weights for Adult Men and Women
Weight with indoor clothing and shoes weighing 3 pounds (1.4 kg).

Women

Height ft/in (cm)	Small Frame lb (kg)	Medium Frame lb (kg)	Large Frame Lb (kg)
4'10" (147)	102-111 (46-50)	109-121 (49-55)	118-131 (54-59)
4'11" (150)	103-113 (47-51)	111-123 (50-56)	120-134 (54-61)
5'0" (152)	104-115 (47-52)	113-126 (51-57)	122-137 (55-62)
5'1" (155)	106-118 (48-54)	115-129 (52-59)	125-140 (56-64)
5'2" (157)	108-121 (49-55)	118-132 (54-60)	128-143 (58-65)
5'3" (160)	111-124 (50-56)	121-135 (55-61)	131-147 (59-67)
5'4" (163)	114-127 (52-58)	124-138 (56-63)	134-151 (61-68)
5'5" (165)	117-130 (53-59)	127-141 (58-64)	137-155 (62-70)
5'6" (168)	120-133 (54-60)	130-144 (59-65)	140-159 (64-72)
5'7" (170)	123-136 (56-62)	133-147 (60-67)	143-163 (65-74)
5'8" (173)	126-139 (57-63)	136-150 (62-68)	146-167 (66-76)
5'9" (175)	129-142 (59-64)	139-153 (63-69)	149-170 (68-77)
5'10" (178)	132-145 (60-66)	142-156 (64-71)	152-173 (69-78)
5'11" (180)	135-148 (61-67)	145-159 (66-72)	155-176 (70-80)
6'0" (183)	138-151 (63-68)	148-162 (67-73)	158-179 (72-81)

Men

Height ft/in (cm)	Small Frame lb (kg)	Medium Frame lb (kg)	Large Frame lb (kg)
5'2" (157)	128-134 (58-61)	131-141 (59-64)	138-150 (63-68)
5'3" (160)	130-136 (59-62)	133-143 (60-65)	140-153 (64-69)
5'4" (163)	132-138 (60-63)	135-145 (61-66)	142-156 (64-71)
5'5" (165)	134-140 (61-64)	137-148 (62-67)	144-160 (65-73)
5'6" (168)	136-142 (62-65)	139-151 (63-68)	146-164 (66-74)
5'7" (170)	138-145 (63-66)	142-154 (64-70)	149-168 (68-76)
5'8" (173)	140-148 (64-67)	145-157 (66-71)	152-172 (69-78)
5'9" (175)	142-151 (64-68)	148-160 (67-73)	155-176 (70-80)
5'10" (178)	144-154 (65-70)	151-163 (68-74)	158-180 (72-82)
5'11" (180)	146-157 (66-71)	154-166 (70-75)	161-184 (73-83)
6'0" (183)	149-160 (68-73)	157-170 (71-77)	164-188 (74-85)
6'1" (185)	152-164 (70-74)	160-174 (73-79)	168-192 (76-87)
6'2" (188)	155-168 (70-76)	164-178 (74-81)	172-197 (78-89)
6'3" (191)	158-172 (72-78)	167-182 (76-83)	176-202 (80-92)
6'4" (193)	162-176 (73-80)	171-187 (78-85)	181-207 (82-94)

Adapted from the Metropolitan Life Insurance Company tables (1983).

place a tape measure around your middle, just above your hipbones. Record the measurement of your waist just after you breathe out.

Other measurements you may want to take are of your bust/chest and hips. To measure your bust, place the measuring tape across your nipples and measure around the largest part of your chest. Be sure to keep the tape parallel to the floor. To measure your hips, place the measuring tape across the widest part of your hips and buttocks and measure all the way around while keeping the tape parallel to the floor.

Record these measurements in your diet diary.

Body Temperature

If you have or suspect you have low thyroid function and your normal body temperature is below 98.6° F (37.0° C), take your temperature now to establish a starting point. You should take your temperature orally three times a day and average them to get an accurate number. Take the first temperature about 3 hours after rising in the morning, the second about 3 hours later, and the third about 3 hours after that. For the best accuracy, take readings for at least 5 days. For each day add the readings together and divide by 3 to get the average. For women, body temperature changes during the first few days of the menstrual cycle and the middle day of the cycle, so avoid taking your temperature at these times. Foods can affect the temperature of the mouth, so take the reading before or at least 15 minutes after eating or drinking.

If your temperature readings vary by more than 2 to 3 tenths of a degree, it may indicate a thyroid problem. Readings that fluctuate greatly suggest that the body has difficulty maintaining normal temperatures.

While you are on the ketogenic diet you may want to take your temperature periodically as described above to see if it is becoming more stable and more normal. Since the Coconut Ketogenic Diet can improve thyroid health, you may want to see what other changes may occur. Go to pages 156-157 and make a list of all the low-thyroid symptoms that apply to you. You may be surprised that after being on the diet awhile, you will notice that many of these symptoms subside or completely go away.

Discontinue Medications

Sometimes medications contribute to weight gain by promoting metabolic resistance. If you are metabolically resistant to weight loss, the medications you are taking may be the cause or at least a contributing factor. The worst offenders seem to be psychotropic drugs, like antidepressants, antipsychotics, and tranquilizers. Drugs used for hormone replacement therapy can prevent weight loss. To a lesser extent, nonsteroidal anti-inflammatory drugs (NSAIDs), antibiotics, insulin, and cardiovascular drugs can have an effect. In fact, any medication can make metabolic resistance worse.

One of the fantastic things about this diet is that it corrects so many metabolic defects that you will be able to discontinue many of the medications you may be taking. Don't be afraid of weaning yourself off of drugs you may have been taking for some years. Have your doctor monitor your health and your progress as you go along.

Before jumping into the program, discontinue all non-essential medications. This includes cholesterol-lowering drugs. Cholesterol-lowering medications are not critical for your health and can be stopped abruptly without harm. You may even feel an immediate improvement as soon as you discontinue them. This diet will improve your cholesterol readings far more than drugs can, and without the awful side effects commonly associated with these drugs, which include liver damage, muscle wasting, and memory loss. The diet also balances blood sugar and insulin; so, once you begin the ketogenic portion of the program, diabetic medications and insulin become unnecessary. Even type 1 diabetics who cannot produce normal amounts of insulin can lower and possibly eliminate insulin injections. If you have high blood pressure, it will come down naturally. If you continue taking blood pressure medications while you are on the program, your blood pressure may dip too low. Check with your doctor and have the medication reduced as needed.

One of the most common complaints I hear when people start adding coconut oil to their diet is that it speeds up their metabolism too much and they become hyperthyroid when they were previously hypothyroid. The problem is not with the coconut oil speeding up their thyroid, but with the medication they have been using. It is now too strong and is causing symptoms of hyperthyroidism. Coconut oil will not cause the thyroid to become overactive. It aids the body in restoring normal thyroid function. If after starting the diet you notice symptoms of an overactive thyroid, go to your doctor and have him reduce your thyroid medication. If you still have a functioning thyroid gland (it hasn't been surgically removed or destroyed by radiation), then you can expect to reduce your medication significantly and maybe even completely. If you do not have a functioning thyroid, you may be able to reduce your medication somewhat, but will always need to take it.

Just adding coconut oil into your diet can make a dramatic change. Mable W. says, "My cholesterol was down to 214 [was 328], which is great, since I went off of medicine in April because of liver damage. After [thyroid] surgery I developed diabetes, I have been able to control this with diet and the coconut oil…My doctor could not believe his eyes when he saw me, nor the medical test that he had performed. He told me, 'Keep up with the coconut oil.' And that I have done. I am doing fantastic, I feel good mentally and physically. Before coconut oil, I was taking 15 prescriptions a day. Now I just take vitamins, coconut oil, and my Synthyroid pill…I know that it is an old saying but, coconut oil has given me back my life. I am able to function mentally and physically now. I have all my family taking it. My husband claims that it charges him up for the day. If you miss a serving you do notice it."

If there are some drugs that you feel you must have and are hesitant about stopping, try to gradually wean yourself off them. Have your doctor monitor your progress and adjust the dosages as needed.

Dietary supplementation is recommended, so if you are taking herbs, vitamins, or minerals, you may continue using them. Some supplements contain sugar and starchy fillers, make sure you read the ingredient labels and take into account any carbohydrate other than fiber. Dextrose and high-fructose corn syrup are common additives.

Prepare Your Pantry

One of the downfalls with sticking to the dietary guidelines in this program is succumbing to temptation from easily accessible restricted foods. Just knowing a favorite treat is sitting and waiting to be eaten can be too overpowering to resist. Removing the temptation is the simplest and best solution.

If possible, all foods that need to be eliminated from your diet should be removed from the house or at least from easy access. Give all the high-carb foods to friends or neighbors or just throw them away. If there are other people living in the house who have no dietary restraints, it will make the diet a bit harder. Perhaps restricted foods can be put in a place where no one except the one who eats them can get to them.

Next, you need to stock your refrigerator and cupboards with the types of foods that are allowed on the diet. Have them available at all times so that there is less of a temptation to resort to seeking restricted foods. Purchase plenty of coconut oil. Have your dietary supplements on hand.

Before starting the program, review acceptable foods and develop several meal plans. Calculate the carb content for each meal and arrange them to fit within the day's total carb allotment. Get into the habit of planning meals and snacks before going to the grocery store so you have everything on hand. If you shop for groceries once a week, it is a good idea to plan each meal for the week before shopping. Otherwise you may find yourself grabbing the first thing you find in the refrigerator or pantry, which may not fit your daily carbohydrate limit.

Get a notebook and start keeping your diet diary. In addition to the foods you eat, you can also include your favorite low-carb recipes and cooking tips, your weight and other body measurements, blood test results, adjustments in the dosage of medications or supplements you are using, and changes in symptoms or the way you feel. Keep it up to date. Your diet diary will become your personal low-carb reference book and progress report.

EVALUATE PROGRESS

You've seen the advertisements: "I lost 50 pounds in 4 weeks" or "I went from a size 18 to a size 8 in 30 days!" All sorts of diets claim to "quickly" lose weight. Unfortunately, advertising claims such as these are generally unrealistic and tend to give people false hope. A pound (0.45 kg) of body fat stores about 3,500 calories. To lose 1 pound using the typical low-fat, calorie-restricted diet, you must reduce your calorie intake by 3,500. Theoretically, a reduction of 500 calories a day (3,500/week) brings about a weight loss of one pound a week. A reduction of 1,000 calories a day equates to a loss of 2 pounds of fat a week. This means that true fat loss takes time. You cannot lose 50 pounds of fat in 6 weeks. Six to 12 pounds is more realistic in this time frame.

Although some people lose weight quickly on this program, it is not designed for quick weight loss. It is designed for fat loss. There is a big difference. This program focuses on removing excess body fat, not simply reducing weight. Most low-fat, weight-loss programs lose weight by loss of water and lean muscle mass, in addition to fat. This is why weight-loss, at first, can be dramatic as well as unhealthy. The Coconut Ketogenic program is designed to take off fat while improving your health. Ketosis helps keep you from losing lean muscle tissue. Drinking throughout the day prevents water loss. So the weight you lose on this plan is nearly all fat.

If you are very overweight, you may lose fat at a slightly faster rate; up to 4 or 6 pounds a week is possible. Realistically, when you start the ketogenic phase of this diet, you can expect to lose anywhere between 1 to 4 pounds a week, with 2 pounds being fairly typical. That may not sound like the hype you hear in fad diet advertisements but it can become very significant. Just 2 pounds of fat loss per week will take off 8 pounds a month, 16 pounds in two months, and 32 pounds in four months. In six months you could be 48 pounds lighter and in a year nearly 100 pounds lighter. The best thing about this is that you can do it while eating steak, eggs, bacon, roast, chops, cheese, gravy, rich sauces, and other delicious foods and eat until you are satisfied.

Don't expect miracles overnight—like you see in the advertisements. Give the diet time to work its magic. You didn't pack on the extra weight overnight, so don't expect to lose it overnight, either. This is not a quick weight loss scheme, it is a sensible fat reduction plan that is meant to help you lose excess body fat and keep it off permanently.

If you want to keep track of your fat loss, use a tape measure. Once every three or four weeks measure your waist, hips and chest and compare them to your starting measurements.

After you have been on the ketogenic portion of the diet for at least two or three months, go back to your doctor and get your blood work redone. Have your blood pressure, fasting glucose, C-reactive protein, HDL, cholesterol ratio, and triglyceride levels measured. Compare these figures with the ones you received just prior to starting the diet. These figures should show substantial improvement, indicating that not only are you losing weight but you are becoming healthier in general. It should be very encouraging. You may want to have your blood work done every few months just to see the continued improvement.

If you have always felt cold, have cold hands and feet, and low body temperature due to low thyroid function, you should notice a greater feeling of warmth, higher body temperature, and more energy. Take your temperature. How does it compare? Revisit the list of low-thyroid symptoms in Chapter 12 and see if you notice any improvements.

You should notice a remarkable improvement in all these measurements indicating that the Coconut Ketogenic Diet is helping to improve your overall health in many ways, besides weight loss.

POSSIBLE SIDE EFFECTS

There are no harmful side effects associated with the ketogenic diet, but there can be some temporary changes you need to be aware of. Some people complain of constipation (68 percent) or diarrhea (23 percent), this is to be expected when dramatic changes occur in the diet. As the digestive system adapts and becomes used to your new way of eating, these symptoms will fade. Generally, when fat consumption dramatically increases, it tends to loosen the bowels for a while until the body has time to adjust to the added fat intake. Some people, however, experience just the opposite and become constipated. There are several reasons why this may happen. Sometimes what people believe is constipation is actually an empty digestive tract. Elimination naturally slows down as food consumption decreases. It is not constipation, but simply a reduction in food volume passing through the digestive tract. Constipation is often a sign of dehydration. Frequently when people start reducing their calorie intake, they also reduce their water intake as well, which can lead to mild dehydration and, consequently, constipation. Paying special attention to drinking adequate amounts water during the day will help prevent constipation. The addition of vitamin C and magnesium will also help prevent constipation.

Another common effect is bad breath (38 percent). When you go into ketosis, excess ketones are excreted in the urine and exhaled in the breath. This is called ketone breath and has a mildly sweet, fruity smell somewhat like the smell of pineapple. This smell is not offensive but pleasant. However, the low-carb, high-fat diet alters body chemistry, stimulating a heightened degree of cleansing and healing. Because toxins will be expelled from the body at an accelerated rate, the breath can take on a putrid smell, completely masking the pleasant fruity smell produced by ketosis. Some people blame ketones for this bad smell, but it is not the ketones, it is the toxins. As the body cleanses itself and heals, the foul breath will fade away. You can tell when your body has purged most of its stored toxins and is on its way to healing when the breath freshens up and smells clean or slightly fruity.

Headaches are another side effect associated with the cleansing process. When someone stops eating sugar, chocolate, and other addictive substances, he or she often experiences withdrawal symptoms. Headaches often accompany the cleansing process and about 60 percent experience at least one headache. Once the body has overcome the addictions, headaches will not be a problem. Dehydration can also cause headaches, so make sure you drink adequate amounts of water.

The most common side effect associated with ketogenic diets is a sudden lack of energy. This symptom is most noticeable if you lead an active lifestyle. If you are a couch potato, it will be less noticeable. You won't feel sleepy, but you will not have as much energy as you used to and will become fatigued sooner while doing your normal tasks. This is especially noticeable if you have a regular exercise program or are involved in physical activities. As soon as you go on the diet, your energy levels will drop. Don't worry, your energy will return to normal in a week or two. Your muscle strength, however, will be the same. There is no decline in strength. Your body has been running almost entirely on sugar probably all your life. It now must adapt and switch to burning fat and ketones. This requires a change in the type of enzymes your body produces. Fat burning enzymes need to replace sugar burning enzymes. It takes a week or two for the body to make this adjustment. Once it is made, you will have the same amount of energy as you did when you were burning sugar, and usually a little more. You will definitely be more mentally alert since the brain functions better burning ketones than it does glucose.

Another frequent side effect is muscle cramps. Lower leg muscles are most commonly affected but cramps can occur anywhere—arms, abdomen, back, toes, jaw, etc. When in ketosis, your body's demand for electrolytes, primarily sodium and magnesium, increases. Most people are magnesium deficient already. When they go into ketosis, the deficiency manifests itself as muscle cramps. Approximately 35 percent of those who go on ketogenic weight loss diets experience some muscle cramping. Adding a magnesium supplement to your daily diet, making sure you get adequate amounts of salt (sodium chloride), and that you are properly hydrated will help reduce cramping. Cramps often occur at night when you are asleep. If you experience a cramp, drink a glass of water along with a magnesium supplement and a pinch of sea salt. Rubbing magnesium oil on the affected muscles will also help bring relief.

Another product I recommend is Electrolyte Powder produced by the Celtic Sea Salt company (www.selinanaturally.com). This powder contains all the major electrolytes (sodium, chloride, sulfate, phosphate, magnesium, and potassium) as well as 60 trace minerals. Each jar comes with a 1 gram

251

scoop. Drinking one or two scoops a day mixed in a little water can help prevent cramps.

Coconut oil is a health-promoting oil and can have a very cleansing and healing effect on some people. The medium chain fatty acids in the oil possess potent antibacterial, antifungal, and antiviral properties. While these fatty acids nourish and feed our cells, they are deadly to potentially harmful microorganisms living in our bodies. When combined with the metabolic stimulating effect of the oil, it can bring on what is known as a Herxheimer reaction. This reaction occurs when a heavy load of dead microbes and toxins are expelled from the body. As the body purges this material a variety of symptoms can occur, which may include skin rash, sinus discharge, fatigue, headache, digestive disturbances, diarrhea, fever, and others. A person will not experience all of these symptoms, only one or two, if any at all. These symptoms are not signs of an infection or illness, but of cleansing. No medications need to be taken. Let the cleanse run its course; the symptoms are only temporary and will go away in few days. Fortunately, most people do not experience any noticeable reaction, but if you do, don't panic, nothing is wrong. You should be happy that these potentially harmful microbes and toxins are being expelled from your body.

WHAT IF YOU HAVE TROUBLE LOSING WEIGHT?

If after following the Coconut Ketogenic Weight Loss Program for several weeks you are not seeing the results you expected, what can you do? Please keep in mind that we are all different and the rate at which you lose weight will be different from that of others. Some will lose weight quickly, others less so. Larger people tend to lose weight quicker than smaller people. You cannot compare your progress with that of someone else.

However, there are a number of reasons why some people appear to have more trouble losing weight. The most common reason is not following the program properly. Are you calculating every gram of carbohydrate you eat? This is the number one stumbling block. Often, people don't bother to take the time to calculate the precise amount of carbohydrate they eat and just make an estimate. Big mistake! Unless you have a lot of experience calculating the carbohydrate content in your foods, you will not be able to make an accurate estimate. People tend to underestimate the volume of the foods they eat, and consequently consume more carbohydrate then they realize. Just a few grams can have a significant effect on your success. When you start this diet you must calculate every gram of carbohydrate you eat. As you gain experience with the carbohydrate content in frequently eaten foods you will be better able to estimate portions.

If you fail to lose weight from the very start and are counting your carbohydrate grams very carefully, you may be metabolically resistant. In this case, you will need to lower your carbohydrate limit to 25 or 20 grams per day. Also, make sure you are getting at least three tablespoons of added oil with each meal. Eating less fat will make the diet less effective.

Jenny first heard about the ketogenic approach to weight loss from a podcast by Jimmy Moore. In the interview Moore described his experience of losing nearly 100 pounds in a year on a low-carb, high-fat, ketogenic diet using coconut oil and other healthy fats. Encouraged by his success, she embarked on a similar diet. After a few weeks she was discouraged, not only had she not lost any weight, but she had gained a couple of pounds. Analyzing her diet it was found that she was consuming between 25 and 30 grams of carbohydrate and about 80 grams of protein a day, and getting approximately 70 percent of her calories from fat. This all looked good, but Jenny was only 5 feet 1 inch (155 cm) tall. Her ideal weight fell in the 115-129 pound (52-59 kg) range. For her size, her protein intake should be limited to 62-71 grams per day. She was getting in excess of 80 grams of protein daily.

As mentioned previously, excess protein can be converted into glucose in the body and act just like carbohydrate, stimulating insulin release. The most common failing with low-carb diets in general is that people tend to overindulge in high-protein foods. They mistakenly believe that simply replacing carbohydrates with meat and eggs will bring about instant weight loss. While such a change can be an improvement, filling up on protein-rich foods can hinder weight loss.

Looking more closely at Jenny's diet we also discovered that each day she would have a couple of cups of coffee sweetened with Splenda—another big mistake! Although coffee, black tea, and green tea can be considered low-carb drinks, they can sabotage your weight loss efforts. Caffeine and artificial sweeteners stimulate an insulin response which triggers fat storage. Regardless of how many or how few calories you consume, any spike in your insulin levels will promote fat synthesis and storage. You can store fat and gain weight eating only 800 calories a day if the foods trigger insulin release. On the other hand, you can lose weight eating 2,000 or more calories a day if your foods do not induce an insulin response. While fat delivers more calories than carbohydrate and protein, it does not raise insulin levels no matter how much of it you eat.

Conditioning your body to burn fat rather than glucose can improve your metabolism so that you can lose excess weight without substantially reducing your total calorie intake, however, if you do limit your calories, you will see faster progress. Since ketosis reduces hunger, limiting calorie consumption is a relatively easy thing to do. Often, we get into the habit of eating at certain times of the day and eating specific quantities of food. You need to break these habits, eat only when hungry and stop eating when you are satisfied, even if there is food left on your plate. Do not finish everything on your plate simply because you don't want to waste food. As a growing child that was a good practice, but now that you are an adult, you don't need all those calories. Since your hunger will be depressed, take advantage of it and skip some meals, eat a small fatty snack instead. It will be just as satisfying.

Normally, we keep eating until our stomach sends a signal to our brain telling us that it is time to stop. This signal is slow. It takes about 20 minutes from the time we begin eating until we receive the signal to stop. If you eat fast, then you can eat twice as much as a slow eater before you feel full.

One thing you can do to avoid this problem is to eat slowly. Have you ever known someone who is a slow eater? You sit down to eat a meal and when everyone else is finished, this person has barely gotten started? What did this person look like? I'll bet you anything he or she was slender. Slow eaters usually don't overeat because they get the signal of fullness before they can finish their meal. In contrast, people who eat fast are often overweight. They eat so fast they can pack in an extra 500 calories before they get the signal to stop. And by all means, when you sense the feelings of fullness, stop eating! Sometimes we enjoy the food so much we keep on eating even though we know we are full and will probably feel gorged for the next 2 hours.

Another way to help keep you from eating too much is to wait at least five or 10 minutes before taking seconds. When you wait like this it gives the stomach time to signal the brain. Have you ever been interrupted in the middle of a meal to answer the phone or the door and came back several minutes later and decided you weren't hungry any longer? This is because your stomach was already full before the interruption. Taking time out allows the signal to reach your brain. If you had continued to sit and eat you would have consumed more calories than your body needed.

Temptation accompanies every diet whether it is low-fat, low-carb, or something else. Any time you eliminate certain cherished (and addictive) foods from your diet, these foods can beckon to you. Even though your hunger on the Coconut Ketogenic Diet will be suppressed and you will have greater resistance, the sight or smell of your favorite carbs when they are placed in front of you can be tempting. Here is where the ketogenic diet has a psychological advantage over other diets. When you go on a ketogenic diet, it takes anywhere from 3 to 6 days to actually get to a level of ketosis where your appetite is noticeably depressed. This pre-ketosis period of time is the hardest part of the entire diet because you will feel hungry, just as you do with any other weight loss diet. Once you get into ketosis it is far easier to ignore temptations. This knowledge can give you a psychological boost to withstand temptation.

With other diets it is too easy to cheat. If you eat some forbidden food when no one is looking, nobody will know and physically you won't feel any difference. You can get away with it. However, on a ketogenic diet, if you cheat and eat a piece of chocolate cake, for example, it could very well throw you out of ketosis, which means that your appetite will return and you have to struggle with hunger pangs for the next several days until you are back into ketosis. The idea that you will suffer with hunger for several days after eating something you shouldn't have, should be enough to motivate you to not cheat. If you are tempted to break your diet with a high-carb treat, think about the discomfort you will have to go through for the next several days because of it. Is it worth it?

MAINTAIN YOUR PROGRESS

On the diet you will lose weight most rapidly in the beginning. As you approach your ideal bodyweight, your rate of weight loss will slow down. Your body will naturally regulate itself. When you start transitioning into the Low-Carb Maintenance Diet you may still lose some weight until you determine your new carbohydrate limit where your weight will remain relatively steady.

Once you are on the maintenance phase of the diet and are no longer in ketosis, you are allowed more carbohydrate. You need to be careful. If you go back to eating the way you used to, even partly so, you will reignite sugar and carb cravings and the weight will come right back. As you increase your carbohydrate intake, you may be tempted to eat some of your old favorite foods even if they can fit within your carbohydrate limit. This is fine as long as you can control your intake of these foods, eating them in small portions and only occasionally. The problem is that a tendency to sugar and carbohydrate addiction never goes away. Once a sugarholic, always a sugarholic. You can break the active addiction to sugar with a ketogenic diet, but the potential for reactivation remains. If you have been struggling with weight problems for several years, chances are, you are a sugarholic. Eating sweets or bread just a few times can be all it takes to reactivate those addictions. I've seen people become addicted to bread and even fruit within just a few days after coming off a low-carb diet. Once these cravings come back, you lose your willpower. It is best to avoid problem foods. However, if you do stumble and find that you have become addicted, don't give up, you can always cut the carbs and go back to the high-fat, ketogenic diet.

You don't have to give up breads and baked goods entirely. Most flours, even nut and soy flours are too high in carbohydrate. A low-carb alternative to wheat and other flours is coconut flour. Coconut flour is made from coconut meat that has been dehydrated, defatted, and ground into a fine powder. It looks and feels just like any other flour and can be used to make a variety of baked goods. The advantage of coconut flour is that it contains far less carbohydrate than any other flour. Coconut flour is naturally very high in fiber and low in digestible carbohydrate. It contains about the same amount of protein as whole wheat flour but is gluten-free, so those people who are sensitive to gluten (wheat protein) can eat it without problem. With coconut flour you can make biscuits, muffins, pancakes, and other baked goods that are truly low-carb.

Because coconut flour contains no gluten and is high in fiber, its baking properties are very different from those of wheat flour. For this reason, you cannot use coconut flour in ordinary recipes designed for wheat flour. The baking properties of coconut flour are so different that these recipes are completely unusable. However, I have created a book of coconut flour recipes titled *Cooking with Coconut Flour: A Delicious Low-Carb, Gluten-Free Alternative to Wheat*. This book includes recipes for quick breads, pancakes, biscuits, muffins, cookies, cakes, and more. Although there are many recipes for "sweet" breads, each recipe includes both a normal sugar version and a low-sugar or no-sugar version as well. Stevia is used as a sweetener in some of the recipes. Even the regular sugar versions contain much less sugar and far less total carbohydrate than those made using wheat flour. For example, the no-sugar muffins have only 1.3 grams of carbohydrate per muffin. The book also includes many savory baked goods like bacon muffins, broccoli cheese muffins, Italian meat loaf, and coconut fried chicken. While many of the recipes can be incorporated into a ketogenic diet, it is most suitable for the Low-Carb Maintenance Diet.

Since eating a very low-carb, high-fat diet is new for most people, preparing meals that follow the Coconut Ketogenic Diet can appear to be a challenge. It really isn't. Meal preparation can be very simple and delicious. With the growing popularity of low-carb dieting, there are many cookbooks now available as well as numerous low-carb recipes on the Internet that can give you guidance. Keep in mind that all so-called "low-carb" foods are not really that low in carbohydrate, so you must select recipes wisely and know how many grams of carbohydrate they have per serving. Pay attention to serving size, as ½ cup is a typical serving.

Eating a low-carb ketogenic diet is really not all that difficult if you focus on eating fresh meats, fish, and fowl and fresh vegetables. You don't need to make it harder than it really is. Often, when people go on low-carb diets they just can't leave their favorite high-carb foods behind, so they make low-carb imitations, like mashed cauliflower (in place of potatoes), wheat-free pizza (using cheese or eggs for the crust), hash browns (fried diced cauliflower), or eggplant lasagna. You can do that if you like, but you don't need to spend all the time, effort, and money to make these concoctions. Some of these foods require a great deal of preparation and don't really taste like the foods they are meant to replace. Simple foods like meat and vegetables are all you really need. Chapter 17 offers you many simple meal ideas to get you started.

Probably the most difficult part of the Coconut Ketogenic Diet is getting your daily allotment of added fat. Three tablespoons of added fat per meal is a lot. Often, you can simply combine the fat with your foods, use it in cooking or add it on afterwards. Fats actually make meat and vegetables taste better. In the following chapter, I have provided a number of recipes for fatty snacks—high-fat foods and drinks that can be consumed by themselves as snacks in place of full meals, or as an accompaniment or "appetizer" to a regular meal to increase the total fat content. A moderate-fat or even a low-fat meal can be transformed into a high-fat meal simply by adding a fatty snack.

Eating out can be a little challenging but has gotten much easier over the years. Because of the popularity of low-carbing, many restaurants now offer low-carb options. Most restaurants that sell hamburgers, including all the popular fast food restaurants, offer bunless hamburgers. These hamburgers include everything you would expect in a regular hamburger but are wrapped in a blanket of lettuce without the bun. Even if this item isn't listed on the menu, most restaurants will be happy to make it for you on request. If you plan on going out, bring some extra oil or mayonnaise with you to increase the fat content of your meal.

If you would like to learn more about the health benefits of coconut oil and other healthy fats visit my website at www.coconutresearchcenter. org. For additional information about the Coco Keto Diet go to www. cocoketodiet.com.

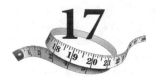

Cooking the Keto Way

At first, learning how to cook the low-carb way may seem like a daunting task. However, it isn't as hard as it may appear. While some low-carb recipes are complicated and time-consuming, much of the cooking is as simple as frying a lamb chop and steaming some zucchini. What could be easier than that?

If you are new to low-carb cooking, I strongly urge you to read this entire chapter. Whether you use any of the recipes or not, this chapter will show you how to make low-carb cooking simple and easy. It will also show you how to incorporate coconut oil into your diet. The recipes provided here are just a few examples of low-carb cooking. For more ideas, check out the books and recipes available at your library, local book stores, and the Internet.

Ideally, fat should comprise at least 60 percent of your total calories. Add as much oil as necessary to your foods to achieve this goal. The amount of fat, as well as the net carbohydrate, protein, and total calories for each serving are listed at the end of each recipe. Note that the fat content is given in grams. One tablespoon of oil equals 14 g (15 ml).

FATTY SNACKS

Fatty snacks are high-fat mini-meals that can be eaten in place of a regular meal or as an appetizer with a full meal. These snacks include 2-3 tablespoons of added oil, generally coconut oil. In essence, they are convenient, palatable ways to eat several tablespoons of fat at one time, while consuming a minimal amount of carbohydrate and total calories.

The fatty snacks can be very simple. Dips, spreads, and fillings can be eaten with sliced vegetables, pork rinds, or wrapped in lettuce leaves, see the following recipes. Soup is an excellent way to add coconut and others oils into your diet. The fatty snack soup recipes described in this section make three to four ½ cup servings. A fatty snack would consist of one ½ cup serving, the remainder of the soup can be refrigerated or frozen, and eaten another day. You can, of course, double the recipe if you like or even eat a larger serving as one of you regular meals. You will notice that the fatty snack soups do not have any added fat listed in the recipes. Oil is added *after* you have made the soup. This way you can add 1, 1½, 2 tablespoons or whatever amount of coconut oil you need for that particular snack or meal. One serving is ½ cup (118 ml) of soup, *plus* the added coconut oil.

Chicken Curry

This is a very simple and tasty low-carb way to get your daily fat allowance. You have two versions to choose from; the first supplies 2 tablespoons of coconut oil and the second, 3 tablespoons.

Version 1
1 ounce (30 g) cooked chicken
2 tablespoons (30 ml) coconut oil
¼ teaspoon curry powder
Salt to taste

Version 2
2 ounces (60 g) cooked chicken
3 tablespoons (45 ml) coconut oil
¼ teaspoon curry powder or to taste
Salt to taste

Cut chicken into small cubes. Combine the chicken with coconut oil, curry powder, and salt into a stovetop safe pan and heat just enough to make the mixture slightly hot. You are not cooking the mixture, just heating it up. The heat melts the coconut oil and brings out the flavor of the curry. Eat warm.

Yield: 1 serving.
Version 1
Per serving: 29 g fat, 0 g net carbs, 9 g protein, 288 calories.

Version 2
Per serving: 44 g fat, 0 g net carbs, 17 g protein, 450 calories.

Coconut Cottage Cheese

This is my favorite fatty snack. As a snack, I usually double or triple this recipe.

1 tablespoon (15 ml) coconut oil
1 tablespoon (14 g) cottage cheese

Put the coconut oil in a small stovetop safe bowl. I use a 1 cup (235 ml) glass bowl. Heat the oil in the bowl on the stove at medium to low heat until the oil is melted or mildly hot (about 150° F/65° C). Scoop in the cottage cheese and using a spoon, blend together until the mixture is smooth but speckled with curds. It is ready to eat. For an added treat, sprinkle 1 or 2 spoonfuls of toasted flaked coconut on top.

The coconut oil and cottage cheese are combined in a 1 to 1 ratio, which makes it easy to modify to get more or less oil. You can easily increase or decrease the amount of fat in this snack by adding 1 or more tablespoons of coconut oil and cottage cheese. Each combination of 1 tablespoon each of coconut oil and cottage cheese gives 14 g fat, 0.5 g net carbs, 2 g protein, and 136 calories.

Yield: 1 serving.

Coconut Cottage Cheese with Berries

This makes an excellent fatty snack or desert. It tastes similar to a warm berry flavored ice cream or pudding, it's actually very good.

2 tablespoons (30 ml) coconut oil
12 blueberries or raspberries or 6 blackberries
2 tablespoons (30 g) cottage cheese
3-4 drops liquid stevia (optional)

Put the coconut oil in a small stovetop safe bowl. I use a 1 cup (235 ml) glass bowl. Heat the oil and the berries in the bowl on the stove at medium to low heat until the oil is melted or mildly hot (about 150° F/65° C). Heating the berries slightly brings out the flavor. Scoop in the cottage cheese, add stevia, and using a spoon, blend together until the mixture is smooth but speckled with curds and berries. It is ready to eat.

Yield: 1 serving.
Per serving: 29 g fat, 3 g net carbs, 4.5 g protein, 291 calories.

Cinnamon Cream Delight

This beverage tastes similar to eggnog, but without the egg.

½ cup (120 ml) heavy cream
¼ teaspoon almond extract
⅛ teaspoon ground cinnamon

Stir all the ingredients together. Drink and enjoy. If you would like to make this beverage into eggnog, simply blend in 1 raw egg.

Yield: 1 serving
Per serving: 44 g fat, 3.5 g net carbs, 2.5 g protein, 420 calories.

Berry Cream Delight

This is a creamy, berry flavored beverage. You can double the recipe and freeze half of it for another day. Tastes good freshly made or frozen.

½ cup (120 ml) heavy cream
⅛ teaspoon almond extract
12 blueberries or raspberries or 6 blackberries (about 0.8 oz/22 g)
1 tablespoon (15 ml) MCT oil or coconut oil (optional)*

Using a food processor or blender, blend cream, almond extract, berries, and MCT oil together for about 15 to 20 seconds. Do not over blend. The cream will be partially whipped giving it a light airy texture. Drink and enjoy.

*If you use coconut oil in place of MCT oil, you will need to add it separately. Place all the ingredients except the coconut oil into the blender or food processor and turn it on. While the mixture is blending, slowly pour in melted coconut oil. Pouring it slowly allows the coconut oil to blend into the beverage without hardening and forming lumps. If you end up with lumps, you poured the coconut oil in too fast.

Yield: 1 serving
Per serving without coconut or MCT oil: 44 g fat, 5.5 g net carbs, 3 g protein, 430 calories.
Per serving with 1 tablespoon of oil: 55 g fat, 5.5 g net carbs, 3 g protein, 556 calories.

Pumpkin Cream Delight

This beverage tastes similar to creamy pumpkin pie filling.

½ cup (120 ml) heavy cream
¼ teaspoon vanilla extract
¼ teaspoon ground pumpkin pie spice mix or allspice

Stir all the ingredients together. Drink and enjoy. Using allspice in place of the pumpkin pie spice mix gives it a little different, but equally good, flavor.

Yield: 1 serving
Per serving: 44 g fat, 3.5 g net carbs, 2.5 g protein, 430 calories.

Sardine Crisps

This is a very yummy and satisfying snack that includes your omega-3 fatty acids. The recipe makes a filling that is spread on crispy pork rinds.

1 can (3.75 oz/109 g) sardines packed in olive oil
¼ cup (60 g) sour cream
2 tablespoons (30 ml) extra virgin olive oil
¼ cup (60 g) finely chopped dill pickle (optional)
Salt and pepper to taste
18 fried pork rinds

Combine the sardines with the sour cream, virgin olive oil, chopped dill pickle, salt, and pepper and mix together. Eat the mixture like a dip using the fried pork rinds.

Yield: Serves 2
Per serving: 29.5 g fat, 1 g net carbs, 18.5 g protein, 343 calories.

Salmon Crisps

This recipe makes a spread that you put on crispy pork rinds.

2 ounces (57 g) cooked salmon
3 tablespoons (42 g) mayonnaise (page 270)
½ ounce (14 g) sharp cheddar cheese, chopped or shredded
1 tablespoon (15 g) finely chopped dill pickle (optional)
Dash paprika
Salt and pepper to taste
9 fried pork rinds

Take one 6 ounce (170 g) can of salmon and divide the contents in thirds. Put two-thirds of the salmon in an airtight container and store in the refrigerator for later use. Combine the remaining salmon (2 oz/57 g) with mayonnaise, cheese, dill pickle, paprika, salt, and pepper and mix together. Eat the mixture like a dip using the fried pork rinds, celery sticks, or other vegetables.

Yield: 1 serving
Per serving: 42.5 g fat, 0 g net carbs, 21.5 g protein, 468 calories.

Chicken Salad Crisps

You can put this spread on crispy pork rinds or wrap it in a lettuce leaf.

2 ounces (57 g) cooked chicken, chopped
3 tablespoons (42 g) mayonnaise (page 270)

2 tablespoons (30 g) finely chopped celery
2 tablespoon (30 g) finely chopped red bell pepper or pimento
⅛ teaspoon onion powder
Salt and pepper to taste
9 fried pork rinds

Combine chicken, mayonnaise, celery, bell pepper, onion powder, salt, and pepper and mix together. Eat the mixture like a dip using the fried pork rinds.

Yield: 1 serving
Per serving: 40 g fat, 1 g net carbs, 23 g protein, 456 calories.

Avocado Bacon Salad Sandwich

This is a delicious, easy-to-make sandwich. It makes a convenient mini-lunch you can take to work. If you do not eat it immediately, you might add in a few drops of lemon juice or citric acid powder (vitamin C) to prevent the avocado from turning brown.

½ avocado
2 strips bacon, crumbled
2 or 3 dashes of chili powder
2 or 3 dashes of onion powder
Salt to taste
Lettuce leaf

To make the filling, mash ½ avocado with chili powder, onion powder, and salt. Mix in crumbled bacon. Spread mixture on a leaf of lettuce and eat like an open faced sandwich or roll the lettuce leaf around the filling and eat like a burrito. Feel free to add chopped scallions, garlic, tomato, or other herbs or vegetables.

Yield: 1 serving
Per serving: 22.5 g fat, 2 g net carbs, 8.5 g protein, 244 calories.

Peanut Butter Celery Sticks

2 tablespoons (32 g) peanut butter
2 tablespoons (30 ml) coconut oil, melted
1 stalk celery, medium long (8 in/20 cm)

Mix together peanut butter and melted coconut oil and put into the refrigerator for about 5 minutes. Once the peanut butter mixture begins to harden, yet not completely hard, remove from the refrigerator, stir, and spread on a stalk of celery. Add salt if desired.

Yield: 1 serving
Per serving: 44 g fat, 5 g net carbs, 8 g protein, 448 calories.

Cream Cheese Celery Sticks
3 tablespoons (45 g) cream cheese
2 tablespoons (30 ml) coconut oil, melted
1 stalk celery, medium long (8 in/20 cm)

Mix together cream cheese and melted coconut oil and put into the refrigerator for about 5 minutes. Once the cream cheese mixture begins to harden, yet not completely hard, remove from the refrigerator, stir, and spread on a stalk of celery. Add salt if desired.

Yield: 1 serving
Per serving: 43 g fat, 2.5 g net carbs, 3 g protein, 409 calories.

Rollups
Rollups can be prepared in advance and make an excellent mini-lunch to go. They also make tasty snacks or a quick breakfast.

1 slice (1 oz/28 g) meat
1 slice (1 oz/28 g) cheese
2 tablespoons (28 g) mayonnaise (page 270)
½ ounce (14 g) sliced pickle
½ ounce (14 g) mixed sprouts (optional)

You can use most any type of thinly sliced meat (ham, beef, corned beef, chicken, turkey) and thinly sliced hard cheese (cheddar, Colby, Edam, Monterey jack, Swiss, mozzarella, Muenster). To make the basic rollup, layer one thinly sliced piece of cheese on top of a thinly sliced piece of meat followed by the mayonnaise, pickle, and sprouts. Roll it into a log with the meat on the outside and sprouts on the inside. Eat and enjoy.

Yield: 1 serving
Per serving: 31.5 g fat, 1.5 g net carbs, 24 g protein, 385 calories.

Variations: A variety of rollups can be created by wrapping other ingredients in the center of the log. You can use any one or more of the following: mustard, mayonnaise, cream cheese, bacon, guacamole, avocado, pickle, chopped eggs, cucumber, sauerkraut, sweet or hot peppers, scallions, and Vinaigrette dressing (page 272).

Meat Bowl

Primitive cultures knew the value of eating fat. Eskimos living off the land in the arctic ate their meat by dipping each bite into seal oil to assure they would get adequate fat. The American Indians ate every speck of fat on the game they killed and would live for months at a time (especially during the winter or when traveling) on pemmican—a mixture of approximately equal portions of chopped dried meat and fat. This Meat Bowl recipe mimics the high-fat diet of these ancient cultures. You can use any type of meat, such as beef, buffalo, venison, chicken, fish, shrimp, and lamb, and any cut of meat, including chopped steak, ground beef, and sausage. The oil can be coconut oil or any other oil or combination of oils. Feel free to adjust the amount of meat and oil used to meet your needs.

2 ounces (56 g) chopped or ground meat (raw or cooked)
3 tablespoons (45 ml) oil
Salt and pepper to taste

Combine meat with oil. If the meat is raw, sauté in the oil until cooked to your preference. If the meat is precooked, heat the two together just until hot. Add salt and pepper to taste. Eat and enjoy. Eat all of the oil.

Yield: 1 serving
Per serving: 54 g fat, 0 g net carbs, 14 g protein, 542 calories.

Beef Soup

6 ounces (170 g) ground beef
¾ cup (80 g) chopped vegetables*
1¼ cups (300 ml) water
¼ teaspoon onion powder
¼ teaspoon paprika
¼ teaspoon marjoram
Salt and pepper to taste

Put ground beef, vegetables, and water in a quart saucepan. Bring to a boil, reduce heat and simmer for about 15 minutes. While cooking, break ground beef into small pieces. Add onion powder, paprika, and marjoram, cook for 1 minute and remove from heat. Add salt and pepper to taste. Let cool slightly. Dish out 1 serving and add 1-3 tablespoons of oil before eating. Put the remainder of the soup, without any added oil, in an airtight container in the refrigerator to eat later. Add your desired amount of oil to each serving just before eating.

*Use two or more of the following vegetables: onion, carrot, mushroom, celery, green beans, bell peppers, okra, turnips, and asparagus.

Yield: 4 ½-cup/118 ml servings
Per serving: 9 g fat, 0 g net carbs, 10.5 g protein, 123 calories. Add 14 grams of fat and 120 calories for every 1 tablespoon of oil added.

Beef Salsa Soup
6 ounces (170 g) ground beef
½ cup (60 g) chopped vegetables*
1¼ (300 ml) cups water
2 tablespoons (30 ml) salsa
Salt and pepper to taste

Put ground beef, vegetables, water, and salsa in a quart saucepan. Bring to a boil, reduce heat and simmer for about 15 minutes. While cooking, break ground beef into small pieces. Remove from heat and add salt and pepper to taste. Let cool slightly. Dish out 1 serving and add 1-3 tablespoons of oil before eating. Put the remainder of the soup, without any added oil, in an airtight container and store in the refrigerator to eat later. Add desired amount of oil to each serving just before eating.

*Use two or more of the following vegetables: onion, carrot, mushroom, celery, green beans, bell peppers, okra, turnips, and asparagus.

Yield: 4 ½-cup/118 ml servings
Per serving: 9 g fat, 1 g net carbs, 10.5 g protein, 127 calories. Add 14 grams of fat and 120 calories for every 1 tablespoon of oil added.

Chicken Soup
1 cup (135 g) chopped chicken
½ cup (60 g) chopped vegetables*
1¼ (300 ml) cups water
⅛ teaspoon celery seed
¼ teaspoon ground sage
Salt and pepper to taste

Put chicken, vegetables, and water in a quart saucepan. Bring to a boil, reduce heat and simmer for about 15 minutes. Add celery seed and sage, cook for 1 minute, and remove from heat. Add salt and pepper to taste. Let cool slightly. Dish out 1 serving and add 1-3 tablespoons of oil before eating. Put the remainder of the soup, without any added oil, in an airtight container and store in the refrigerator to eat later. Add your desired amount of oil to each serving just before eating.

*Use two or more of the following vegetables: onion, carrot, mushroom, celery, green beans, bell peppers, okra, turnips, and asparagus.

Yield: 3 ½-cup/118 ml servings
Per serving: 2 g fat, 0 g net carbs, 14.5 g protein, 76 calories. Add 14 grams of fat and 120 calories for every 1 tablespoon of oil added.

Creamy Ham Soup

This is a low-carb version of ham and potato soup. Chopped turnip is used in place of the potato. When cooked, turnips become sweeter to the taste and have a texture very similar to boiled potatoes, making them good low-carb substitutes for potatoes.

1 cup (135 g) chopped ham
½ cup (60 g) chopped turnips
½ cup (60 g) chopped celery
1 garlic clove, chopped
¾ cup (180 ml) chicken broth or water
½ cup (120 ml) heavy cream
⅛ teaspoon onion powder
⅛ teaspoon salt
⅛ teaspoon black pepper
Butter

Put ham, turnips, celery, garlic, and broth in a saucepan. Bring to a boil, reduce heat and simmer for about 15 minutes or until turnips are tender. Add cream and seasonings, simmer for 1-2 minutes, and remove from heat. Let cool slightly. Dish out 1 serving and add 1-2 tablespoons of butter before eating. Put the remainder, without any added oil or butter, in an airtight container and store in the refrigerator to eat later. Add desired amount of butter to each serving just before eating.

Yield: 4 ½-cup /118 ml servings
Per serving: 16 g fat, 3 g net carbs, 7 g protein, 184 calories. Add 12 grams of fat and 108 calories for every 1 tablespoon of butter added.

Creamy Chicken Soup

1 cup (135 g) chicken, chopped
½ cup (60 g) chopped vegetables*
¾ cup (180 ml) chicken broth or water
½ cup (120 ml) heavy cream

⅛ teaspoon onion powder
⅛ teaspoon celery seed
¼ teaspoon thyme
⅛ teaspoon salt
⅛ teaspoon black pepper

Put chicken, vegetables, and broth in a saucepan. Bring to a boil, reduce heat and simmer for about 15 minutes or until vegetables are tender. Add cream and seasonings, simmer for 1-2 minutes, and remove from heat. Let cool slightly. Dish out 1 serving and add 1-2 tablespoons of coconut oil or another oil before eating. Put the remainder, without any added oil, in an airtight container and store in the refrigerator to eat later. Add desired amount of oil to each serving just before eating.

*Use two or more of the following vegetables: onion, carrot, mushroom, celery, green beans, bell peppers, okra, turnip, and asparagus.

Yield: 3 ½-cup/118 ml servings
Per serving: 17 g fat, 1.5 g net carbs, 15 g protein, 219 calories. Add 14 grams of fat and 120 calories for every 1 tablespoon of oil added.

Tomato Beef Soup
6 ounces (170 g) ground beef
1 cup (235 ml) water
⅓ cup (80 ml) tomato sauce
⅛ teaspoon celery seed
¼ teaspoon onion powder
⅛ teaspoon garlic powder
⅛ teaspoon paprika
¼ teaspoon salt
⅛ teaspoon black pepper
1 teaspoon lemon juice

Combine first nine ingredients into a saucepan, bring to a boil, reduce heat and simmer for 10 minutes. Remove from heat and add lemon juice. Let cool slightly. Dish out 1 serving and add 1-3 tablespoons of coconut oil or another oil before eating. Put the remainder, without any added oil, in an airtight container and store in the refrigerator to eat later. Add desired amount of oil to each serving just before eating.

Yield: 4 ½-cup/118 ml servings
Per serving: 9 g fat, 1 g net carbs, 11 g protein, 129 calories. Add 14 grams of fat and 120 calories for every 1 tablespoon of oil added.

Cream of Broccoli with Cheese

1 cup (240 ml) chicken broth
¾ cup (90 g) chopped broccoli
1 cup (135 g) chopped cooked chicken
½ cup (120 ml) heavy cream
¼ teaspoon salt
⅛ teaspoon black pepper
¼ cup (25 g) freshly grated Parmesan cheese
1 teaspoon scallion, chopped

In a covered saucepan, simmer chicken broth and broccoli for 20 minutes until broccoli is soft. Remove from heat, put into a blender and blend until smooth. Add back to saucepan along with chicken, cream, salt, pepper, and cheese. Heat to a simmer and cook 1-2 minutes. Remove from heat. Serve with freshly chopped scallion sprinkled on top. Let cool slightly. Dish out 1 serving and add 1-3 tablespoons of coconut oil or another oil before eating. Put the remainder, without any added oil, in an airtight container and store in the refrigerator to eat later. Add desired amount of oil to each serving just before eating.

Yield: 4 ½-cup/118 ml servings
Per serving: 14.5 g fat, 1 g net carbs, 14 g protein, 190 calories. Add 14 grams of fat and 120 calories for every 1 tablespoon of oil added.

LOW-CARB SALAD DRESSINGS

Tossed green salads make a good addition to any low-carb or ketogenic diet and, when combined with an oil-based dressing, can supply a sufficient amount of fat in a single meal. Salads can be made with a number of ingredients and dressings that can give you a variety of tastes and flavors. Don't limit yourself to the common iceberg lettuce—try butterhead lettuce, red leaf, romaine, and other varieties. Vegetables that go well with salads include cucumber, bell peppers, banana peppers, tomatoes, avocado, parsley, onion, shallots, scallions, radishes, jicama, parsley, cilantro, watercress, sprouts, celery, celery root (celeriac), bok choy (Chinese cabbage), napa cabbage, red and green cabbage, broccoli, cauliflower, spinach, chard, kale, carrots, Jerusalem artichoke, sauerkraut, chicory, endive, and snow peas. Salads don't always have to include lettuce. You can make a variety of lettuce-free salads with all these vegetables.

Toppings add spark to salads. Low-carb toppings include hard boiled eggs, ham, crumbled bacon, beef, chicken, turkey, pork, fish (salmon, sardines, etc.), crab, shrimp, nori, hard cheeses (cheddar, Monterey, Munster, etc.), soft cheeses (feta, cottage, etc.), nuts, olives, and pork rinds.

The dressing is perhaps the most important part of the salad. It is what makes the salad stand out and gives the other ingredients zing. Most commercially prepared dressings are made using a base of soybean or canola oils and often include sugar, high fructose corn syrup, MSG, and other undesirable additives. Many of them are promoted as low-calorie or low-fat, but few are low-carb. A better choice is a homemade low-carb salad dressing using healthier ingredients. The following are a few such recipes.

Mayonnaise

Most vegetable oils can be used to make mayonnaise. Olive oil produces a mayonnaise that is far healthier than the type you get in the store that is made from polyunsaturated oils. Extra virgin olive oil, however, gives mayonnaise a very strong, olive oil flavor that can overpower the foods it is combined with. Another type of oil called "extra light" olive oil has a mild flavor and makes excellent mayonnaise.

2 egg yolks
2 tablespoons (30 ml) apple cider vinegar
1 teaspoon prepared mustard
¼ teaspoon paprika
½ teaspoon salt
1 cup (240 ml) extra light olive oil

Have all ingredients at room temperature before beginning. Combine egg yolk, mustard, paprika, salt, and ¼ cup (60 ml) oil in blender or food processor. Blend for about 60 seconds. While machine is running, pour in the remaining oil *very slowly*, drop by drop at first and gradually building to a fine, steady stream. The secret to making good mayonnaise is to add the oil in slowly. Mayonnaise will thicken as oil is added. Taste and adjust seasonings as needed. Store the mayonnaise in an airtight container in the refrigerator. It will keep in the refrigerator for several weeks.

Yield: about 20 tablespoons (280 g)
Per tablespoon: 11 g fat, 0 g net carbs, 0 g protein, 99 calories.

Coconut Mayonnaise

Make the mayonnaise recipe as directed above but replace ½ cup of extra light olive oil with ½ cup of coconut oil. Make sure coconut oil is at room temperature and liquid before using. I prefer the milder tasting expeller pressed coconut oil over virgin coconut oil for making mayonnaise.

You can make mayonnaise using only coconut oil, without any olive oil, but you must use it all immediately. Because coconut oil hardens when chilled, if you store the mayonnaise in the refrigerator it will harden and become generally unusable. Mixing the oils allows the mayonnaise to remain soft and creamy when chilled.

Vinegar and Coconut Oil Dressing
¼ cup (60 ml) coconut oil, melted*
¼ cup (60 ml) extra light olive oil
2 tablespoons (30 ml) water
¼ cup (60 ml) apple cider vinegar
⅛ teaspoon salt
⅛ teaspoon white pepper

Put all ingredients into a Mason jar or similar container. Cover and shake vigorously until well blended. Let stand at room temperature until ready to use. It can be stored in the cupboard for several days without refrigeration. If the dressing is to be stored for more than a week, put it into the refrigerator. When chilled, the oil will tend to solidify. To liquefy, take it out of the refrigerator at least 1 hour before using.
  *You may also use MCT oil in place of coconut oil. If desired, you may replace both coconut and extra light olive oils with an equal amount of extra virgin olive oil.

Yield: 14 tablespoons (210 ml)
Per tablespoon: 8 g fat, 0 g net carbs, 0 g protein, 72 calories.

Asian Almond Dressing
½ cup (120 ml) coconut oil
¼ cup (25 g) slivered almonds
1 tablespoon (15 ml) extra light olive oil
2 tablespoons (30 ml) tamari sauce
1 tablespoon (15 ml) apple cider vinegar
¼ teaspoon ground ginger
¼ teaspoon salt

Put coconut oil in small saucepan. At medium to low heat, sauté slivered almonds until lightly browned. Remove from heat and let cool to room temperature. Stir in remaining ingredients. As the dressing sits, the oil will separate to the top and the almonds will sink to the bottom. Stir just before using. Spoon dressing onto salad, making sure to include the almonds. Dressing may be stored in cupboard for several days without refrigeration. If it is to be stored for more than a week, put it into the refrigerator.

Yield: 14 tablespoons (210 ml)
Per tablespoon: 10 g fat, 0 g net carbs, 0.5 g protein, 92 calories.

Vinaigrette

¼ cup (60 ml) red or white wine vinegar
¼ teaspoon salt
⅛ teaspoon white pepper
¾ cup (180 ml) extra virgin olive oil

In a bowl, mix vinegar, salt, and pepper with a fork. Add oil and mix vigorously until well blended.

Yield: 16 tablespoons (240 ml)
Per tablespoon: 10.5 g fat, 0 g net carbs, 0 g protein, 94 calories.

Garlic Herb Dressing

2 cloves garlic, peeled and crushed
1 teaspoon tarragon
1 teaspoon marjoram
1 teaspoon powdered mustard
½ teaspoon salt
¼ teaspoon black pepper
½ cup (120 ml) extra virgin olive oil
¼ cup (60 ml) red or white wine vinegar

Put all ingredients in a pint Mason jar or similar container. Screw on lid and shake contents to mix. Let stand at room temperature at least 1 hour. Shake again just before using.

Yield: 12 tablespoons (180 ml)
Per tablespoon: 9 g fat, 0 g net carbs, 0 g protein, 81 calories.

Ranch Dressing

This dressing is made using sour cream. It tastes best freshly made so the recipe below uses small portions.

3 tablespoons (45 g) sour cream
1 tablespoon (15 ml) heavy cream
⅛ teaspoon onion powder
⅛ teaspoon dill
⅛ teaspoon salt
Dash black pepper

Mix all the ingredients together and serve on a salad.

Yield: 4 tablespoons (60 ml)
Per tablespoon: 3 g fat, 0.5 g net carbs, 0.g protein, 29 calories.

MEALS FOR BREAKFAST, LUNCH, AND DINNER

For most people, breakfast is the most difficult part of the low-carb diet. Traditionally, breakfast consists of high-carb foods such as hot or cold cereal, pancakes, waffles, French toast, hash brown potatoes, muffins, bagels, donuts, toaster pastries, toast and jelly, orange juice, cocoa, and such. The only traditional low-carb breakfast foods are eggs, bacon, ham, and sausage. You can do a lot with eggs. Serve them fried, scrambled, poached, hard or soft boiled, deviled, or as omelets and soufflés, and you already have a great variety. Adding meats and vegetables increases the serving possibilities further. One of the advantages of egg-based meals is that a full meal along with meat and vegetables generally contains fewer than 5 grams of carbohydrate. This allows for a larger amount of carbohydrate to be eaten at lunch and dinner. Several egg dishes are provided below.

As tasty and nutritious as eggs are, it is still nice to have variety for breakfast. Therefore, you should experiment with eating foods not generally considered a part of the traditional breakfast such as salads, soups, beef, chicken, fish, and vegetables. The following recipes can be used for breakfast, lunch, or dinner.

Most of the recipes below specify the use of coconut oil, but you may use butter, bacon drippings, red palm oil, or any other cooking oil you desire. You may also use a combination of oils. Coconut oil is specified in most recipes since this is one of the best ways to add coconut oil into the diet.

You don't have to be a gourmet chef to make delicious low-carb meals. Other than tossed salads, the easiest low-carb meals consist simply of a piece of cooked meat (roasted, fried, baked, grilled, poached, stir-fried) and a vegetable or two. The vegetables can be sautéed, steamed, roasted, poached, or raw. Easier still is to combine the meat and vegetables into a single skillet, crock pot, or baking dish and cook them together. The advantage to this is that it simplifies cooking, requires less cleanup, and, best of all, the meat drippings, especially when combined with seasoned salt or other spices, give the vegetables a wonderful flavor. Below you will find several single skillet recipes to show you how simple and tasty this way of cooking can be.

In most of the recipes provided below you can use more oil than indicated. If you want to make sure you get your daily dose. Calculate this so that you know exactly how much coconut oil is in the dish. When meat is cooked in coconut oil, the oil takes on the flavor of the meat drippings. Use the drippings like a sauce and pour it over your meat and vegetables. Fatty cuts of meat and chicken with the skins on produce the best-tasting drippings.

Easy Omelet

Omelets are easy to make and, with different ingredients, can be made into a dozen or more variations. Omelets made in the traditional French manner can be a bit complicated. This recipe is a simplified version that tastes just as good and allows for multiple variations. These directions are for a plain omelet.

2 tablespoons (30 ml) coconut oil
4 eggs
¼ teaspoon salt
⅛ teaspoon black pepper

Melt coconut oil in skillet over medium heat. Whisk together eggs, salt and pepper in a bowl. Pour mixture into the hot skillet, cover, and cook without stirring until the top of the omelet is set, about five minutes. Remove omelet from pan and serve hot.

Yield: 2 servings
Per serving: 24 g fat, 1 g net carbs, 12 g protein, 268 calories.

Cheese Omelet

Follow the directions for making the Easy Omelet, but after pouring the egg mixture into the hot skillet, sprinkle ¾ cup (84 g) of shredded cheese over the top. Cover and cook without stirring until the omelet is set and the cheese is melted.

Yield: 2 servings
Per serving: 37.5 g fat, 1 g net carbs, 30.5 g protein, 463 calories.

Sausage, Mushroom, and Tomato Omelet

This is a good example of how to prepare an omelet that is combined with meats and vegetables. See the many variations below.

2 tablespoons (30 ml) coconut oil
¼ pound (120 g) sausage
2 mushrooms, sliced
3 eggs
¼ teaspoon salt
½ cup (90 g) chopped tomato

Heat coconut oil in a skillet. Add sausage and mushrooms and cook until sausage is browned. Whisk together eggs and salt in a bowl. Pour mixture into the hot skillet over the sausage and mushrooms, cover, and cook without stirring until the top of the omelet is set, about five minutes. Add tomato, cover, and cook 1 minute. Remove omelet from pan and serve hot.

Yield: 2 servings
Per serving: 42.5 g fat, 3 g net carbs, 19 g protein, 466 calories.

274

Variations: A variety of omelets can be made using many different ingredients including ham, bacon, chicken, sausage, ground beef, ground lamb, shrimp, crab, onions, eggplant, zucchini, garlic, sweet or hot peppers, tomatoes, avocado, asparagus, broccoli, cauliflower, spinach, and mushrooms. The meats and most of the vegetables are cooked before combining with the egg mixture. Tomato, avocado, and garnishes such as cilantro and chives are best used raw and added after cooking. Sour cream can be used as a garnish as well. Cheese can be melted on top during the cooking of the eggs. Any one or more of these ingredients can be combined. You need to make note of the quantities of each ingredient used so that you can calculate the net carbs and fat content.

Simple Soufflé

Soufflés are similar to omelets. This version starts on the stovetop like an omelet but is finished off in the oven, giving it a unique taste and texture. Use eggs at room temperature; this will give them better volume. It is important to use a pan that is both stovetop and oven safe.

4 eggs, separated
¼ teaspoon salt
⅛ teaspoon black pepper
3 tablespoons (45 ml) coconut oil

Preheat oven to 350° F (180° C or gas mark 4). Beat egg yolks, salt, and pepper lightly with a fork. In a separate bowl, beat egg whites until stiff peaks form. Gently mix one-fourth of the egg whites into the yolks. Fold remaining whites into the yolk mixture. Do not over mix. Heat oil in an oven safe pan on the stovetop. Pour egg mixture into hot pan and cook for 1 minute. Transfer pan to oven and cook uncovered for 15 minutes or until soufflé is puffy and delicately browned. Remove from oven, divide in half with a spatula, and serve.

As with all the recipes in this chapter, you can add more oil to increase the fat content. You can also increase fat content by adding cheese, sausage, and other fatty ingredients.

Yield: 2 servings
Per serving: 31 g fat, 0.75g net carbs, 12 g protein, 329 calories.

Cheese Soufflé

In this recipe you first make a cheese sauce which is then mixed into the egg whites. Use a pan that is both stovetop and oven safe.

275

2 tablespoons (30 ml) butter
½ cup (120 ml) heavy cream
1¼ cups (150 g) sharp cheddar cheese, shredded
3 eggs, separated
¼ teaspoon salt
⅛ teaspoon black pepper
1 tablespoon (15 ml) coconut oil

Melt butter in a saucepan over moderate heat. Add cream and cheese, stirring until cheese is melted. Beat egg yolks, salt, and pepper lightly with a fork. Blend about ¼ cup (60 ml) of hot cheese sauce into the yolks. Immediately stir the yolk mixture into the cheese sauce. Cook the sauce over low heat, stirring constantly, for 1-2 minutes. Remove from heat and let cool to room temperature. Meanwhile, preheat oven to 350 ° F (180° C or gas mark 4). In a separate bowl, beat egg whites until stiff peaks form. Gently mix one-fourth of the egg whites into the sauce. Fold the remaining whites into the sauce. Do not over mix or your soufflé will become flat. Heat coconut oil in an oven safe pan on the stovetop. Pour egg mixture into hot pan and cook for 1 minute. Transfer pan to oven and cook uncovered for 18-20 minutes or until soufflé is puffy and delicately browned. Remove from oven, divide in half with a spatula, and serve.

Yield: 2 servings
Per serving: 74 g fat, 3 g net carbs, 28 g protein, 790 calories.

Variations: Prepare Cheese Soufflé as directed but before cooling cheese sauce, mix in ¼ to ½ cup (25-50 g) of any of the following: cooked ham or sausage, crisp crumbled bacon, minced sautéed chicken livers, deviled ham, minced sautéed mushrooms, minced cooked fish or shellfish, minced cooked vegetables (pimiento, asparagus, spinach, broccoli, cauliflower, cabbage, Brussels sprouts, or onions). Adjust net carbs to account for additional ingredients.

Sausage Pancakes
This is a type of egg dish made with coconut flour, sausage, and cheese. Coconut flour is a low-carb flour that can be used to make low-carb baked goods.

6 ounces (170 g) pork sausage
4 eggs
¼ teaspoon onion powder
¼ teaspoon salt
2 tablespoons (16 g) coconut flour

2 teaspoons finely chopped jalapeno pepper
2 ounces (56 g) shredded cheddar cheese
3 tablespoons (45 ml) coconut oil

Brown sausage in a skillet, remove from heat, and let cool. In a bowl, whisk together eggs, onion powder and salt. Add coconut flour and whisk until smooth. Stir in jalapeno pepper, sausage, and cheese. Melt coconut oil in skillet. Spoon batter into hot skillet, making a dozen 2½-inch (6 cm) diameter pancakes. Cook until the underside of the pancakes are browned, turn and cook the other side (about 5 minutes each side, depending on the temperature of the skillet).

Yield: 12 pancakes
Per pancake: 10 g fat, 0.5 g net carbs, 5 g protein, 112 calories.

No Sugar Blueberry Muffins

Blueberry muffins on a low-carb diet, is it possible? Yes, if you use coconut flour and low-carb ingredients. This recipe shows you how it's done. Each muffin contains only 2.2 g of net carbohydrate. Three muffins provide the equivalent of 3 tablespoons of fat. Don't expect these muffins to be highly sweetened like ordinary high-carb muffins. The mild sweetness comes from the berries and a little stevia. Other sweeteners are not recommended. The sweetness of these muffins is tame enough to give you a treat, yet not reactivate your sweet tooth. This recipe makes six muffins.

3 eggs
¼ cup (60 ml) heavy cream
5 tablespoons (70 g) butter, melted
¼ teaspoon almond extract
¼ teaspoon salt
30 drops liquid stevia
¼ cup (32 g) coconut flour
¼ teaspoon baking powder
⅓ cup (50 g) fresh blueberries

Preheat oven to 400° F (200° C or gas mark 6). Using a whisk, blend together eggs, cream, butter, almond extract, salt, and stevia. Combine coconut flour with baking powder and thoroughly mix into batter until there are no lumps left. The batter will be slightly stiff and will stiffen up even more if left to sit, so immediately fold in blueberries. Blueberries should be dry. If they have been rinsed, dry them off before adding to batter. Spoon the batter into muffin tin. Bake for 18-20 minutes. Remove from the oven and cool before eating.

More low-carb coconut flour recipes can be found in my book *Cooking with Coconut Flour: A Delicious Low-Carb, Gluten-Free Alternative to Wheat*.

Yield: 6 muffins
Per muffin: 18.5 g fat, 2.5 g net carbs, 4.5 g protein, 194 calories.

Bratwurst and Cabbage

This delicious single skillet meal can be enjoyed for breakfast or for dinner.

2 tablespoons (30 ml) coconut oil
1 bratwurst
¼ cup (40 g) chopped onion
¼ cup (40 g) chopped bell pepper
1½ cups (112 g) chopped cabbage
Salt and black pepper to taste

Heat coconut oil in skillet. Add bratwurst, onions, and bell pepper. Sauté until the vegetables are crisp and tender and bratwurst is lightly browned. Stir in cabbage, cover, and cook until tender. Add salt and black pepper to taste and serve. Pour meat drippings over vegetables.

Yield: 1 serving
Per serving: 48 g fat, 7.5 g net carbs, 11.5 g protein, 504 calories.

Pork Chops and Green Beans

2 tablespoons (30 ml) coconut oil or butter
2 pork chops
½ cup (80 g) onion, chopped
3 cups (300 g) green beans
4 mushrooms, sliced
Salt and black pepper to taste

Skillet method: Heat coconut oil in skillet. Add pork chops and cook until browned on one side. Turn pork chops over and add onion and green beans. Cover and cook until chops are browned on second side and vegetables are tender. Stir in mushrooms and cook until tender, about 2 minutes. Remove from heat. Add salt and pepper and serve. Pour meat drippings over vegetables.

Oven method: Preheat oven to 350° F (180° C or gas mark 4). Place chops, onion, green beans, and mushrooms in a baking dish, cover, and cook for 60 minutes. Remove from oven. Add butter or coconut oil, salt, and pepper just before serving.

Yield: 2 servings
Per serving: 33 g fat, 12 g net carbs, 27.5 g protein, 455 calories.

Hamburger Steak, Mushrooms, and Onions

Ground beef is cooked like a steak alongside mushrooms and onions. This single-dish meal can be cooked in a skillet or in the oven.

3 tablespoons (45 ml) coconut oil or butter
8 ounces (230 g) ground beef
8 ounces (230 g) sliced mushrooms*
2 ounces (60 g) cheese
½ medium onion, sliced and separated
Salt and black pepper to taste

Skillet method: Heat the oil in a skillet. Divide ground beef into two patties and place in the hot skillet. Add the onions. Cook the meat until one side is browned and flip over. Add mushrooms and continue to cook until second side of beef patty is cooked and mushrooms are tender. Divide the cheese equally and put half on top of each beef patty. Cook until the cheese begins to melt. Add salt and pepper to taste. Pour drippings over meat and vegetables.

Oven method: Preheat oven to 350° F (180° C or gas mark 4). Place patties, mushrooms, and onion in a baking dish, cover, and cook for 45-50 minutes. Put cheese on top of each patty and continue cooking for about 5 minutes or until cheese begins to melt. Remove from oven. Add butter, salt, and pepper just before serving.

*In addition to the mushrooms you can add broccoli, cauliflower, green beans, or other vegetables of your choice.

Yield: 2 servings
Per serving: 54 g fat, 7 g net carbs, 39 g protein, 670 calories.

Chicken and Broccoli

¼ cup (60 ml) coconut oil or butter
8 ounces (230 g) chicken parts (breast, thigh, or leg)
8 ounces (230 g) broccoli, divided into stalks
½ medium onion, sliced and separated
Salt and black pepper to taste

Skillet method: Heat coconut oil in a large skillet over medium heat. Place chicken, skin side down, in hot skillet, cover, and cook for 20-25 minutes. Turn chicken over, cover, and continue to cook for 15 minutes. Add broccoli and onion, cover, and cook another 10 minutes or until vegetables are tender and chicken is completely cooked. Add salt and pepper to taste. Pour meat drippings over broccoli.

Oven method: Preheat oven to 350° F (180° C or gas mark 4). Place chicken, broccoli, and onion in a baking dish, cover, and cook for 60 minutes. Add butter, salt, and pepper just before serving.

Yield: 2 servings
Per serving: 33 g fat, 5 g net carbs, 39 g protein, 473 calories.

Lamb Chops and Asparagus

3 tablespoons (45 ml) coconut oil or butter
2 lamb chops* (8 oz/230 g)
1 pound (450 g) asparagus
Salt and black pepper to taste

Skillet method: Heat oil in a skillet, add chops, cover, and cook until one side is browned. Flip chops and add asparagus, cover and cook until asparagus is tender and chops thoroughly cooked. Remove from heat and add salt and pepper to taste. Pour meat drippings over asparagus.

Oven method: Preheat oven to 350° F (180° C or gas mark 4). Place chops and asparagus in a baking dish, cover, and cook for 60 minutes. Add butter, salt, and pepper just before serving.

*May also use pork chops or beefsteak.

Yield: 2 servings
Per serving: 41 g fat, 7.5 g net carbs, 32.5 g protein, 529 calories.

Chicken Stir-Fry

¼ cup (60 ml) coconut oil
½ pound (225 g) chicken, cut into bite size pieces
½ cup (80 g) chopped onion
½ cup (80 g) snow peas, cut in half
½ cup (80 g) chopped bok choy
½ cup (80 g) chopped bell pepper
4 mushrooms, sliced
½ cup (80 g) bamboo shoots
1-3 teaspoons (5-15 ml) rice vinegar (optional)
Salt to taste

Heat coconut oil in a skillet. Sauté chicken and vegetables until vegetables are tender and chicken is cooked. Turn off heat, add rice vinegar and salt to taste.

Yield: 2 servings
Per serving: 33 g fat, 6 g net carbs, 37 g protein, 469 calories.

Fillet of Sole in Coconut Milk

2 tablespoons (30 ml) coconut oil
½ medium onion, chopped
½ cup bell pepper, chopped
2 cups (200 g) chopped cauliflower
2 cloves garlic, chopped
2 sole fillets*
1 teaspoon garam masala**
¾ cup (180 ml) coconut milk
Salt and black pepper to taste

Heat coconut oil in skillet and sauté onion, pepper, cauliflower, and garlic until tender. Push vegetable to side of skillet and add sole. Stir garam masala into coconut milk and add to skillet. Cover and simmer for about 8 minutes. Add salt and pepper.

*You may use any type of fish in this recipe.

**Garam masala is a blend of spices commonly used in Indian cuisine and similar to curry powder. It's available in the spice section of most grocery stores. If you don't have garam masala, you can use curry powder.

Yield: 2 servings
Per serving: 33 g fat, 9 g net carbs, 14 g protein, 349 calories.

Appendix

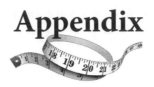

Nutrient Counter

This table lists the number of grams of energy producing nutrients—net carbohydrate, fat, and protein—as well as the calorie content of a variety of basic foods. Net carbohydrate is the carbohydrate in foods that provides calories and affects blood sugar. It is derived by subtracting the fiber content from the total carbohydrate content of each food.

The information in this table is derived primarily from databases of nutritive values of foods published by United States Department of Agriculture (USDA). There are many factors that can influence the amounts of nutrients in foods, including the climate and growing conditions, the method of processing, genetics, the diet of animals, the type of fertilizers used on crops, the season of the year, methods of analysis, methods of storage, and methods of cooking. The values reported in the USDA databases are often presented as single numbers, when in reality, the numbers are actually an average of a range of values based on the samples analyzed. As a consequence, nutrient values reported in various reliable sources may differ slightly. This is why you may see different values for the same type of food from separate sources.

Some nutrient tables list values to the tenth of a gram. This gives the appearance of a highly precise measurement, but in reality gives a false impression of accuracy. All nutrient values are averages and can differ from one source to another by as much as several grams. Therefore, nutrient tables that report values to a tenth of a gram can be misleading and make calculating total nutrient intake more cumbersome without any additional accuracy.

All nutritive values listed in this table are given to the nearest half gram as reported on the USDA databases. Values for many foods not found in this list, including prepared, packaged foods and popular restaurant foods may be found at www.calorieking.com.

Food	Amount	Net Carbs (g)	Fat (g)	Protein (g)	Calories (kcal)
Vegetables					
Alfalfa sprouts	1 cup/33 g	0.5	1	0	11
Artichoke, boiled	1 medium/120 g*	6.5	5.5	0.5	86
Arugula	1 cup/20 g	0.5	0	0.5	5
Asparagus, raw	4 spears/1 cup/60 g	2	0	2	15
Avocado (Haas)	1 each/173 g*	3.5	28	4	282
Bamboo shoots, canned	1 cup/131 g	2.5	0.5	2	23
Beans, boiled, drained					
black	1 cup/172 g	26	1	15	173
black-eyed peas	1 cup/172 g	15	1	13	121
garbanzo (chickpeas)	1 cup/164 g	34	4	15	232
great northern	1 cup/177 g	26	1	15	173
green beans, fresh	1 cup/100 g	7	0	2	40
kidney	1 cup/170 g	27	1	14	173
lentils	1 cup/198 g	30	1	18	201
lima	1 cup/172 g	24	1	14	161
navy	1 cup/182 g	32	1	16	201
pinto	1 cup/898 g	24	1	14	161
soybeans	1 cup/172 g	12	15	29	298
Bean sprouts (mung)					
boiled	1 cup/124 g	2	0	3	20
raw	1 cup/104 g	3	0	3	24
Beets (sliced), raw	1 cup/170 g	8	0	1	36
Beet greens, boiled	1 cup/144 g	5	0	4	36
Broccoli, raw, chopped	1 cup/88 g	2	0	3	20
Brussels sprouts, boiled	1 cup/156 g	8	1	6	65
Cabbage, green, shredded					
cooked	1 cup/150 g	3	0.5	1	20
raw	1 cup/70 g	2	0	0.5	10
Cabbage, red, shredded					
cooked	1 cup/150 g	3	0	1	16
raw	1 cup/70 g	2	0	1	12
Chinese cabbage (bok choy)					
cooked	1 cup/170 g	1	0	2.5	14
raw	1 cup/170 g	1	0	1	8
Carrot					
boiled, chopped	1 cup/156 g	10	0	1.5	46
raw, whole	1 medium/72 g	5	0	0.5	22
raw, shredded	1 cup/110 g	8	0	2	40
juice	1 cup/246 g	18	1	2	89

*The amount indicated is for the edible portion, less skin, core, pit, seeds, etc.

Food	Amount	Net Carbs (g)	Fat (g)	Protein (g)	Calories (kcal)
Cauliflower					
boiled	1 cup/124 g	1.5	0.5	2	19
raw, chopped	1 cup/100 g	2.5	0	2	18
Celery					
raw, whole	8 in long/40 g	1	0	0	6
raw, diced	1 cup/120 g	2	0	0.5	10
Chard					
boiled	1 cup/175 g	3.5	0	3	26
raw	1 cup/36 g	1.5	0	0.5	7
Chives, chopped	1 tbsp/6 g	0	0	0	1
Collards					
boiled, drained	1 cup/190 g	4	0.5	4	36
raw	1 cup/37 g	0.5	0	1	6
Cucumber, sliced					
raw with peel	1 cup/119 g	3	0	0	14
Daikon, raw	4 in/10 cm long	6	0	2	33
Eggplant, raw	1 cup/82 g	2	0	1	12
Escarole, raw	1 cup/50 g	0.5	0	1	6
Garlic, raw	1 clove	1	0	0	4
Jerusalem artichoke, raw	1 cup/150 g	24	0	3	104
Jicama, raw	1 cup/130 g	5	0	1	24
Kale, chopped, boiled	1 cup/130 g	3	1	3	33
Kelp, raw	1 oz/28 g	2	0	1	12
Kohlrabi					
cooked, sliced	1 cup/140 g	7	0	2	36
raw, sliced	1 cup/165 g	9	0	3	48
Leeks, raw	1 cup/104 g	13	0	2	60
Lettuce					
butterhead	2 leaves/15 g	0	0	0	1
iceberg	1 wedge/135 g	1	0	1	8
iceberg, shredded	1 cup/56 g	0.5	0	0.5	4
loose leaf, chopped	1 cup/56 g	0.5	0	0.5	4
romaine, chopped	1 cup/56 g	0.5	0	0.5	4
Mushrooms (button)					
boiled	1 cup/156 g	4	0.5	3.5	34
raw, sliced	1 cup/70 g	2.5	0	2.5	20
raw	3 mushrooms	1	0	1	9
Mustard greens					
raw	1 cup/60 g	1	0	1.5	10
boiled	1 cup/140 g	0.5	0	3	14
Okra, raw, sliced	1 cup/184 g	12	0	4	64

Food	Amount	Net Carbs (g)	Fat (g)	Protein (g)	Calories (kcal)
Onion					
raw, sliced	1 cup/115 g	8	0	1	36
raw, chopped	1 cup/160 g	11	0	2	52
raw, whole medium	2.5 in/6.4 cm dia	10	0	1	46
Parsley					
raw, chopped	1 tbsp/4 g	0	0	0	1
Parsnips					
raw, chopped	1 cup/110 g	17.5	0.5	1.5	80
Peas					
edible-pod, cooked	1 cup/160 g	7	0.5	5.5	54
green, boiled	1 cup/160 g	7	0	4	44
split, boiled	1 cup/196 g	31	1	16	197
Peppers					
hot red chili, raw	½ cup/68 g	3	0	1	17
jalapeno, canned	½ cup/68 g	1	0	1	8
sweet (bell), raw,	1 cup/50 g	2	0	1	10
sweet (bell), raw	1 medium	4	0	1	20
Potatoes					
baked, with skin	1 medium/202 g	46	0	5	204
baked, without skin	1 medium/156 g	32	0	3	140
mashed, with milk	1 cup/210 g	34	1	4	162
hash brown					
cooked in oil	1 cup/156 g	41	18	5	344
Pumpkin, canned	1 cup/245 g	15	0.5	2.5	75
Radish, raw	10 radishes/45 g	1	0	0	7
Rhubarb, raw, copped	1 cup/122 g	3.5	0	1	18
Rutabaga, chopped,					
cooked	1 cup/170 g	12	0	2	58
Sauerkraut, canned					
with liquid	1 cup/236 g	6	0	2	32
Scallions					
raw, chopped	½ cup/50 g	3	0	1	16
raw, whole	4 in/10 cm long	1	0	0	5
Shallots, raw, minced	1 tbsp/10 g	1	0	0	7
Spinach					
cooked, drained	1 cup/180 g	3	0	5	32
raw, chopped	1 cup/56 g	1	0	2	13
Sprouts, see Alfalfa					
Squash, winter verities					
crookneck, raw, sliced	1 cup/180 g	5	1	2	36
scallop, raw sliced	1 cup/113 g	3	0	1	18
zucchini, raw sliced	1 cup/180 g	3	0	1	16

Food	Amount	Net Carbs (g)	Fat (g)	Protein (g)	Calories (kcal)
Squash, summer varieties					
acorn, baked, mashed	1 cup/245 g	29	0	3	128
butternut, baked,					
mashed	1 cup/245 g	19	0	2	84
Hubbard, baked,					
mashed	1 cup/240 g	20	1	6	113
spaghetti, baked	1 cup/155	6	0	1	28
Sweet potato, baked	1 med,4 oz/114 g	25	0	2.5	110
Taro					
root, cooked, sliced	1 cup/104 g	24	0	2	104
leaves, raw, chopped	1 cup/28 g	1	0	1	9
Tofu	½ cup/126 g	1	5	10	88
Tomato					
cooked/stewed	1 cup/240 g	10	1	3	61
raw, chopped	1 cup/180 g	5	0	2	28
raw, sliced	0.25 in/0.6 cm thick	1	0	0	4
raw, whole	1 med, 4.3 oz/123 g	4	0	1	22
raw	1 lg, 6.4 oz/181 g	5	0	2	28
cherry	2 med, 1.2 oz/34 g	1	0	0	6
Italian	1 med, 2.2 oz/62 g	2	0	1	11
juice	1 cup/244 g	8	0	2	42
paste	½ cup/131 g	19	1	5	105
sauce	½ cup/122 g	7	0	3	40
Turnips, raw	1 med	6	0	1	28
Turnip greens, raw	1 cup/55g	1.5	0	0.5	12
Water chestnuts, sliced	½ cup/70 g	7	0	0.5	30
Watercress, raw chopped	½ cup/17 g	0	0	0	2
Yam, baked	1 cup/150 g	36	0	2	152

Fruit

Food	Amount	Net Carbs (g)	Fat (g)	Protein (g)	Calories (kcal)
Apples					
raw	1 each/138 g*	18	0	0.5	76
juice	1 cup/248 g	29	0	0	116
applesauce,					
unsweetened	1 cup/244 g	24	0	0	98
Apricots					
raw	1 each	3	0	0.5	16
canned, in syrup	1 cup/258 g	51	0	1.5	213
Banana	1 each/114 g*	25	0.5	1	109
Blackberries, fresh	1 cup/144 g	8	1	1	45
Blueberries, fresh	1 cup/145 g	17	1	1	83

Food	Amount	Net Carbs (g)	Fat (g)	Protein (g)	Calories (kcal)
Boysenberries, frozen	1 cup/132 g	9	0	1	40
Cantaloupe	½ each/267 g	19	1	2	94
Cherries, sweet, raw	10 each/68 g	9.5	0	0.5	40
Cranberry					
Raw	1 cup/95 g	7	0	0	44
Sauce, whole berry					
canned	1 cup/277 g	102	0	1	410
Dates, raw					
whole without pits	10 each/83 g	54	0	2	228
chopped	1 cup/178 g	116	1	4	489
Elderberries, raw	1 cup/145 g	16.5	0.5	1	75
Figs	10 each/187 g	101	2	6	446
Gooseberries, raw	1 cup/150 g	9	1	1	49
Grapefruit, raw	1 half/91 g	7	0	1	34
Grapes					
Thompson seedless	10 each/50 g	8	0	0	35
American (slip skin)	10 each/50 g	4	0	0	18
juice, canned	1 cup/236 ml	37	0	0	150
juice, from					
frozen concentrate	1 cup/236 ml	31	0	0	126
Honeydew	1 cup/6 oz/170 g*	14	0	1	60
Kiwi, raw	1 each/76 g*	8	0.5	1	38
Lemon, raw	1 each	4	0	0.5	18
Lemon Juice	1 tbsp/15 ml	1	0	0	4
Lime, raw	1 each	3	0	0	12
Lime Juice	1 tbsp/15 ml	1	0	0	4
Loganberries, frozen	1 cup/147 g	11	0.5	2	57
Mandarin orange					
canned, juice pack	1 cup/250 g	22	0	1.5	94
canned, light syrup	1 cup/250 g	39	0	1	160
Mango, raw	1 each/207 g*	28	1	1	125
Mulberries, raw	1 cup/138 g	11	0.5	2	57
Nectarines, raw	1 each/136 g*	13	0.5	1.5	63
Olives					
black	10 each	2	4	0	44
green	10 each	1	5	0	49
Oranges, raw	1 each/248 g*	12	0	1	52
Juice, fresh	1 cup/236 ml	25	0.5	1.5	110
Juice, from					
frozen concentrate	1 cup/236 ml	27	0	12	115
Papayas, raw, sliced	1 cup/140 g*	12	0	1	52

*The amount indicated is for the edible portion, less skin, core, pit, seeds, etc.

Food	Amount	Net Carbs (g)	Fat (g)	Protein (g)	Calories (kcal)
Peaches					
raw, whole	1 each/87 g*	8	0	1	37
raw sliced	1 cup/153 g	14	0.5	1.5	66
canned, heavy syrup	1 cup/256 g	48	0	1	196
canned, juice packed	1 cup/248 g	26	0	2	112
Pears					
raw	1 each/166 g*	20	0.5	1	89
canned, heavy syrup	1 cup/255 g	45	0	1	184
canned, juice packed	1 cup/248 g	28	0	1	116
Persimmon, raw	1 each	8.5	0	0	34
Pineapple,					
fresh, cubed	1 cup/155 g	17	1	1	81
crushed/cubed, packed					
in heavy syrup	1 cup/255 g	50	0	1	204
crushed/cubed,					
juice packed	1 cup/250 g	37	0	1	152
Plantains, cooked, sliced	1 cup/154 g*	41	0	1	168
Plums, raw	1 each/66 g*	7.5	0	0.5	34
Prunes					
dried	10 each/84 g	45	0	2	188
juice	1 cup/236 ml	42	0	2	176
Raisins	1 cup/145 g	106	1	5	431
Raspberries, raw	1 cup/123 g	6	0.5	1	33
Strawberries					
raw, whole	1 each	1	0	0	3
raw, halves	1 cup/153 g	8	0	1	36
raw, sliced	1 cup/167 g	9	0	1	41
Tangerines, fresh	1 each/84 g*	7.5	0	0.5	32
Watermelon					
sliced	1 inch/2.5 cm	33	0.5	3	149
balls	1 cup/160 g	11	0	1	47
Nuts and Seeds					
Almonds					
sliced or slivered	1 cup/95 g	9	47	20	539
whole	1 oz/28 g	3	15	6	171
almond butter	1 tbsp/16 g	2	9	2	97
Brazil nuts	1 oz/28 g	1.5	19	4	193
Cashew					
halves and whole	1 cup/137 g	37	63	21	799
whole	1 oz/28 g	6	14	5	170
cashew butter	1 tbsp/16 g	3	8	3	94

Food	Amount	Net Carbs (g)	Fat (g)	Protein (g)	Calories (kcal)
Coconut					
fresh	2 x 2 in/5 x 5 cm	2	15	2	153
fresh, shredded	1 cup/80 g	3	27	3	267
dried, unsweetened	1 cup/78 g	7	50	5	498
dried, sweetened	1 cup/93 g	35	33	3	449
Filberts (hazelnuts)					
whole	1 oz/28 g	2	18	4	186
whole	1 cup/118 g	11	72	15	752
Macadamia					
whole	1 oz/28 g	1.5	22	2	212
whole or halves	1 cup/134 g	7	102	10.5	988
Peanuts					
oil roasted	1 cup/144 g	14	71	38	846
oil roasted	1 oz/28 g	3	14	7	164
peanut butter	1 tbsp/16 g	2	8	4	94
Pecans					
halves, raw	1 cup/108 g	5	73	8	709
halves, raw	1 oz/28 g	3	19	2	191
Pine nuts					
whole	1 oz/28 g	3	17	3	177
Pistachio					
Whole, roasted	1 oz/28 g	6	14	6	174
Whole, roasted	1 cup/128 g	21	68	19	772
Pumpkin seeds					
whole	1 oz/28 g	3	12	9	154
whole	1 cup/227 g	11	50	39	650
Sesame seeds					
whole	1 tbsp/9.5 g	1	4.5	1.5	51
sesame butter (tahini)	1 tbsp/15 g	2	8	3	92
Soy nuts, roasted	1 oz/28 g	5	5	9	101
Sunflower seeds					
whole, hulled	1 tbsp/8.5 g	1	4	2	47
Walnuts					
Black	1 oz/28 g	1	16	7	176
black, chopped	1 cup/125 g	4	71	30	775
English	1oz/28 g	3	18	4	190
English, chopped	1 cup/120 g	8	74	17	766

Grains and Flours

Food	Amount	Net Carbs (g)	Fat (g)	Protein (g)	Calories (kcal)
Amaranth, whole grain	1 cup/192 g	100	13	28	629
Arrowroot flour	1 tbsp/8.5 g	7	0	0	27

Food	Amount	Net Carbs (g)	Fat (g)	Protein (g)	Calories (kcal)
Barley					
pearled, uncooked	1 cup/200 g	127	2	16	590
pearled, cooked	1 cup/157 g	40	1	4	183
flour	1 cup/124 g	95	2	15	458
Buckwheat					
whole grain	1 cup/175 g	112	4	23	576
flour	1 cup/98 g	73	4	15	388
Bulgur					
whole grain, cooked	1 cup/182 g	23	0	6	116
flour	1 cup/140 g	75	2	17	386
Coconut flour	1 cup/114 g	24	16	24	336
Corn					
whole kernel	1 cup/210 g	38	1	5	181
ear, small	6 in/15 cm long	12	1	3	69
ear, medium	7 in/18 cm long	15	1	3	81
ear, large	8.5 in/22 cm long	23	2	5	90
grits, uncooked	1 cup/156 g	122	2	14	562
grits, cooked with water	1 cup/240 g	30	1	3	140
cornmeal, dry	1 cup/122 g	81	4	10	400
corn starch	1 tbsp/8.5 g	7	0	0	28
popcorn, air popped	1 cup/8.5 g	5	0	1	24
hominy, canned	1 cup/260 g	20	2	2	106
Millet					
uncooked	1 cup/200 g	129	7	22	667
cooked	1 cup/240 g	54	2	8	266
Oats					
oatmeal, cooked	1 cup/234 g	21	2	6	126
oatmeal, uncooked	1 cup/100 g	46	5	11	269
oat bran, uncooked	¼ cup/25 g	13	2	4	86
Quinoa					
uncooked	1 cup/170 g	98	10	24	578
cooked	1 cup/184 g	34	4	8	204
Rice					
brown, cooked	1 cup/195 g	42	2	5	206
white, cooked	1 cup/205 g	56	1	6	257
instant, cooked	1 cup/165 g	34	1	3	157
wild rice, cooked	1 cup/164 g	32	1	4	153
brown rice flour	1 cup/159 g	114	4	11	536
white rice flour	1 cup/159 g	123	2	9	546
Rye flour	1 cup/102	64	2	10	314
Semolina flour, enriched	1 cup/167 g	115	2	21	562

Food	Amount	Net Carbs (g)	Fat (g)	Protein (g)	Calories (kcal)
Soy flour	1 cup/88 g	24	6	41	314
Tapioca					
pearl dry	1 cup/152 g	133	0	3	544
flour	1 tbsp/8 g	7	0	0	26
Wheat					
white, flour	1 cup/128 g	92	1	13	429
white, flour	1 tbsp/8 g	6	0	1	28
whole wheat flour	1 cup/120 g	72	2	16	370
whole wheat flour	1 tbsp/7.5 g	5	0	1	24
wheat bran	½ cup/30 g	11	1	5	73

Bread and Baked Goods

Food	Amount	Net Carbs (g)	Fat (g)	Protein (g)	Calories (kcal)
Bagels					
white enriched	1 ea (3.7 oz/105 g)	57	2	12	294
whole grain	1 ea (4.5 oz/128 g)	64	3	14	339
Bread					
rye	1 slice	13	1	3	73
whole wheat	1 slice	11	1	4	69
white	1 slice	12	1	2	65
raisin bread	1 slice	13	1	2	69
hamburger bun	1 roll	20	2	4	114
hot dog bun	1 roll	20	2	4	114
hard/Kaiser roll	1 roll	29	2	6	158
Crackers					
Saltine	1 each	2	0	0	9
wheat	1 each	1	0	0	5
cheese	1 each	1	0	0	5
English muffin	1 each	24	1	4	121
Pancake	1 ea (4 in/10 cm dia)	13	5	3	108
Pita					
white	1 each	32	1	5	157
whole wheat	1 each	31	2	6	166
Tortilla					
corn	1 ea (6 in/15 cm)	11	1	2	61
flour	1 ea (8 in/20 cm)	22	4	4	140
flour	1 ea (10.5 in/27 cm)	34	5	6	205
Wonton wrappers	1 ea (3.5 in/9 cm)	5	0	1	23

Pasta

Food	Amount	Net Carbs (g)	Fat (g)	Protein (g)	Calories (kcal)
Macaroni, cooked					
white, enriched	1 cup/140 g	38	1	8	193

Food	Amount	Net Carbs (g)	Fat (g)	Protein (g)	Calories (kcal)
whole wheat	1 cup/140 g	35	1	8	181
corn	1 cup/140 g	32	1	4	153
Noodles, cooked					
cellophane					
(mung bean)	1 cup/190 g	39	0	1	160
egg	1 cup/160 g	36	2	8	194
soba	1 cup/113 g	19	0	6	100
rice	1 cup/175 g	42	0	2	176
Spaghetti, cooked					
white, enriched	1 cup/140 g	38	1	7	189
whole wheat	1 cup/140 g	32	1	7	165
corn	1 cup/140 g	32	1	4	153

Dairy

Food	Amount	Net Carbs (g)	Fat (g)	Protein (g)	Calories (kcal)
Almond milk	1 cup/236 ml	7	3	1	59
Butter	1 tbsp/14 g	0	12	0.5	110
Buttermilk	1 cup/236 ml	12	8	8	152
Cheese (hard)					
American, sliced	1 oz/28 g	0.5	9	6	107
Cheddar, sliced	1 oz/28 g	0.5	9	7	111
Cheddar, shredded	1 cup/113 g	1.5	37	28	451
Colby, sliced	1 oz/28 g	0.5	9	7	111
Colby, shredded	1 cup/113 g	3	36	27	444
Edam, sliced	1 oz/28 g	0.5	8	7	101
Edam, shredded	1 cup/113 g	1.5	29	26	371
Gruyere, sliced	1 oz/28 g	0	9	8	113
Gruyere, shredded	1 cup/113 g	0.5	35	32	445
Monterey, sliced	1 oz/28 g	0	9	7	108
Monterey, shredded	1 cup/113 g	1	34	28	421
mozzarella, sliced	1 oz/28 g	0.5	6	6	80
mozzarella, shredded	1 cup/113 g	2.5	25	25	335
Muenster, sliced	1 oz/28 g	0	8	7	100
Muenster, shredded	1 cup/113 g	1	33	26	405
Parmesan, sliced	1 oz/28 g	1	7	10	107
Parmesan, grated	1 tbsp/5 g	0	2	2	25
Swiss, sliced	1 oz/28 g	1.5	8	8	110
Swiss, shredded	1 cup/113 g	6	30	29	305
Cheese (soft)					
Brie	1 oz/28 g	1	8	6	100
Camembert	1 oz/28 g	0	7	6	87
cottage, non-fat	1 cup/226 g	9.5	0.5	15	102
cottage, 2% fat	1 cup/226 g	8	4	31	192

Food	Amount	Net Carbs (g)	Fat (g)	Protein (g)	Calories (kcal)
cream cheese, plain	1 tbsp/14 g	0.5	5	1	51
cream cheese, low-fat	1 tbsp/14 g	1	3	1.5	37
feta, crumbled	1 oz/28 g	1	6	4	75
ricotta, whole milk	1 oz/28 g	1	3.5	3	44
ricotta, whole milk	1 cup/246 g	7.5	31.5	27.5	424
ricotta, part skim	1 oz/28 g	1.5	2	3	36
ricotta, part skim	1 cup/246 g	12.5	19	27.5	331
Coconut milk, canned	1 cup/236 ml	7	50	5	498
Coconut milk beverage, carton	1 cup/236 ml	7	5	1	77
Cream					
heavy whipping	1 cup/236 ml	6.5	89	5	847
half and half	1 cup/236 ml	10.5	28	7	322
sour	1 tbsp/28 g	0.5	2.5	0.5	26
Goat milk	1 cup/236 ml	11	10	9	170
Milk					
skim, non-fat	1 cup/236 ml	12	0.5	8.5	86
1%	1 cup/236 ml	12	2.5	8.5	104
2%	1 cup/236 ml	11.5	4.5	8	119
whole, 3.3% fat	1 cup/236 ml	11	8	8	148
Kefir	1 cup/236 ml	9	5	9	117
Rice milk					
plain	1 cup/236 ml	23	3	1	123
vanilla	1 cup/236 ml	26	3	1	135
Soy milk	1 cup/236 ml	7	4	6	88
Yogurt					
plain, fat-free	1 cup/227 g	19	0.5	14	136
plain, low-fat	1 cup/227 g	16	3	12	139
plain, whole milk	1 cup/227 g	12	8.5	9	160
vanilla, low-fat	1 cup/227 g	31	3	11	195
fruit added, low-fat	1 cup/227 g	43	2.5	10	234

Meat and Eggs

Food	Amount	Net Carbs (g)	Fat (g)	Protein (g)	Calories (kcal)
Beef	3 oz/85 g	0	18	21	246
Eggs	1 large	0.5	5	6	71
Egg yolk	1 large	0.5	5	3	59
Egg white	1 large	0	0	4	17
Fish					
bass	3 oz/85 g	0	3	21	111
cod	3 oz/85 g	0	1	19	87
flounder	3 oz/85 g	0	1	21	93

Food	Amount	Net Carbs (g)	Fat (g)	Protein (g)	Calories (kcal)
haddock	3 oz/85 g	0	1	19	87
Pollock	3 oz/85 g	0	1	20	89
salmon	3 oz/85 g	0	5	17	113
sardines, canned, drained	3 oz/85 g	0	11	21	183
trout	3 oz/85 g	0	4	22	124
tuna, canned, water packed	3 oz/85 g	0	1	25	109
Lamb chop	3 oz/85 g	0	20	25	280
Poultry					
chicken, dark meat	1 cup/140 g	0	14	38	278
chicken, dark meat	3 oz/85 g	0	8	23	164
chicken, light meat	1 cup/140 g	0	6	43	226
chicken, light meat	3 oz/85 g	0	4	26	140
duck	½ duck/221 g	0	108	73	1264
turkey, dark meat	3 oz/85 g	0	6	24	150
turkey, light meat	3 oz/85 g	0	3	25	127
turkey, ground	3 oz/85 g	0	12	21	192
Pork					
bacon, cured	3 pieces	0.5	13	10	159
Canadian-style bacon	2 pieces	1	4	11	84
chops	3 oz/85 g	0	19	24	267
fresh side (uncured bacon)	3 oz/85 g	0	13	10	157
ham	3 oz/85 g	1	14	18	202
Sausage					
frankfurter, beef/pork	1 ea/57 g	1	17	6	181
frankfurter, chicken	1 ea/45 g	3	9	6	117
frankfurter, turkey	1 ea/45 g	1	8	6	100
bratwurst	1 ea/70 g	2	20	10	228
kielbasa	1 ea/26 g	1	7	3	79
Polish	1 ea/28 g	0	8	4	88
pork, link (large)	1 ea/68 g	1	21	9	229
pork, link (small)	1 ea/13 g	0	4	3	48
salami, beef/pork	2 pices/57 g	1	11	8	135
Shellfish					
clams, canned	3 oz/85 g	4	2	22	122
crab, cooked	1 cup/135 g	0	2	27	126
lobster, cooked	1 cup/145 g	2	1	30	137
mussels, cooked	1 oz/28 g	2	1	7	45
oysters, raw	1 cup/248 g	10	6	18	166

Food	Amount	Net Carbs (g)	Fat (g)	Protein (g)	Calories (kcal)
scallops	3 oz/85 g	1	1	20	93
shrimp, cooked	3 oz/85 g	0	1	18	81
Venison	3 oz/85 g	0	3	26	131

Miscellaneous

Food	Amount	Net Carbs (g)	Fat (g)	Protein (g)	Calories (kcal)
Baking soda	1 tsp/9 g	0	0	0	0
Catsup					
regular	1 tbsp/15 g	4	0	0	15
low-carb	1 tbsp/15 g	1	0	0	5
Fats and oils	1 tbsp/14 g	0	14	0	122
Gelatin, dry	1 envelope/7 g	0	0	6	23
Fish sauce	1 tbsp/15 ml	0.5	0	1	11
Herbs and spices	1 tbsp/5 g	2	0	0	9
Honey	1 tbsp/21 g	17	0	0	68
Horseradish, prepared	1 tbsp/15 g	1.5	0	0	5
Maple syrup	1 tbsp/15 ml	13.5	0	0	54
Mayonnaise	1 tbsp/14 g	0	10	0	90
Molasses	1 tbsp/20 g	15	0	0	58
Molasses, blackstrap	1 tbsp/20 g	12	0	0	47
Mustard					
yellow	1 tbsp/15 g	0	1	1	12
Dijon	1 tbsp/15 g	0	0	0	5
Pancake syrup	1 tbsp/15 g	15	0	0	58
Pickles					
dill, medium	1 pickle/65 g	3	0	1	12
dill, slice	1 (0.2 oz/6 g)	1	0	0	5
sweet, medium	1 pickle/35 g	11	0	0	44
pickle relish, sweet	1 tbsp/15 g	5	0	0	20
Tartar sauce	1 tbsp/15 g	2	8.5	0	85
Salsa	1 tbsp/15 g	1	0	0	5
Soy sauce	1 tbsp/15 ml	1	0	1	8
Sugar					
white, granulated	1 tbsp/11 g	12	0	0	48
brown, unpacked	1 tbsp/8 g	9	0	0	35
powdered	1 tbsp/8 g	8	0	0	32
Vinegar					
apple cider	1 tbsp/15 ml	0	0	0	3
balsamic	1 tbsp/15 ml	2	0	0	8
red wine	1 tbsp/15 ml	0	0	0	3
rice	1 tbsp/15 ml	0	0	0	3
Worcestershire sauce	1 tbsp/15 ml	3	0	0	12

References

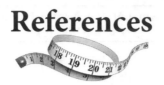

Chapter 1—The Undiet Diet
1. McGee, C.T. *Heart Frauds: Uncovering the Biggest Health Scam in History*. Piccadilly Books, Ltd: Colorado Springs, CO, 2001.
2. Prior, I.A., et al. Cholesterol, coconuts, and diet on Polynesian atolls: a natural experiment: the Pukapuka and Tokelau Island studies. *Am J Clin Nutr* 1981;34:1552.

Chapter 2—Big Fat Lies
1. Vigilante, K. and Flynn, M. *Low-Fat Lies: High-Fat Frauds and the Healthiest Diet in the World*. Life Line Press: Washington, DC, 1999.

Chapter 3—Are You In Need of An Oil Change?
1. Cleave, T.L. *The Saccharine Disease*. Keats Publishing: New Canaan, CT, 1973.
2. Raloff, J. Unusual fats lose heart-friendly image. *Science News* 1996;150(6):87.
3. Kummerow, F.A. *Federation Proceedings* 1975;33:235.
4. Mensink, R.P. and Katan, M.B. Effect of dietary trans fatty acids on high-density and low-density lipoprotein cholesterol levels in healthy subjects. *N Eng J Med* 1990;323(7):439.
5. *Science News*. Trans fats: worse than saturated? 1990;138(8):126.
6. Willett, W.C., et al. Intake of trans fatty acids and risk of coronary heart disease among women. *Lancet* 1993;341(8845):581.
7. Thampan, P.K. *Facts and Fallacies About Coconut Oil*. Asian and Pacific Coconut Community: Jakarta, 1994.
8. Booyens, J. and Louwrens, C.C. The Eskimo diet. Prophylactic effects ascribed to the balanced presence of natural cis unsaturated fatty acids and to the absence of unnatural trans and cis isomers of unsaturated fatty acids. *Med Hypoth* 1986;21:387.
9. Kritchevsky, D., et al. *Journal of Atherosclerosis Research* 1967;7:643.
10. Gutteridge, J.M.C. and Halliwell, B. 1994. *Antioxidants in Nutrition, Health, and Disease*. Oxford University Press: Oxford, 1994.

11. Addis, P.B. and Warner, G.J. *Free Radicals and Food Additives*. Aruoma, O.I. and Halliwell, B. eds. Taylor and Francis: London, 1991.

12. Loliger, J. 1991. *Free Radicals and Food Additives*. Aruoma, O.I. and Halliwell, B. eds. Taylor and Francis: London, 1991.

Chapter 4: Cholesterol and Saturated Fat

1. White, P.D. *Prog. Cardiovascular Dis* 1971;14:249.

2. *Statistical Abstracts of the United States*. United States Department of Commerce. Cited by McGee, C.T. *Heart Frauds: Uncovering the Biggest Health Scam in History*. Piccadilly Books, Ltd: Colorado Springs, CO, 2001.

3. McCully, K.S. *The Homocysteine Revolution*. Keats Publishing: New Canaan, CT, 1997.

4. McGee, C.T. *Heart Frauds: Uncovering the Biggest Health Scam in History*. Piccadilly Books, Ltd: Colorado Springs, CO, 2001.

5. Liebman, B. Solving the diet-and-disease puzzle. *Nutrition Action Health Letter* 1999:26(4):6.

6. Rosenberg, H. *The Doctor's Book of Vitamin Therapy*. G.P. Putnam's Sons: New York, 1974.

7. Krumholz, H.M. Lack of association between cholesterol and coronary heart disease and morbidity and all-cause mortality in persons older than 70 years. *JAMA* 1994;272:1335.

8. Addis, P.B. and Warner, G.J. *Free Radicals and Food Additives*. Aruoma, O.I. and Halliwell, B. eds. Taylor and Francis: London, 1991.

9. Gutteridge, J.M.C. and Halliwell, B. 1994. *Antioxidants in Nutrition, Health, and Disease*. Oxford University Press: Oxford, 1994.

10. Napier, K. Partial absolution. *Harvard Health Letter* 1995;20(10):1.

11. Siri-Tarino, P.W., et al. Meta-analysis of prospective cohort studies evaluating the association of saturated fat with cardiovascular disease. *Am J Clin Nutr* 2010;91:535-546.

12. Ramsden, C.E., et al. Use of dietary linoleic acid for secondary prevention of coronary heart disease and death: evaluation of recovered data for the Sydney Diet Heart Study and updated meta-analysis. *BMJ* 2013 Feb 4;346:e8707. doi:10.1136/bmj.e8707.

13. Calder, P.C. Old study sheds new light on the fatty acids and cardiovascular health debate. *BMJ* 2013 Feb 4;346:f493. doi:10.1136/bmj.f493.

14. Chowdhury, R., et al. Association of dietary, circulating, and supplement fatty acids with coronary risk: a systematic review and meta-analysis. *Ann Intern Med* 2014;160:398-406.

15. Watkins, B.A. and Seifert, M.F. Food lipids and bone health *Food Lipids and Health*, R.E. McDonald and D.B. Min (eds). Marcel Dekker, Inc.: New York, NY, 1996.

16. Corliss, R. Should you be a vegetarian? *Time Magazine*, July 15, 2002.

17. Kabara, J..J. *The Pharmacological Effects of Lipids*. The American Oil Chemist's Society: Champaign, IL, 1978.

18. Cohen, L.A., et al. Dietary fat and mammary cancer. II. Modulation of serum and tumor lipid composition and tumor prostaglandins by different dietary fats: association with tumor incidence patterns. *J Natl Cancer Inst* 1986;77:43.

19. Nanji, A.A., et al. Dietary saturated fatty acids: a novel treatment for alcoholic liver disease. *Gastroenterology* 1995;109(2):547-54.

20. Cha, Y.S. and Sachan, D.S. Opposite effects of dietary saturated and unsaturated fatty acids on ethanol-pharmacokinetics, triglycerides and carnitines. *J Am Coll Nutr* 1994;13(4):338-43.

21. Carroll, K.K. and Khor, H.T. Effects of level and type of dietary fat on incidence of mammary tumors induced in female sprague-dawley rats by 7, 12-dimethylbenzanthracene. *Lipids* 1971;6:415.

22. Fife, B. *Stop Alzheimer's Now! How to Prevent and Reverse Dementia, Parkinson's, ALS, Multiple Sclerosis, and Other Neurodegenerative Disorders*. Piccadilly Books, Ltd.: Colorado Springs, CO, 2011.

23. Yamori, Y., et al. Pathogenesis and dietary prevention of cerebrovascular diseases in animal models and epidemiological evidence for the applicability in man. In: Yamori Y., Lenfant C. (eds.) *Prevention of Cardiovascular Diseases: An Approach to Active Long Life*. Elsevier Science Publishers: Amsterdam, the Netherlands, 1987.

24. Ikeda, K.., et al. Effect of milk protein and fat intake on blood pressure and incidence of cerebrovascular disease in stroke-prone spontaneously hypertensive rats (SHRSP). *J Nutr Sci Vitaminol* 1987;33:31.

25. Kimura, N. Changing patterns of coronary heart disease, stroke, and nutrient intake in Japan. *Prev Med* 1985;12:222.

26. Omura, T., et al. Geographical distribution of cerebrovascular disease mortality and food intakes in Japan. *Soc Sci Med* 1987;24:40.

27. McGee, D., et al. The relationship of dietary fat and cholesterol to mortality in 10 years. *Int. J. Epidemiol.* 1985;14:97.

28. Gillman, M. W., et al. Inverse association of dietary fat with development of ischemic stroke in men. *JAMA* 1997;278(24):2145.

Chapter 5: Good Carbs, Bad Carbs

1. Applel, L.J., et al. Effects of protein, monounsaturated fat, and carbohydrate intake on blood pressure and serum lipids: results of the OmniHeart randomized trial. *JAMA* 2005;294:2455-2464.

2. Hu, F.B. and Malik, V.S. Sugar-sweetened beverages and risk of obesity and type 2 diabetes: epidemiologic evidence. *Physiol Behav* 2010;100:47-54.

3. Stranahan, A.M., et al. Diet-induced insulin resistance impairs hippocampal synptic plasticity and cognition in middle-aged rats. *Hippocampus* 2008;18:1085-1088.

4. Cao, D., et al. Intake of sucrose-sweetened water induces insulin resistance and exacerbates memory deficits and amyloidosis in a transgenic mouse model of Alzheimer disease. *J Biol Chem* 2007;282:36275-36282.

5. Sanchez, A., et al. Role of sugars in human neutrophilic phagocytosis. *Am J Clin Nurt* 1973;26:1180-1184.

6. Higginbotham, S., et al. Dietary glycemic load and risk of colorectal cancer in the Women's Health Study. *Journal of the National Cancer Institute* 2004;96:229-233.

7. Reiser, S., et al. 1985. Indices of copper status in humans consuming a typical American diet containing either fructose or starch. *Am. J. Clin. Nutr* 42(2):242-251.

8. Forristal, L.J. The murky world of high fructose corn syrup. *Wise Traditions* 2001;2(3):60-61.

9. Ouyang, X., et al. Fructose consumption as a risk factor for non-alcoholic fatty liver disease. *J Hepatol* 2008;48:993-999.

10. Abdelmalek, M.F., et al Increased fructose consumption is associated with fibrosis severity in patients with nonalcoholic fatty liver disease. *Hepatology* 2010;51:1961-1971.

11. Bocarsly, M.E., et al. High-fructose corn syrup causes characteristics of obesity in rats: increased body weight, body fat and triglyceride levels. *Pharmacol Biochem Behav* 2010;97:101-106.

12. Stoddard, M.N. *The Deadly Deception*. Aspartame Consumer Safety Network, http://www.aspartamesafety.com.

13. Qin, X. What made Canada become a country with the highest incidence of inflammatory bowel disease: Could sucralose be the culprit? *Can J Gastroenterol* 2011;25:511.

14. Roberts, J.J. *Aspartame (NutraSweet), Is it Safe?* Aspartame Consumer Safety Network, http://www.aspartamesafety.com/

Chapter 6: Carbohydrates Make You Fat

1. Swithers, S.E. and Davidson, T.L. A role for sweet taste: calorie predictive relations in energy regulation by rats. *Behav Neurosci* 2008;122:161-173.

2. Davidson, T.L., et al. Intake of high-intensity sweeteners alters the ability of sweet taste to signal caloric consequences: implications for the learned control of energy and body weight regulation. *Q J Exp Psychol (Hove)* 2011;64:1430-1441.

3. Swithers, S.E., et al. High-intensity sweeteners and energy balance. *Physiol Behav* 2010;100:55-62.

4. Magalle, L., et al. Intense sweetness surpasses cocaine reward. *PLoS One* 2007;8:e698.

5. Gearhardt, A.N., et al. Neural correlates of food addiction. *Arch Gen Psychiatry* 2011;68:808-816.

Chapter 7: Not All Calories are Equal

1. Allee, G.I., et al. Metabolic consequences of dietary medium chain triglycerides in the pig. *Proc Soc Exp Biol Med* 1972;139:422-427.

2. Takase, S., et al. Long-term effect of medium-chain triglyceride in hepatic enzymes catalyzing lipogenesis and cholesterogenesis in rats. *J Nutr Sci Vitaminol* 1977;23:43-51.

3. Bocarsly, M.E., et al. High-fructose corn syrup causes characteristics of obesity in rats: increased body weight, body fat and triglyceride levels. *Pharmacol Biochem Behav* 2010;97:101-106.

4. Alzamendi A., et al. Fructose-rich diet-induced abdominal adipose tissue endocrine dysfunction in normal male rats. *Endocrine* 2009;35:227–232.

5. Melanson K.J., et al. High-fructose corn syrup, energy intake, and appetite regulation. *Am J Clin Nutr* 2008;88:1738S–1744S.

6. Shapiro A., et al. Fructose-induced leptin resistance exacerbates weight gain in response to subsequent high-fat feeding. *Am J Physiol Regul Integr Comp* Physiol 2008;295:R1370–1375.

7. http://en.wikipedia.org/wiki/Walter_Hudson_(1944%E2%80%931991).

Chapter 8: Eat Fat and Grow Slim

1. Pennington, A.W. Obesity. *Times* 1952;80:389-398.

2. Kekwick, A. and Pawan, G.L.S. Calorie intake in relation to body weight changes in the obese. *Lancet* 1956;2:155.

3. Kekwick, A. and Pawan, G.L.S. Metabolic study in human obesity with isocaloric diets high in fat, protein or carbohydrate. *Metabolism* 1957;6:447-460.

4. Benoit, F., et al. Changes in body composition during weight reduction in obesity. *Archives of Internal Medicine*, 1965;63:604-612.

5. Vigilante, K. and Flynn, M. *Low-Fat Lies: High-Fat Frauds and the Healthiest Diet in the World.* Life Line Press: Washington, DC, 1999.

6. Eyton, A. *The F-Plan Diet.* Crown Publishers, Inc.: New York, NY, 1983.

7. Rolls, B.J. and Miller, D.L. Is the low-fat message giving people a license to eat more? *Journal of the American College of Nutrition* 1997;16:535.

8. Furuse, M., et al. Feeding behavior in rats fed diets containing medium chain triglyceride. *Physiol Behav* 1992;52:815.

9. Rolls, B.J., et al. Food intake in dieters and nondieters after a liquid meal containing medium-chain triglycerides. *Am J Clin Nutr* 1988;48:66-71.

10. Stubbs, R.J. and Harbron, C.G. Covert manipulation of the ration of medium- to long-chain triglycerides in isoenergetically dense diets: effect on food intake in ad libitum feeding men. *Int J Obes* 1996;20:435-444.

11. Van Wymelbeke, V., et al. Influence of medium-chain and long-chain triacylglycerols on the control of food intake in men. *Am J Clin Nutr* 1998;68:226-234.

12. St-Onge, M.P. and Jones, P.J. Physiological effects of medium-chain triglycerides: potential agents in the prevention of obesity. *J Nutr* 2002;132:329-332.

13. McManus, K., et al. A randomized controlled trial of a moderate-fat, low-energy diet compared with a low-fat, low-energy diet for weight loss in overweight adults. *Int. J Obes Relat Metab Disord* 2001;25(10):1503-11.

14. Gardner, C.D., et al. Comparison of the Atkins, Zone, Ornish, and LEARN diets for change in weight and related risk factors among overweight premenopausal women: the A to Z weight loss study: A randomized trial. *JAMA*, 2007;297:969-977.

15. Yancy, W.S. Jr., et al. A low-carbohydrate, ketogenic diet versus a low-fat diet to treat obesity and hyperlipidemia: a randomized, controlled trial. *Ann Intern Med* 2004;140:769-777.

16. Westman, E.C., et al. Low-carbohydrate nutrition and metabolism. *Am J Clin Nutr* 2007;86:276-284.

17. Sharman, M.J., et al. Very low-carbohydrate and low-fat diets affect fasting lipids and postprandial lipemia differently in overweight men. *J Nutr* 2004;134:880-885.

Chapter 9: Dietary Ketosis

1. Leiter, L.A. and Marliss, E.B. Survival during fasting may depend on fat as well as protein stores *JAMA* 1982;248:2306-2307.

2. Reger, M.A., et al. Effects of beta-hydroxybutyrate on cognition in memory-impaired adults. *Neurobiol Aging* 2004;25:311-314.

3. VanItallie, T.B., et al. Treatment of Parkinson disease with diet-induced hyperketonemia: a feasibility study. *Neurology* 2005;64:728-730.

4. Duan, W., et al. Dietary restriction normalizes glucose metabolism and BDNF levels, slows disease progression, and increases survival in huntingtin mutant mice. *Proc Natl Acad Sci USA* 2003;100:2911-2916.

5. Zhao, Z., et al. A ketogenic diet as a potential novel therapeutic intervention in amyotrophic lateral sclerosis. *BMC Neuroscience* 2006;7:29.

6. Veech, R.L. The therapeutic implications of ketone bodies: the effects of ketone bodies in pathological conditions: ketosis, ketogenic diet, redox states, insulin resistance, and mitochondrial metabolism. *Prostaglandins, Leukotrienes and Essential Fatty Acids* 2004;70:309-319.

7. Kashiwaya, Y., et al Substrate signaling by insulin: a ketone bodies ratio mimics insulin action in heart. *Am J Cardiol* 1997;80:50A-60A.

8. Yancy, W.S., et al. A low-carbohydrate, ketogenic diet versus a low-fat diet to treat obesity and hyperlipidemia: a randomized, controlled trial. *Ann Intern Med* 2004;140:769-777.

9. Cahill, G.F. Jr. and Veech, R.L. Ketoacids? Good Medicine? *Transactions of the American Clinical and Climatological Association* 2003;114:149-163.

10. Heinbecker, P. Studies on the metabolism of Eskimos. *J Biol Chem* 1928;80:461-475.

11. McClellan, W.S. and DuBois, E.F. Clinical calorimetry. XLV. Prolonged meat diets with a study of kidney function and ketosis. *J Biol Chem* 1930;87:651-667.

12. Stefansson, V. *Human Nutrition Historic and Scientific, Monograph III.* International Universities Press: NY, 1960.

13. Westman, E.C., et al. Low-carbohydrate nutrition and metabolism. *Am J Clin Nutr* 2007;86:276-284.

14. Maki, K.C., et al. Effects of a reduced-glycemic-load diet on body weight, body composition, and cardiovascular disease risk markers in overweight and obese adults. *Am J Clin Nutr* 2007;85:724-734.

15. Boden, G., et al. Effect of a low-carbohydrate diet on appetite, blood glucose levels, and insulin resistance in obese patients with type 2 diabetes. *Ann Intern Med* 2005;142:403-411.

16. Nickols-Richardson, S.M., et al Perceived hunger is lower and weight loss is greater in overweight premenopausal women consuming a low-carbohydrate/high-protein vs high-carbohydrate/low-fat diet. *J Am Diet Assoc* 2005;105:1433-1437.

17. Velasquez-Mieyer, P.A., et al. Suppression of insulin secretion is associated with weight loss and altered macronutrient intake and preference in a subset of obese adults. *Int J Obes Relat Metab Disord* 2003;27:219-226.

18. Patel, A., et al. Long-term outcomes of children treated with the ketogenic diet in the past. *Epilepsia* 2010;51:1277-1282.

19. Sharman, M.J., et al. Very low-carbohydrate and low-fat diets affect fasting lipids and postprandial lipemia differently in overweight men. *J Nutr* 2004;134:880-885.

20. Yancy, W.S., Jr., et al. A low-carbohydrate, ketogenic diet versus a low-fat diet to treat obesity and hyperlipidemia: a randomized, controlled trial. *Ann Intern Med* 2004;140:769-777.

21. Westman, E.C., et al. Low-carbohydrate nutrition and metabolism. *Am J Clin Nutr* 2007;86:276-284.

22. Westman, E.C., et al. A review of low-carbohydrate ketogenic diets. *Curr Atheroscler Rep* 2003;5:476-483.

23. Westman, E.C., et al. The effect of a low-carbohydrate, ketogenic diet versus a low-glycemic index diet on glycemic control in type 2 diabetes mellitus. *Nutr Metab (Lond)* 2008;5:36.

24. Sharman, M.J., et al. Very low-carbohydrate and low-fat diets affect fasting lipids and postprandial lipemia differently in overweight men. *J Nutr* 2004;134:880-885.

25. Gardner, C.D., et al. Comparison of the Atkins, Zone, Ornish, and LEARN diets for change in weight and related risk factors among overweight premenopausal women: The A to Z Weight Loss Study: A randomized trial. *JAMA* 2009;297:969-977.

26. Volek, J.S. and Sharman, M.J. Cardiovascular and hormonal aspects of very-low-carbohydrate ketogenic diets. *Obes Res* 2004;12 Suppl 2:115S-123S.

27. Foster, G.D., et al. Weight and metabolic outcomes after 2 years on a low-carbohydrate versus low-fat diet: A randomized trial. *Ann Intern Med* 2010;153:147-157.

28. Schwartzkroin, P.A. Mechanisms underlying the anti-epileptic efficacy of the ketogenic diet. *Epilepsy Res* 1999;37:171-180.

29. Fife, B. *Stop Autism Now! A Parent's Guide to Preventing and Reversing Autism Spectrum Disorders*. Piccadilly Books, Ltd: Colorado Springs, CO, 2012.

30. Husain, A.M., et al. Diet therapy for narcolepsy. *Nuerology* 2004;62:2300-2302.

31. Reger, M.A., et al. Effects of beta-hydroxybutyrate on cognition in memory-impaired adults. *Neurobiol Aging* 2004;25:311-314.

32. VanItallie, T.B., et al. Treatment of Parkinson disease with diet-induced hyperketonemia: a feasibility study. *Neurology* 2005;64:728-730.

33. Duan, W., et al. Dietary restriction normalizes glucose metabolism and BDNF levels, slows disease progression, and increases survival in huntingtin mutant mice. *Proc Natl Acad Sci USA* 2003;100:2911-2916.

34. Zhao, Z., et al. A ketogenic diet as a potential novel therapeutic intervention in amyotrophic lateral sclerosis. *BMC Neuroscience* 2006;7:29.

35. Prins, M.L., et al. Increased cerebral uptake and oxidation of exogenous βHB improves ATP following traumatic brain injury in adult rats. *J Neurochem* 2004;90:666-672.

36. Suzuki, M., et al. Beta-hydroxybutyrate, a cerebral function improving agent, protects rat brain against ischemic damage caused by permanent and transient focal cerebral ischemia. *Jpn J Phamacol* 2002;89:36-43.

37. Yeh, Y.Y. and Zee, P. Relation of ketosis to metabolic changes induced by acute medium-chain triglyceride feeding in rats. *J Nutr* 1976;106:58-67.

38. Tantibhedhyangkul, P., et al. Effects of ingestion of long-chain and medium-chain triglycerides on glucose tolerance in man. *Diabetes* 1967;16:796-799.

39. Kashiwaya, Y., et al Substrate signaling by insulin: a ketone bodies ratio mimics insulin action in heart. *Am J Cardiol* 1997;80:50A-60A.

40. Fife, B. *Coconut Cures: Preventing and Treating Common Health Problems with Coconut*. Piccadilly Books, Ltd: Colorado Springs, CO, 2005.

41. Poplawaki, M.M., et al. Reversal of diabetic nephropathy by a ketogenic diet. *PLoS ONE* 2011;6:e18604.

42. Lardy, H.A. and Phillips, P.H. Studies of fat and carbohydrate oxidation in mammalian spermatozoa. *Arch Biochem* 1945;6:53-61.

43. Mavropoulos, J.C., et al. The effects of a low-carbohydrate, ketogenic diet on the polycystic ovary syndrome: a pilot study. *Nutrition and Metabolism (London)* 2005;2:35.

44. Seyfried, T.N., et al. Role of glucose and ketone bodies in the metabolic control of experimental brain cancer. *British Journal of Cancer* 2003;89:1375-1382.

45. Nebeling, L.C., et al. Effects of a ketogenic diet on tumor metabolism and nutritional status in pediatric oncology patients: two case reports. *J Am Coll Nutr* 1995;86:202-208.

46. Kashiwaya, Y., et al Substrate signaling by insulin: a ketone bodies ratio mimics insulin action in heart. *Am J Cardiol* 1997;80:50A-60A.

47. Fontana, L. Neuroendocrine factors in the regulation of inflammation: excessive adiposity and calorie restriction. *Exp Gerontol* 2009;44:41-45.
48. Veech, R.L., et al. Ketone bodies, potential therapeutic uses. *IUBMB Life* 2001;51:241-247.
49. Chance, B., et al. Hydroperoxide metabolism in mammalian organs. *Physiol Rev* 1979;59:527-605.

Chapter 10: Is Your Thyroid Making You Fat?

1. Derry, D.M. *Breast Cancer and Iodine*. Trafford Publishing: Victoria, BC, 2001.
2. Wolfe. W.S. and Campbell, C.C. Food pattern, diet quality, and related characteristics of school children in New York State. *J Am Diet Assoc* 1993;93:1280-1284.
3. Fernandez-Real, J.M., et al. Thyroid function is intrinsically linked to insulin sensitivity and endothelium-dependent vasodilation in healthy euthyroid subjects. *J Clin Endocrinol Metab* 2006;91:3337-3343.
4. Roos, A., et al. thyroid function is associated with components of the metabolic syndrome in euthyroid subjects. *J Clin Endocrinol Metab* 2007;92:491-496.
5. Gobatto, C.A, et al. The monosodium glutamate (MSG) obese rat as a model for the study of exercise in obesity. *Res Commun Mol Pathol Pharmacol* 2002;111:89-101.
6. Peat, R. *Ray Peat's Newsletter* 1997, p.2-3.
7. Sarandol, E., et al. Oxidative stress and serum paraoxonase activity in experimental hypothyroidism: effect of vitamin E supplementation. *Cell Biochem Funct* 2005;23:1-8.
8. Karatas, F., et al. Determination of free malondialdehyde in human serum by high-performance liquid chromatography. *Anal Biochem* 2002;311:76-79.
9. Arthur, J.R., et al. Selenium deficiency, thyroid hormone metabolism, and thyroid hormone deiodinases. *Am J Clin Nutr* 1993;57 Suppl:236S-239S.
10. Ullrich, I.H., et al. Effect of low-carbohydrate diets high in either fat or protein on thyroid function, plasma insulin, glucose, and triglycerides in healthy young adults. *J Am Coll Nutr* 1985;4:451-459.
11. Deshpande, U.R., et al. Effect of antioxidants (vitamin C, E and turmeric extract) on methimazole induced hypothyroidism in rats. *Indian J Exp Biol* 2002;40:735-738.
12. Inouse, A., et al. Unesterified long-chain fatty acids inhibit thyroid hormone binding to the nuclear receptor. Solubilized receptor and the receptor in cultured cells. *Eur J Biochem* 1989;183:565-572.
13. Duntas, L.H. and Orgazzi, J. Vitamin E and thyroid disease: a potential link that kindles hope. *Biofactors* 2003;19:131-135.
14. Sondergaard, D. and Olsen, P. The effect of butylated hydroxytoluene (BHT) on the rat thyroid. *Toxicol Lett* 1982:10:239-244.

Chapter 11: Iodine and Your Health

1. Anderson, M., et al. Current global iodine status and progress over the last decade towards the elimination of iodine deficiency. *Bulletin of the World Health Organization* 2005;83:518-525.
2. Stadel, B.V. Dietary iodine and risk of breast, endometrial and ovarian cancer. *Lancet* 1976;1:890-891.
3. Venturi, S., et al. Role of iodine in evolution and carcinogenesis of thyroid, breast, and stomach. *Adv Clin Path* 2000;4:11-17.
4. Foster, H.D. The iodine-selenium connection: Its possible roles in intelligence, cretinism, sudden infant death syndrome, breast cancer and multiple sclerosis. *Medical Hypothesis* 1993;40:61-65.
5. Bretthauer, E. Milk transfer comparisons of different chemical forms of radioiodine. *Health Physics* 1972;22:257.
6. Derry, D.M. *Breast Cancer and Iodine*. Trafford Publishing, Victoria, BC, 2001.
7. Eskin, B.A. Iodine and mammary cancer. *Adv Exp Med Biol* 1977;91:293-304.
8. http://www.thyroid.org/.
9. Hollowell, J.E., et al. Iodine nutrition in the United States. Trends and public health implications: Iodine excretion data from National Health and Nutrition Examination Surveys I and III (1971-74 and 1988-94). *J Clin Endocrinol Metab* 1998;83:3401-3408.
10. Pavelka, S. Metabolism of bromide and its interference with the metabolism of iodine. *Physiol Res* 2004;53 Supple 1:S81-S90.
11. Hattersley, J.G. Fluoridation's defining moment. *J Orthomol Med* 1999;14:1-20.
12. Lu, Y., et al. Effect of high fluoride water on intelligence in children. *Fluoride* 2000;33:74-78.
13. Kimura, S., et al. Development of malignant goiter by defatted soybean with iodine-free diet in rats. *Gann* 1976;67:763-765.
14. Chorazy, P.A., et al. Persistent hypothyroidism in an infant receiving a soy formula: case report and review of the literature. *Pediatrics* 1995;96:148-150.
15. Pinchers, A., et al. Thyroid refractoriness in an athyreotic cretin fed soybean formula. *New Eng J Med* 1965;265:83-87.
16. Ishizuki, Y., et al. The effects on the thyroid gland of soybeans administered experimentally to healthy subjects. *Nippon Naibunpi Gakkai Zasshi* 1991;67:622-629.
17. Divi, R.L., et al. Identification, characterization and mechanisms of anti-thyroid activity of isoflavones from soybean. *Biochem Pharmacol* 1997;54:1087-1096.
18. Fort, P., et al. Breast and soy-formula feedings in early infancy and the prevalence of autoimmune thyroid disease in children. *J Am Clin Nutr* 1990;9:164-167.

19. Nagata, C., et al. Decreased serum total cholesterol concentration is associated with high intake of soy products in Japanese men and women. *J Nutr* 1998;128:209-213.
20. Samuels, M.H., et al. Variable effects of nonsteroidal antiinflammatory agents on thyroid test results. *Journal of Clinical Endocrinology and Metabolism* 2003;88:5710-5716.
21. Aceves, C. Is iodine a gatekeeper of the integrity of the mammary gland? *J of Mammary Gland Biol and Neoplasia* 2005;10:189-196.
22. Berson, S.A., et al. Quantitative aspects of iodine metabolism. The exchangeable organic iodine pool and the rates of thyroidal secretion, peripheral degradation and fecal excretion of endogenously synthesized organically bound iodine. *J Clin Invest* 1954;33:1533-1552.
23. Abraham, G.E., et al. Orthoiodosupplementation: Iodine sufficiency of the whole human body. *The Original Internist* 2002;9:30-41.
24. Sang, Z., et al. Exploration of the safe upper level of iodine intake in euthyroid Chinese adults: a randomized double-blind trial. *Am J Clin Nutr* 2012;143:2038-2043.
25. http://www.nutridesk.com.au/iodine-and-breast-health.phtml.
26. Brownstein, D. *Iodine: Why You Need It, Why You Can't Live Without It,* 2nd Ed. Medical Alternatives Press: West Bloomfield, MI, 2006.
27. Abraham, G.E. Iodine supplementation markedly increases urinary excretion of fluoride and bromide. *Townsend Letter* 2001;238:108-109.
28. Abraham, G.E. The historical background of the iodine project. *The Original Internist* 2005;12:57-66.

Chapter 12: Thyroid System Dysfunction
1. Samuels, M.H. and McDaniel, P.A. Thyrotropin levels during hydrocortisone infusions that mimic fasting-induced cortisol elevations: a clinical research center study. *J Clin Endocrinol Metab* 1997;82:3700-3704.
2. Opstad, K. Circadian rhythm of hormones is extinguished during prolonged physical stress, sleep and energy deficiency in young men. *Eur J Endocrinol* 1994;131:56-66.

Chapter 13: Supercharge Your Metabolism
1. Fushiki, T. and Matsumoto, K. Swimming endurance capacity of mice is increased by chronic consumption of medium-chain triglycerides. *Journal of Nutrition* 1995;125:531.
2. Applegate, L. Nutrition. *Runner's World* 1996;31:26.
3. Ogawa A., et al. Dietary medium-and long-chain triacylglycerols accelerate diet-induced thermogenesis in humans. *Journal of Oleo Science* 2007; 6: 283-287.
4. Baba, N. Enhanced thermogenesis and diminished deposition of fat in response to overfeeding with diet containing medium chain triglyceride. *Am J of Clin Nutr* 1982;35:678-682.

5. Papamandjaris, A.A., et al. Endogenous fat oxidation during medium chain versus long chain triglyceride feeding in healthy women. *Int J Obes Relat Metab Disord* 2000;24:1158-1166.

6. Murry, M.T. *American Journal of Natural Medicine* 1996;3(3):7.

7. Hill, J.O., et al. Thermogenesis in man during overfeeding with medium chain triglycerides. *Metabolism* 1989;38:641-648.

8. Seaton, T.B., et al. Thermic effect of medium-chain and long-chain triglycerides in man. *Am J Clin Nutr* 1986;44:630-634.

9. Scalfi, L., et al. Postprandial thermogenesis in lean and obese subjects after meals supplemented with medium-chain and long-chain triglycerides. *Am J Clin Nutr* 1991;53:1130-1133.

10. Dulloo, A.G., et al. Twenty-four-hour energy expenditure and urinary catecholamines of humans consuming low-to-moderate amounts of medium-chain triglycerides: a dose-response study in human respiratory chamber. *Eur J Clin Nutr* 1996;50:152-158.

11. St-Onge, M.P., et al. Medium-chain triglycerides increase energy expenditure and decrease adiposity in overweight men. *Obes Res* 2003;11:395-402.

12. Tsuji, H., et al. Dietary medium-chain triacylglycerols suppress accumulation of body fat in a double-blind, controlled trial in healthy men and women. *J Nutr* 2001;131:2853-2859.

13. St-Onge, M.P. and Bosarge, A. Weight-loss diet that includes consumption of medium-chain triacylglycerol oil leads to a greater rate of weight and fat mass loss than does olive oil. *Am J Clin Nutr* 2008;87:621-626.

14. St-Onge, M.P., et al. Medium-versus long-chain triglycerides for 27 days increases fat oxidation and energy expenditure without resulting in changes in body composition in overweight women. *Int J Obes Relat Metab Disord* 2003;27:95-102.

15. Crozier, G., et al. Metabolic effects induced by long-term feeding of medium-chain triglycerides in the rat. *Metabolism* 1987;36:807-814.

16. Geliebter, A., et al. Overfeeding with medium-chain triglyceride diet results in diminished deposition of at. *Am J Clin Nutr* 1983;37:1-4.

17. Lavau, M.M. and Hashim, S.A. Effect of medium chain triglycende on lipogenesis and body fat in the rat. *J Nutr* 1978;108:613-620.

18. Baba, N., et al. Enhanced thermogenesis and diminished deposition of fat in response to overfeeding with diet containing medium chain triglyceride. *Am J Clin Nutr* 1982;35:678-682.

19. St-Onge, M.P. and Jones, P.J. Physiological effects of medium-chain triglycerides: potential agents in the prevention of obesity. *J Nutr* 2002;132:329-332.

20. Seaton, T.B., et al. Thermic effect of medium-chain and long-chain triglycerides in man. *Am J Clin Nutr* 1986;44:630-634.

21. Papamandjaris, A.A., et al. Medium chain fatty acid metabolism and energy expenditure: obesity treatment implications. *Life Sci* 1998;62:1203-1215.

307

22. Han, J.R., et al. Effects of dietary medium-chain triglyceride on weight loss and insulin sensitivity in a group of moderately overweight free-living type 2 diabetic Chinese subjects. *Metabolism* 2007;56:985-991.

23. Kasai, M., et al. Effect of dietary medium - and long ± chain triacylglycerols (MLCT) on accumulation of body fat in healthy humans. *Asia Pacific J Clin Nutr* 2003;12(2):151-160.

24. St-Onge M.P., et al. Medium-chain triglycerides increase energy expenditure and decrease adiposity in overweight men. Obesity Research 2003;11:395-402.

25. Beermann, C., et al. Short term effects of dietary medium-chain fatty acids and n-3 long-chain polyunsaturated fatty acids on the fat metabolism of healthy volunteers. *Lipids Health Dis* 2003;2:10.

26. St-Onge M.P. and Jones, P.J.H. Greater rise in fat oxidation with medium-chain triglyceride consumption relative to long-chain triglyceride is associated with lower initial body weight and greater loss of subcutaneous adipose tissue. *International Journal of Obesity* 2003;27:1565-1571.

27. St-Onge M.P. and Bosarge, A. Weight-loss diet that includes consumption of medium-chain triacylglycerol oil leads to a greater rate of weight and fat mass loss than does olive oil. *Am J Clin Nutr* 2008;87:621-626.

28. Xue, C., et al. Consumption of medium- and long-chain triacylglycerols decreases body fat and blood triglyceride in Chinese hypertriglyceridemic subjects. *Eur J Clin Nutr* 2009;63:879-886.

29. Rollisco, C.C. and Carlos-Raboca, J. The effect of virgin coconut oil on weight and lipid profile among overweight, healthy individuals. *Phil J Inter Med* 2008;46:45-44.

30. Assuncao, M.L., et al. Effects of dietary coconut oil on the biochemical and anthropometric profiles of women presenting abdominal obesity. *Lipids* 20090;44:593-601.

31. Nagao, K. and Yanagita, T. Medium-chain fatty acids: functional lipids for the prevention and treatment of the metabolic syndrome. *Pharmacol Res* 2010;61:208-212.

32. Turner, N., et al. Enhancement of muscle mitochondrial oxidative capacity and alterations in insulin action are lipid species-dependent: Potent tissue-specific effects of medium chain fatty acids. *Diabetes* 2009;58:2547-2554.

33. St-Onge, M.P. and Jones P.J.H. Psysiological effects of medium-chain triglycerides: potential agents in the prevention of obesity. *J Nutr* 2002;132:329-332.

34. Alvarez, J.A. and Ashraf, A. Role of vitamin D in insulin secretion and insulin sensitivity for glucose homeostasis. *Int J Endocrinol* 2010;2010:351385.

35. Roos, P.A. Light and electromagnetic waves: the health implications. *Journal of the Bio-Electro-Magnetics Institute.* 1991;3(2):7-12.

36. Garland, F.C., et al. Occupational sunlight exposure and melanoma in the U.S. Navy. *Archives of Environmental Health.* 1990;45:261-267.

37. Editorial. Excessive sunlight exposure, skin melanoma, linked to vitamin D. *International Journal of Biosocial and Medical Research.* 1991;13(1):13-14.
38. Ahuja, K.D.K., et al. Effects of chili consumption on postprandial glucose, insulin, and energy metabolism. *Am J Clin Nutr* 2006;84:63-69.
39. Chaiyasit, K., et al. Pharmacokinetic and the effect of capsaicin in Capsicum frutesscens on decreasing plasma glucose level. *J Med Assoc Thai* 2009;92:108-113.
40. Yoshioka, M., et al. Effects of red pepper on appetite and energy intake. *Br J Nutr* 1999;82:115-123.

Chapter 14: Drink More, Weigh Less

1. Kleiner, S.M. Water: an essential but overlooked nutrient. *American Dietetic Association Journal* 1999;99(2):200-206.
2. Dauterman, K.W., et al. Plasma specific gravity for identifying hypovolemia. *J Diarrhoeal Dis. Res.* 1995;13:33-38.
3. Ershow, A.G., et al. Intake of tapwater and total water by pregnant and lactating women. *Am. J. Public Health* 1991;81:328-334.
4. Dauterman, K.W., et al. Plasma specific gravity for identifying hypovolaemia. *J Diarrhoeal Dis. Res.* 1995;13:33-38.
5. Torranin, C., et al. The effects of acute thermal dehydration and rapid rehydration on isometric and isotonic endurance. *J. Sports Med. Phys. Fitness* 1979;19:1-9.
6. Armstrong, L.E., et al. Influence of diuretic-induced dehydration on competitive running performance. *Med. Sci. Sports Exerc.* 1985;17:456-461.
7. Sawka, M.N. and Pandolf, K.R. Effects of body water loss on physiological function and exercise performance. In: Gisolfi C.V. and Lamb, D.R. eds. *Fluid Homeostasis During Exercise.* Benchmark Press: Carmel, Ind, 1990.
8. Sansevero, A.C. Dehydration in the elderly: strategies for prevention and management. *Nurse Pract.* 1997;22(4):41-42, 51-57, 63-66 passim.
9. Sagawa, S., et al. Effect of dehydration on thirst and drinking during immersion in men. *J. Appl. Physiol.* 1992;72:128-134.
10. Gopinathan, P.M., et al. Role of dehydration in heat stress-induced variations in mental performance. *Arch Environ Health* 1988;43:15-17.
11. Torranin, C., et al. The effects of acute thermal dehydration and rapid rehydration on isometric and isotonic endurance. *J Sports Med Phys Fitness* 1979;19:1-9.
12. Armstrong, L.E., et al. Influence of diuretic-induced dehydration on competitive running performance. *Med Sci Sports Exerc* 1985;17:456-461.
13. Sagawa, S., et al. Effect of dehydration on thirst and drinking during immersion in men. *J Appl Physiol* 1992;72:128-134.
14. Curhan, G.C. and Curhan, S.G. Dietary factors and kidney stone formation. *Comp Ther* 1994;20:485-489.

15. Goldfarb, S. The role of diet in the pathogenesis and therapy of nephrolithiasis. *Endocrinol Metab Clin North Am* 1990;19:805-820.

16. Stamford, B. Muscle cramps: untying the knots. *Phys Sportsmed* 1993;21:115-116.

17. Boschmann, M., et al. Water-induced thermogenesis. *JCEM* 2003;88:6015.

18. Miller, W.D. Extrathyroidal benefits of iodine. *J Am Physicians Surgeons* 2006;11:106-110.

19. Stolarz-Skrzypek, K., et al. Fatal and nonfatal outcomes, incidence of hypertension, and blood pressure changes in relation to urinary sodium excretion. *JAMA* 2011;4:1777-1785.

20. Garg, R., et al. Low-salt diet increases insulin resistance in healthy subjects. *Metabolism Clinical and Experimental* 2011;60:965-968.

21. O'Donnell, M.J., et al. Urinary sodium and potassium excretion and risk of cardiovascular events. *JAMA* 2011;306:2229-2238.

22. Stolarz-Skrzypek, K., et al. Fatal and nonfatal outcomes, incidence of hypertension, and blood pressure changes in relation to urinary sodium excretion *JAMA* 2011;305:1777-1785.

23. Elliott, P. Commentary: role of salt intake in the development of high blood pressure. *International Journal of Epidemiology* 2005;34:975-978.

24. Rauws, AG. Pharmacokinetics of bromine ion—an overview. *Food Chem Toxicol* 1983;21:379-382.

25. Sensenbach, W.J. Bromide intoxication. *AMA Journal* 1944;125:769-772.

Chapter 15: Low-Carb, High-Fat Eating Plan

1. Gordon, N. and Newton, R.W. Glucose transporter type 1 (GLUT) deficiency. *Grain Dev* 2003;25:477-480.

2. Brighenti, F., et al. Effect of neutralized and native vinegar on blood glucose and acetate responses to a mixed meal in healthy subjects. *Eur J Clin Nutr* 1995;49:242-247.

3. Johnston, C.S., et al. Vinegar improves insulin sensitivity to a high-carbohydrate meal in subjects with insulin resistance or type 2. diabetes. *Diabetes Care* 2004;27:281-282.

4. Hollis, J.F., et al. Weight loss during the intensive intervention phase of the weight-loss maintenance trial. *Am J Prev Med* 2008;35:118-126.

5. Naylor, G.J., et al. A double blind placebo controlled trial of ascorbic acid in obesity. *Nutr Health* 1985;4:25-28.

Index

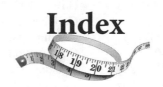

Acesulfame K, 56
Acetoacetic acid (AcAc), 103, *see* also Ketones
Acetone, 103, *see* also Ketones
Addis, Paul, 39
Antioxidants, 21, 37, 131, 132, 133-134
Advanced glycation end products (AGEs), 50
Agave, 51
Alcohol, 199
Aluminium, 144
Alzheimer's disease, 49, 72, 104
Amyloid plaque, 49
Anderson, Karsen, 107-108
Apoptosis, 134
Arthritis, 193
Artificial sweeteners, 55-58, 68, 70, 253
Aspartame, 55, 57
Atherosclerosis, 28, 30, 36-37, 39, 129, 242
Atkins, Robert, 92, 104, 238
Autoimmune thyroiditis, 123

Barnes, Broda, 89-90, 160
Basal metabolic rate (BMR), 78, 80, 89, 165, 170
Batmanghelidj, Fereydoon, 192

Benoit, Frederick, 92
Beriberi, 128
Beta-carotene, 21, 47, 129, 131
Beta-hydroxybutyric acid (BHB), 103, *see* also Ketones
Beverages, 219-220
Blaylock, Russell, 57
Blood glucose, 23, 50, 52, 53, 62, 65, 196
Blood pressure, 136, 202-203
Blood sugar, *see* Blood glucose
Body mass index (BMI), 171-172, 244
Body temperature, 68-69, 124, 154, 156-164, 246
Bomb calorimeter, 82
Breads and grains, 218-219
Breast Cancer and Iodine, 123
Bromide, 137-140, 142, 148, 203
Brominated vegetable oil, 139
Bromine, *see* Bromide
Brownstein, David, 137, 143, 145-147
Butter, 135, 136
Butylatedhydroxytoluene (BHT), 132
Butylhydroxyanisol (BHA), 132

Cadmium, 148

Caffeine, 198-200, 219, 253
Calcium, 22, 37, 42
Calories, 17-18, 20, 77-84, 183
Calories Don't Count, 89
Cancer, 19, 50-51, 72, 119, 129,
  132, 133-134, 144-146, 182-183,
  195
Candida, 60
Canola, 140
Capsaicin, 187
Carbohydrate
  complex, 45-47, 66
  fiber, 45-47, 48, 72, 94-95, 209
  net, 209
  sensitivity, 64-66, 103, 208
  simple, 45-47, 66
  source, 45
  starch, 45, 50, 64, 66, 72, 125
  sugar, 45-60, 64, 66-76, 83, 220-
  221
  vegetables, 47-48
  weight loss, 91, 61-76
Castelli, William, 7
Center for Disease Control and
  Prevention (CDC), 17, 54, 137
Chloride, 137-140, 202-204
Chlorine, *see* Chloride
Cholesterol, 24, 28, 33-41, 88, 104,
  113-115, 241-243
Cholesterol hypothesis, 34, 36,
  38-40
Cholesterol ratio, 114-115
Chili peppers, 187-188
Chromium, 126, 225
Cirrhosis, 54
Cocaine, 69
Coconut Cures, 11, 12
Coconut flour, 255-256
Coconut oil, 8, 10-12, 25, 97-98,
  117, 167-180, 207-208, 227-228,
  252
The Coconut Oil Miracle, 11, 12

Coffee, 199, 253
Collagen, 53
Condiments, 220
Constipation, 195
Cooking with Coconut Flour, 256
Copper, 131
Copra, 227
Cortisol, 159
Cramps, 196, 202, 204, 251
C-reactive protein, 44, 51, 104, 119,
  241-242
Cream, 135
Crisco, 27
Cruciferous vegetables, 140
Cyclamate, 56

Dairy, 213-214
DeBakey, Michael, 39
Dehydration, 192-196, 251
Dental disease, 51, 58
Derry, David, 123
Diabetes, 29, 49-50, 52-53, 65, 71,
  104, 115, 118, 129, 173, 174, 188
Dietary supplements, 224-226
Diet diary, 209, 222-224, 232, 248
Diet-induced obesity, 80, 85
Disaccharide, 46
Distilled water, 204
Dr. Atkins New Diet Revolution, 92
Drugs, 142-143, 178-180, 246-248
DuBois, Eugene, 108
DuPont, 88, 139

Electrolytes, 202-204
Empty stomach syndrome, 66-67
Enig, Mary, 29
Enzymes, 156, 159, 167, 181, 182,
  197, 232
Epilepsy, 104
Eskimo, 107, 208
Essential fatty acids, 21
Exercise, 183-185

Exercise performance, 23, 167-168
Excitotoxins: The Taste That Kills, 58

Fasting, 92
Fasting blood sugar, 50, 65
Fats
  athletic performance, 23
  bad, 214
  benefits of, 19-23
  blood sugar regulation, 23
  bone health, 23
  building blocks, 19-20
  definition, 24
  deposition, 171-174
  energy storage, 20
  ketosis, 208, 104-105
  leptin, 71, 83, 119
  lipid, 24
  mobilizing substance, 91
  non-preferred, 214
  nutrition, 20-22, 54
  preferred, 214
  protein metabolization, 106-108
  satiety, 23, 96-98, 108-111
  skin, 23
  source, 45
  storage, 62-64
  traditional, 26
  weight management, 23, 83
Fatty acids, 20, 25, 27, 62-64, 102
Fatty snacks, 221-222, 257-259
Field, Meira, 53
Flechas, Jorge, 149
Fluoride, 137-140, 142, 148, 203-204
Fluorine, *see* Fluoride
Flynn, Mary, 22, 93
Food additives, 130-132
Fractionated coconut oil, 173
Free radicals, 21, 30-32, 38, 50, 119, 131, 134

Fructose, 37, 46, 52-55, 83
Fruit, 217

Ghrelin, 83
Gillman, Matthew, 44
Glucose, 52, 53, 62, 72, 102, 105, 116, 126-127
Glycerol, 64
Glycogen, 62, 83
Goiter, 122, 133, 135-137, 140-143
Goiterogens, 140-143
Graves' disease, 123
Gum disease, 51

Halides, *see* Halogens
Halogens, 137-140, 148, 203
Hashimoto's disease, 123
Heart attack, 37, 43
Heart disease, 29, 34-37, 38-44, 53, 92, 115, 129, 173, 203
Heart Frauds, 22, 138
Heavy metals, 148
Herxheimer reaction, 252
Hoebel, Bart, 54
Hormones, 19
Hudson, Walter, 84
Hunger, 23, 66-67, 96-98, 108-111
Hydrogenation, 27-30, 130
Hyperthyroidism, 122-123, 138, 147-148
Hypothalamus, 123, 181
Hypothyroidism, 122-132, 133, 137, 138, 140-151, 181
Hypothyroidism: The Unsuspecting Illness, 160

Immune function, 19, 36, 50, 133
Inflammation, 36, 38, 50, 51, 104, 119, 242
Insulin, 29, 53, 62-66, 72, 104, 110, 115, 126, 174, 219

Insulin resistance, 50, 52, 64-66, 71, 72, 119, 174, 181, 188, 196-197, 203, 220
Iodine, 129, 133-151
Iodine load test, 149-151
Iodine: Why You Need it, Why You Can't Live Without It, 137
Iodolipids, 134
Iodoral, 145, 149
Irritable bowel disease, 57

Japanese, 146, 147, 203

Kedwick, Alan, 91
Keeton, Robert W. 89
Ketoacidosis, 104, 115-116
Ketogenic diet, 104-105, 208
Ketones, 102-121, 208, 229
Ketone test strips, 116-117
Ketosis, 103-105, 116-117
Keys, Ancel, 34
Kidney stones, 195
Kossoff, Eric, 113
Krumholz, Harlan, 39

Lactose, 45, 46
Lard, 25
Lead, 148
Legumes, 140
Leptin, 71, 83, 119
Levothyroxine, 122, 143, 152, 155, 163
Linoleic acid, 37, 93
Lipase, 232
Lipid, 24, 134
Lipoproteins, 167
Liquid coconut oil, 229
Liver disease, 53-54
Long chain fatty acids (LCFAs), 167
Long chain triglycerides (LCTs), 25, 167-174
Low-calorie diets, 78
Low-carb diets, 105

Low-fat diets, 16-19, 21, 22, 98-100
Low-Fat Lies, 92
Lugol, Jean, 145
Lugol's solution, 144-146
Lycopene, 47, 131

Magnesium, 37, 204, 251
Magnesium oil, 204
Malnutrition, 125-132, 158, 159, 166
Margarine, 28, 136
McGee, Charles, 22, 38
McCully, Kilmer, 40
MCT oil, 173, 228-229
Meat, 212-213
Medium chain fatty acids (MCFAs), 167
Medium chain triglyceride oil, *see* MCT oil
Medium chain triglycerides (MCTs), 11, 25, 97-98, 117, 167-174
Melanoma, 182-183
Mercury, 148
Metabolic resistance, 238
Metabolic syndrome, 54
Metabolism, 68-69, 78-81, 89, 110, 124, 128, 154, 156-160, 165-190, 199
Minerals, 37, 201-204
Monosaccharide, 46
Monosodium glutamate (MSG), 130
Monounsaturated fatty acids, 25, 29
Moore, Jimmy, 253
Multiple enzyme dysfunction, 156, 157

Net carbohydrate, 209
Nutrasweet, *see* Aspartame
Nutrition Facts, 209
Nuts and seeds, 218

Obesity, 49, 80
Olive oil, 25

Omega-3, 20
Omega-6, 20
Oxidation, 26-28, 31, 37, 53, 131-32, 144

Palm kernel oil, 25
Pancreas, 62, 66
Parkinson's disease, 49, 72, 104
Pawan, Gaston L.S., 91
Pellagra, 128
Pennington, Alfred W., 87
Perchlorate, 139-140, 148
Phagocytosis, 50
Pituitary gland, 123, 154
Polysaccharide, 46
Potassium bromide, 136, 139
Potassium iodide, 136, 139, 145
Pritikin, Nathan, 22
Prostaglandins, 19, 37
Protein, 45, 64, 91, 95-96, 105-108, 208, 253
Protein poisoning, 107
Pukapuka, 11
Phytonutrients, 47-48

Rabbit starvation, 107
RBD coconut oil, 227-228

Saccharide, 46
Saccharin, 56, 68
Salt, 136-137, 144, 186, 201-204, 251
Satiety, 93-98, 108-111, 188
Saturated fat, 41-44, 107-108, 113
Saturated fatty acids, 25, 41-44
Scurvy 51, 107-108, 127-128
Seafood, 135
Seaweed, 144
Seasonal affective disorder (SAD), 181
Selenium, 131
Side effects, 250-252
Soda, 198-200

Soy, 140-141
Splenda, *see* Sucralose
Staessen, Jan, 202
Starch, 45, 50, 64, 66, 72, 125
Stefensson, Vilhjalmur, 107-108, 128
Stevia, 59-60
Stroke, 43-44, 104
Subclinical disease, 51
Subclinical malnutrition, 37, 125-132, 159, 166
Sucralose, 56
Sucrose, 37, 46, 51-52, 54
Sugar, 45-47, 48-60, 64, 66-76, 220-221
Sugar addiction, 69-70, 72-75
Sugar alcohols, 57-59, 70
Sunlight, 180-183
Synthroid, *see* Levothyroxine

Taller, Herman, 85-89
Tea, 138, 199
Tert-butylhydroquinone (TBHQ), 132
Thyroid, 119, 122-132, 133-151, 152-164, 181
Thyroid stimulating hormone (TSH), 123, 154
Thyroid gland disorder, 154-155
Thyroid system disorder, 152-164
Thyroxin (T4), 122, 129, 133, 154-155, 159, 162-164
Tofu, 140-141
Tokelau, 11
Trace minerals, 144, 204, 251
Trans fatty acids, 28-30, 130
Triglycerides, 24-25, 104, 113, 115, 241, 243
Triiodothyronine (T3), 122, 133, 154-155, 159, 162-164
Tyrosine, 129

Ulcer, 192

Vegetable oils, 26, 29, 126, 132
Vegetables, 47-48, 214-216
Vigilante, Kevin, 92-93
Vinegar, 220
Vitamin A, 129
Vitamin B12, 129
Vitamin B deficiency, 37
Vitamin C, 36, 51, 126-128, 225
Vitamin D, 37, 181-183

Waist size, 173, 244
Warner, Gregory, 39
Water, 191-206, 251
Wheat, 72
Whitaker, Julian, 170
White, Paul Dudley, 34

Willett, Walter, 28, 99
Wilson, Denis, 155, 160-161
Wilson's temperature syndrome, *see*
Wilson's thyroid syndrome
Wilson's thyroid syndrome, 152-164, 175
World Health Organization (WHO), 134

Xylitol, 58

Your Body's Many Cries for Water, 193
Yo-yo effect, 80, 101

Zinc, 131

COCONUT CURES
Preventing and Treating
Common Health Problems with Coconut

You've heard about the healing power coconut oil but did you know that the entire coconut is a virtual medicine chest? Coconut meat, milk, and water all have medicinal as well as nutritional value. The health benefits of the entire coconut are explained in *Coconut Cures: Preventing and Treating Common Health Problems with Coconut*.

"I consider this book an amazing contribution to people who are in the quest for optimal health."

—Jean Rosales, M.D.

"Excellent book. It is very helpful for those seeking to improve their health using natural medicine. I am actively conducting clinical trials and medical research using coconut oil and have seen very positive results with my patients."

—Marieta Jader-Onate, M.D.

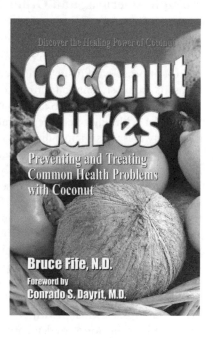

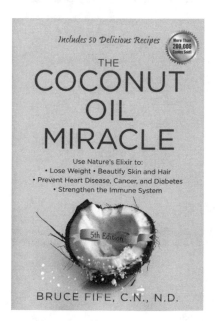

THE COCONUT OIL MIRACLE

"Dr. Bruce Fife should be commended for bringing together in this very readable book the positive health benefits of coconut oil. The inquiring reader will have a new and more balanced view of the role of fat and especially saturated fats in our diet."—Jon Kabara, Ph.D. Michigan State University

"He does a fabulous job of documenting how coconut oil, a saturated fat, is actually beneficial to your heart...Fife's book explains in great detail many of the other healing aspects of this forgotten oil. I heartily recommend you get a copy of the book and study it for yourself."

—William Campbell Douglass, M.D., *Second Opinion*

STOP ALZHEIMER'S NOW!

How to Prevent and Reverse Dementia, Parkinson's, ALS, Multiple Sclerosis, and Other Neurodegenerative Disorders

By Bruce Fife, ND, Foreword by Russell L. Blaylock, MD

More than 35 million people have dementia today. Each year 4.6 million new cases occur worldwide—one new case every 7 seconds. Alzheimer's disease is the most common form of dementia. Parkinson's disease, another progressive brain disorder, affects about 4 million people worldwide. Millions more suffer with other neurodegenerative disorders. The number of people affected by these destructive diseases continues to increase every year.

Dementia and other forms of neurodegeneration are *not* a part of the normal aging process. The brain is fully capable of functioning normally for a lifetime, regardless of how long a person lives. While aging is a risk factor for neurodegeneration, it is not the cause! Dementia and other neurodegenerative disorders are disease processes that can be prevented and successfully treated.

This book outlines a program using ketone therapy and diet that is backed by decades of medical and clinical research and has proven successful in restoring mental function and improving both brain and overall health. You will learn how to prevent and even reverse symptoms associated with Alzheimer's disease, Parkinson's disease, amyotrophic lateral sclerosis (ALS), multiple sclerosis (MS), Huntington's disease, epilepsy, diabetes, stroke, and various forms of dementia.

The information in this book is useful not only for those who are suffering from neurodegenerative disease but for anyone who wants to be spared from ever encountering one or more of these devastating afflictions. These diseases don't just happen overnight. They take years, often decades, to develop. In the case of Alzheimer's disease, approximately 70 percent the brain cells responsible for memory are destroyed *before* symptoms become noticeable.

You *can* stop Alzheimer's and other neurodegenerative diseases before they take over your life. The best time to start is now.

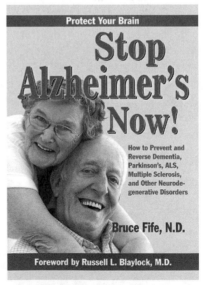

COOKING WITH COCONUT FLOUR
A Delicious Low-Carb, Gluten-Free Alternative to Wheat
By Bruce Fife, N.D.

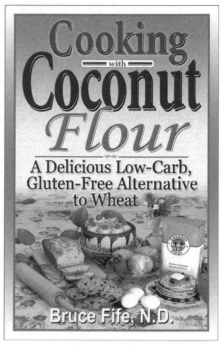

Do you love breads, cakes, pies, cookies, and other wheat products but can't eat them because you are allergic to wheat or sensitive to gluten? Perhaps you avoid wheat because you are concerned about your weight and need to cut down on carbohydrates. If so, the solution for you is coconut flour. Coconut flour is a delicious, healthy alternative to wheat. It is high in fiber, low in digestible carbohydrate, and a good source of protein. It contains no gluten so it is ideal for those with celiac disease.

Coconut flour can be used to make a variety of delicious baked goods, snacks, desserts, and main dishes. It is the only flour used in most of the recipes in this book. These recipes are so delicious that you won't be able to tell that they aren't made with wheat. If you like foods such as blueberry muffins, cheese crackers, and chicken pot pie, but don't want the wheat, you will love the recipes in this book!

These recipes are designed with your health in mind. Every recipe is completely free of wheat, gluten, soy, trans fats, and artificial sweeteners. Coconut is naturally low in carbohydrate and recipes include both regular and reduced sugar versions. Coconut flour provides many health benefits. It can improve digestion, help regulate blood sugar, protect against diabetes, help prevent heart disease and cancer, and aid in weight loss.

"This book is absolutely chock full of easy to understand information on the use of coconut flour and its benefits." --*Book Review Cafe*

Visit Us on the Web
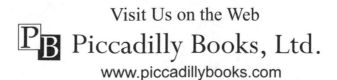

Piccadilly Books, Ltd.
www.piccadillybooks.com